Printed in the United States
By Bookmasters

Participatory Health Research

Michael T. Wright • Krystyna Kongats
Editors

Participatory Health Research

Voices from Around the World

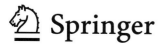
Springer

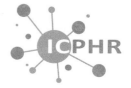

Editors
Michael T. Wright
Catholic University of Applied Sciences
Institute for Social Health
Berlin, Germany

Krystyna Kongats
School of Public Health
University of Alberta
Edmonton, AB, Canada

ISBN 978-3-030-06378-8   ISBN 978-3-319-92177-8   (eBook)
https://doi.org/10.1007/978-3-319-92177-8

Cover illustration: Different fabrics waving in the wind a metaphor for the voices of the world, all different in width and length and strength. Together they form an interesting colourful whole.
Created by artist Janine Schrijver.
This resonates with the cover of the Springer companion book entitled *Participatory Research for Health and Social Well-being*.

Printed on acid-free paper

This Springer imprint is published by the registered company Springer Nature Switzerland AG.
The registered company address is: Gewerbestrasse 11, 6330 Cham, Switzerland

Preface: The Need for Participatory Health Research

A wealth of international studies have documented that health is distributed in society according to a social gradient, with those of higher social status living longer and healthier than those of lower social status. Finding means to explain and remedy this disparity has become a central focus of public health research and practice (Marmot 2011; Jakab and Marmot 2012). The field of health promotion in particular is concerned with effecting change in the social environment for the purpose of improving health, particularly the health of socially marginalized groups. Here the necessity of addressing complex social processes at the collective level (community, neighborhood, society) has become apparent. Also issues of health care access and delivery involve factors which need to be examined in terms of collective mechanisms, such as social exclusion (Green 2006; Kemm 2006; Trickett 2011).

Participatory health research (PHR) is gaining increased attention as a way to generate data leading to action for addressing social disparities in health outcomes. In PHR, the goal is to maximize the participation of those whose life or work is the subject of the research in all stages of the research process (International Collaboration for Participatory Health Research 2013). This type of participation is the defining principle of PHR, and it is what sets this type of research apart from other approaches in the health field. In PHR, research is not done "on" people as passive subjects providing "data" but "with" them to provide relevant information for improving their lives. As this book documents, reaching a deep level of participation in health research is very challenging, but it provides a unique opportunity for transformative change in health systems and in the lives of the people engaged in the research process.

Participatory forms of research have achieved recognition in several fields including education, social work, management, and community development; however, the application of participatory approaches to health research is relatively new. Health research is dominated by the biomedical model which follows a positivist paradigm consistent with the natural sciences, thus privileging experimental designs and quantitative data. The focus is on acquiring an "objective" knowledge which is influenced neither by the particular context in which the data are collected nor by the particularities of the lives of the study participants. Through various means related to design, data collection, and statistical analysis, the researchers seek to isolate and measure specific causal mechanisms and intervention effects as precisely as possible. The knowledge thus generated is sorted hierarchically into "classes of evidence" according to the principles of evidenced-based medicine (EBM), with the results of experimental studies being judged as providing the strongest proof for mechanisms of disease causation and for the efficacy of interventions to ameliorate health problems.

Although the biomedical paradigm has been shown to have severe limitations regarding social (as opposed to clinical) aspects of health (McQueen and Anderson 2001, 2004; Greenhalgh et al. 2014), alternatives such as qualitative and participatory forms of research have a difficult time being accepted by some as constituting sufficient evidence for effective action in public health (Denzin 2017; Mays and Pope 2000). As documented in this volume, PHR as practiced in many different countries indeed provides unique contributions to improving the health of communities which cannot be achieved by other research approaches.

This book provides a first look at PHR from an international perspective. Until recently, participatory health researchers have been relatively isolated, focused on structures and issues at the local or regional level. Through the work of the International Collaboration for Participatory Health Research (ICPHR) and the growing number of national and regional networks, participatory health researchers have been able to come together to exchange their experience and ideas about what PHR is and what it can be. The chapters in this book document the work of the ICPHR, while highlighting issues of international and regional importance.

Overview of Chapters

This book is divided into two parts: "Central Themes" and "Regional Perspectives."

Part I provides insight into some of the core issues currently facing participatory health researchers. PHR draws from various traditions in different countries; Chapter 1 identifies several characteristics which these traditions have in common. Chapter 2 moves into a discussion on the development and progression of the International Collaboration for Participatory Health Research (ICPHR) over the past decade, highlighting the issues raised in bringing together researchers from the various traditions. Chapter 3 explores the challenges of evaluating PHR projects in light of their complex structure, diversity of stakeholders, and multiple outcomes. Chapter 4 reflects on the unique requirements for teaching health and social work professionals how to conduct PHR in higher education settings, with a focus on ways to provide a transformative learning experience. The topic of research impact has become an important issue worldwide. Demonstrating the impact of PHR poses specific challenges which are examined in Chapters 5 and 6, including issues related to building a systematic and dynamic evidence base for the field. Chapter 7 looks at the emerging role of children as co-researchers in PHR projects from theoretical and practical perspectives, based on the work of the international network Kids in Action, a project of the ICPHR.

Part II of the book builds off the central themes presented in Part I using regional case studies from around the globe including: Germany, India, Latin America, the Netherlands, North America, Portuguese-speaking countries, South Africa, and the United Kingdom. Each chapter "sets the stage" by outlining the influence of the regional context on conducting PHR. Through these chapters, the reader will not only gain a better understanding of how PHR differs depending on political and cultural context but also of the similarities in terms of challenges and core principles. Chapter 8 provides an account of the German research consortium PartKommPlus, sharing some of the challenges and opportunities in scaling up PHR to address national policy priorities. Chapter 9 looks at the central role nongovernmental organizations in India have played in health promotion at the local level, drawing on the practice of participatory health research, and how this practice challenges existing research agendas. Chapter 10 reflects on the rich and diverse history of PHR in Latin America, exploring the current status of PHR in this region with a particular focus on chronic noncommunicable diseases. Chapter 11 provides an account of PHR in the Netherlands, focusing on older people and how historical and cultural differences between generations influence research practice. Chapters 12 and 13 both describe PHR from a North American perspective, the former presenting results from a qualitative literature review of PHR in health organizations and the latter reflecting on the evolution of PHR from the "pre-health promotion" to the "evidence-based practice" era. Chapter 14 is a reflexive, comparative analysis of PHR across Portuguese-speaking countries including Angola, Brazil, Cape Verde, and Portugal. Chapter 15 looks at PHR in the South African context, discussing action-oriented and policy-focused approaches in the face of dramatic social and health inequities in the post-apartheid years. Finally, Chapter 16 closes with a reflection on the historical development of PHR in the UK, highlighting the inherent political tensions in top-down initiatives vs. grassroots ownership and the new opportunities which the current moment provides.

Join Us!

This book is the result of nearly a decade of cooperation and exchange within the International Collaboration for Participatory Health Research. We hope readers will find encouragement and a sense of community in seeing some of their own challenges mirrored in the work presented here, and be inspired by new possibilities for participatory health research in their own countries and communities. The book is an invitation to join with the ICPHR as it seeks to promote participatory health research in its myriad forms as a means for addressing the pressing health problems of our world.

Berlin, Germany   Michael T. Wright
Edmonton, AB, Canada   Krystyna Kongats

References

Denzin, N. K. (2017). Critical qualitative inquiry. *Qualitative Inquiry, 23*(1), 8–16.

Green, L. W. (2006). Public health asks of system science: to advance our evidence-based practice, can you held us get more practice-based evidence? *American Journal of Public Health, 96,* 1–5.

Greenhalgh, T., Howick, J., & Maskrey, N. (2014). Evidence based medicine: a movement in crisis? *BMJ, 348,* g3725.

International Collaboration for Participatory Health Research (2013) 'Position Paper 1: What is participatory health research?'. Berlin: International Collaboration for Participatory Health Research Report. Available at: http://www.icphr.org/uploads/2/0/3/9/20399575/ichpr_position_paper_1_defintion_-_version_may_2013.pdf.

Jakab, Z., & Marmot, M. (2012). Social determinants of health in Europe. *Lancet, 379*(9811), 103–105.

Kemm, J. (2006). The limitations of 'evidence-based' public health. *Journal of Evaluation and Clinical Practice, 12,* 319–324.

Marmot, M. (2011). Global action on social determinants of health. *Bulletin of the World Health Organisation, 89*(10): 702.

Mays, N., & Pope, C. (2000). Qualitative research in health care: Assessing quality in qualitative research. *BMJ: British Medical Journal, 320*(7226), 50.

McQueen, D. V., & Anderson, L. M. (2001) What counts as evidence: issues and debates. *WHO regional publications. European series, 92,* 63–81.

McQueen, D.V., & Anderson, L. M. (2004) Utiliser des données probantes pour évaluer l'efficacité de la promotion de la santé: quelques enjeux fondamentaux. *Promotion & Education, 11(1), suppl., 11–16.*

Trickett, E. J., Beehler, S., Deutsch, C., Green, L. W., Hawe, P., McLeroy, K., Miller, R. L., Rapkin, B. D., Schensul, J. J., Schulz, A. J. & Trimble, J. E. (2010). Advancing the Science of Community-Level Interventions. *American Journal of Public Health, 101*(8), 1410–1419.

Contents

Part I
Central Themes

Chapter 1
What Is Participatory Health Research?

Michael T. Wright, Jane Springett, and Krystyna Kongats

Introduction

The theory and practice of participatory health research (PHR) is very diverse, particularly when taking into account the international literature as a whole. Minkler and Wallerstein (2008) acknowledge the plurality of motivations and "ideological commitments" operative among participatory researchers in the USA but insist on an underlying "participatory research paradigm" which unites all. A similar argument is brought by Reason and Bradbury (2001) in their volume on action research, which includes examples of participatory research from various countries. The plurality is described in terms of a "family" of research approaches united by a common "participatory worldview." The remarkable variety of work presented by Reason and Bradbury draws attention, however, to the dramatic differences which exist between participatory researchers at the theoretical and operational levels—not just in the health field. Various approaches such as pragmatism, critical theory, feminism, and constructivism are applied to varying degrees in the conduct of participatory research, impacting data production and interpretation as well as questions of internal and external validity in different ways. This lack of coherence gives credence to the critics of PHR who claim that participatory researchers are united more by a common (political) purpose, than by common scientific criteria. As

M. T. Wright (✉)
Catholic University of Applied Sciences, Institute for Social Health, Berlin, Germany
e-mail: michael.wright@khsb-berlin.de

J. Springett
School of Public Health, University of Alberta, Edmonton, Alberta, Canada
e-mail: jane.springett@ualberta.ca

K. Kongats
School of Public Health, University of Alberta, Edmonton, Alberta, Canada
e-mail: krystyna.kongats@ualberta.ca

© Springer International Publishing AG, part of Springer Nature 2018
M. T. Wright, K. Kongats (eds.), *Participatory Health Research*,
https://doi.org/10.1007/978-3-319-92177-8_1

3

Lukesch and Zecha (1978) observed early in the participatory research movement in Germany (p. 41): "Action researchers are apparently less interested in generating scientific knowledge than in creating social change—that is, in taking political action." Many call into question the scientific merit of PHR, which has made it difficult for this approach to receive the same level of recognition as other forms of research (Conchelos and Kassam 1981; von Unger et al. 2007).

The variety of methodological and theoretical approaches among studies calling themselves "community-based" or "participatory" is not a problem in itself. The complexity of public health and particularly of health promotion requires a diversity of approaches. The problem is, rather, that PHR has yet to achieve a clear scientific profile to serve as a basis for debating in what ways PHR can make a unique contribution to building knowledge and theory. This has implications for the advancement of PHR as a whole and for the uptake of the findings produced by way of participatory methods. In our experience, an important reason why it is generally more difficult to receive the approval of local research review boards and to secure funding for PHR research projects is that each proposal needs to be argued on its own terms, unable to reference an internationally recognized body of common scientific principles.

The International Collaboration for Participatory Health Research (ICPHR) was created in 2009 as a place to bring together what we are learning internationally about the application of participatory research approaches to address health issues (Wright et al. 2009, 2010a, 2010b). See Chap. 2 for further discussion on the history and future of the ICPHR. Through consolidating existing knowledge and reaching agreement on common terminology and principles, the ICPHR seeks to strengthen the role of PHR in intervention design and decision-making on health issues and thus to provide a means for people most affected by health problems to influence how these problems are addressed in the society. This includes developing guidelines for conducting and evaluating PHR, describing which forms of theory and evidence are produced by this approach, and finding a means for conducting systematic reviews of the PHR literature in order to contribute to the body of international knowledge on health.

In a first position paper, the ICPHR sought to define the core principles of ICPHR, citing a larger body of international literature (ICPHR 2013). This paper is one contribution, from a particular set of perspectives, to the international discussion on PHR. In such an emerging and diverse field, there is no "definitive" description of this approach. Although qualitative research and PHR are distinct, each is an open-ended project which "resists attempts to impose a single, umbrella-like paradigm over the entire project" (Denzin and Lincoln 2011, p. xiii). PHR, and participatory research more generally, cannot be confined to a narrow set of epistemological principles (Fals-Borda and Rahman 1991). Part of PHR's richness and appeal is the range of paradigms, strategies of inquiry, and methods of analysis that researchers can draw upon and utilize. PHR's multiple disciplinary histories leads to constant tensions and contradictions regarding its methods, findings and interpretations. This inherent plurality is part of PHR's epistemological strength which we strive to recognize in this chapter.

The central characteristics as described by the ICPHR are summarized here for the purpose of dissemination to a larger audience and thus to promote debate and critical reflection on what it means to do health research in a participatory way.

Participatory Health Research Is an Approach, Not a Method

The ICPHR understands PHR as being a research approach rather than a research method. The research approach guides the research process.

Participation as a research *method* means that people are involved in health research in specific ways in order to improve the quality of the research. In recent years there has been a movement in some countries to increase the participation of citizens in health research by consulting them over the course of developing and implementing studies (e.g., Cropper et al. 2010; DoH 1999, 2006; Institute of Medicine 2009; National Health and Medical Research Council 2002). These various ways of increasing the involvement of people affected by the health problem under study has led to improvements, for example, regarding recruitment, retention of participants (less loss-to-follow-up), quality of data, data interpretation, and dissemination of findings.

PHR as a research *approach* means that participation is the defining principle throughout the research process. A research approach or paradigm is the set of underlying assumptions about the world and how it should be studied which serves as the basis for defining what constitutes "good research" (cf. Guba and Lincoln 2005; Kuhn 2012). For PHR, the primary underlying assumption is that participation on the part of those whose lives or work is the subject of the study fundamentally affects all aspects of the research. The engagement of these people in the study is an end in itself and is the hallmark of PHR, recognizing the value of each person's contribution to the co-creation of knowledge in a process that is not only practical, but also collaborative and empowering (Onwuegbuzie et al. 2009). The engagement of others within the research process can also be important, for example, policy makers who can act on the research findings and thus improve the situation of those affected by a health issue.

Characteristics of Participatory Health Research

Although there is a great diversity within PHR, the following principles are emerging as being common to many approaches (cf. Hart and Bond 1995; Waterman et al. 2001; Whitelaw et al. 2003; Israel et al. 1998, 2003; Viswanathan et al. 2004; Ismail 2009; Macaulay et al. 1999; Cargo and Mercer 2008).

PHR Is Participatory

The goal of PHR is to maximize the participation of those whose life or work is the subject of the research in all stages of the research process, including the formulation of the research question and goal, the development of a research design, the selection of appropriate methods for data collection and analysis, the implementation of the research, the interpretation of the results, and the dissemination of the findings. Such participation is the core, defining principle of PHR, setting this type of research apart from other approaches in the health field.

Several generalized "scales" have been created to aid those conducting participatory research to identify the degree to which the various stakeholders are involved, for example, Cornwall (2008) or Wright (2016). Such scales have been complemented by models which describe participation as occurring at different levels within a system, articulating the relationship between "individual" and "organizational" participation (cf. Smithies and Webster 1998; Rifkin 1996). Other authors have drawn the boundaries differently, tying participation more closely to intention (e.g., Blackstock et al. 2007). The appropriateness of any given model is largely dependent on local culture and context, the available resources, and the joint decision-making process in each research team. Using a model helps researchers to be actively aware of the participatory dimensions of the study and to reflect on the purpose and expected impact of these dimensions. Whatever model is used to describe participation in the research process, the goal of PHR is to provide the opportunity for all participants to be equitably involved to the maximum degree possible throughout the research.

PHR Is Locally Situated

PHR is grounded in the reality of daily life and work in a specific place and time. The issue being researched must be located in the social system which is likely to adopt the changes that result from the research process. This is the strength of PHR and results in the further development of local knowledge. The local dimension not only impacts the choice of research focus but also the research methods used, the process of learning from the research, and its impact (cf. Stoecker 2013). The emphasis placed on the local level of knowledge and experience does not mean that PHR projects are necessarily restricted to having a local scope. Increasingly, there are examples of PHR projects which mobilize a large number of people to pool their local knowledge in order to make statements about health issues at the regional, national, or international level (e.g., IPPF et al. 2013; von Unger 2012; Wright 2010; ATHENA and GCWA 2013, Chaps. 8, 9, 10, 11, 12, 13,14, 15, and 16 in Part II of this book).

PHR Is a Collective Research Process

In nonparticipatory forms of health research, the research process is generally under the control of one or more academics who are responsible for all aspects of the study. There is usually a hierarchy among the researchers, with the "principal investigator" assuming primary responsibility. In PHR, the research process is typically conducted by a group representing the various stakeholders taking part in the study. This group often includes engaged citizens, members of civil society (NGOs), health and social welfare professionals, health organizations, academic researchers, and policy makers. Any one of these stakeholders can initiate and lead a study. The title "participatory researcher" or "co-researcher" is not reserved for the academics but rather designates all members of the research group. The leadership role consists of facilitating a shared decision-making group process for developing, implementing, analyzing, and disseminating the research. Through the group process, the participants become co-owners of the research and experience self-efficacy through their influence on the process. An explicit goal of the facilitation is to empower all members to engage actively in the process and thus have control over the research.

PHR Projects Are Collectively Owned

Consistent with the above-named principles, the ownership of the research lies in the hands of the group conducting the study. The group needs to decide how to best report on the findings of the research in order to meet the set goals (Stoecker 2013).

PHR Aims for Transformation Through Human Agency

As in other forms of participatory research, PHR follows the explicit goal of creating positive social change as a result of the research process for those persons whose life or work is the focus of the research. Typical research goals are improving the health of a specific group of people, addressing the social determinants of health by improving living standards, addressing the political determinants of health by changing repressive or restrictive policy, and/or improving the quality of services by addressing organizational issues. Actions to produce social change are embedded in the research process itself and are themselves the topic of the research (in accordance with the tenets of action research, more generally), or the actions to produce change directly follow the completion of the research based on an agenda for action formulated as an outcome of the study.

PHR Promotes Critical Reflexivity

Critical reflexivity means considering how power and powerlessness affect the daily lives and practice of those whose life or work is the focus of the research. In this way, a critical consciousness (conscientization, Freire 1970) is developed among the participants. The micro-politics of everyday experience are recognized, allowing for new links between theory and practice, between "subject" and "object," thus laying groundwork for change.

From the perspective of health and welfare professionals engaged in PHR, critical reflexivity requires a questioning of professional roles and the knowledge of professionals, based on power differentials between themselves and service users and based on the expertise gained through life experiences and the social disadvantages faced by people without professional health qualifications (cf. Schön 1983; Ledwith and Springett 2010; Wright 2012). The critically reflective professional understands the expert role as one in which a partnership is formed with people seeking services for the purpose of promoting empowerment and thus to take action for their health. Health problems are seen as being caused not only by biological but also by social factors which are often not under the control of the person seeking help. The critically reflective professional works with service users to develop not only individual but also collective strategies to address these social determinants.

From the perspective of those engaged in PHR who are not from the health or welfare professions, critical reflexivity can be described using the categories of health literacy defined by Nutbeam (2000). Typically, we think of health research as benefiting people in terms of improving their *functional health literacy* and their *interactive health literacy*. Functional health literacy means the ability to understand the factors which promote health as well as health risks and the knowledge needed to access help in the healthcare system. Interactive health literacy means the ability to seek out actively health information and to appropriate this information for the purpose of improving or preserving one's health. *Critical health literacy* refers to the ability to act together with others to address the social and political factors which impinge on the health of a group as a whole.

Critical reflexivity is perhaps the most challenging aspect of PHR work but lies at the center of issues of authenticity, transparency and transferability, and an explicit values base.

PHR Produces Knowledge Which Is Local, Collective, Co-created, Dialogical, and Diverse

The knowledge typically produced by health research is by and for an academic audience. Often highly technical in both methodology and reporting, the knowledge can be difficult to diffuse to policy makers, practitioners, community leaders, and others who could use the information to make change. This problem has received considerable attention in recent years under such headings as knowledge translation and translational research.

The knowledge produced by PHR is typically local in scope. As in other forms of participatory research, the people whose life or work is being studied have the opportunity to articulate their local knowledge (also known as indigenous or tacit knowledge) and to question and expand on that knowledge through the participatory research process. Local knowledge encompasses all that people know about the subject at hand based on their direct experience and their own empirical investigations. Local knowledge is typically passed on in the form of local theories which define health issues in concrete terms, identifying specific local causes and ways to address those causes (cf. Wright et al. 2010; Brito 2008). In contrast to "general scientific theories," local theories are less abstract and offer different forms of generalizability. As Winter (2002, p. 144) puts it: "…an account of a specific situation that gets sufficiently close to its underlying structure to enable others to see potential similarities with other situations" (cf. Bassey 2001).

The knowledge produced by PHR is co-created and dialogical, incorporating the various perspectives of the participants. The collective research process is conducted in such a way that knowledge is produced in an ongoing dialogue among the participants on all aspects of the research process. The various perspectives of the participants need to be incorporated into this dialogue. PHR, and participatory research more generally, is often misunderstood as being a consensus-oriented process in which the perspective of academic researchers should have little influence. The strength in PHR lies, however, in the ability to uncover and examine different points of view, which may mean presenting a variety of perspectives throughout a study.

PHR Strives for a Broad Impact

A key facet of PHR is its explicit intention of bringing about social change. In PHR, learning and research are not considered separate entities. Social learning (learning together and from each other) is a fundamental dimension of the PHR process, and the continual cycle of "look, reflect, act" underpins the dynamics of developing a connected knowing. This means trying to understand the other person or idea through dialogue from relations of trust and empathy (Goldberger et al. 1996). Everyone learns as co-researcher to differing degrees. Ideally, the process should engage the participants in transformative learning, i.e., changes in the way they see the world and themselves (Freire 1970; Mezirow et al. 1990), through interactive processes which address both the personal and the collective. In turn, this generates an intention of being able to act based on the research findings, thus having a wider impact beyond the scientific community in the narrow sense. On the whole, how social change is defined is largely determined by whether the approach is pragmatic (i.e., focused on issues of practical utilization) or emancipatory (where the focus is on changing the way people think and act in their world)—or an attempted combination of both (Johansson and Lindhult 2008; Mercer 2002).

PHR Produces Local Evidence Based on a Broad Understanding of Generalizability

The primacy of the local context in PHR has implications for the generalization of the results of PHR studies. As Greenwood and Levin (2005) argue, cogenerative, context-centered knowledge requires a revision of traditional notions of generalization. Nonparticipatory forms of health research are often focused on generating representational knowledge which can be used to develop standardized interventions for similar local settings. The question of scaling up from this perspective is thus one of replicating interventions on a large scale which have been shown to be effective under scientifically controlled conditions at the local level. The goal of PHR is developing interventions for a specific time and place, giving primacy to the local context. The result is the generation of local evidence which can be accumulated over time by local participants for the purpose of strengthening their ability to take effective action on health issues (cf. Brandão 1987; Wright et al. 2013). The transfer of interventions from one locality to the next is about understanding the contextual conditions in the new setting, how they differ from the setting in which the knowledge was produced, and reflecting on the consequences (Macaulay et al. 2011). Through PHR, a deep understanding of the essence of a particular situation can be gained and communicated to others who can then judge the relevance of the findings for their own situation (cf. Winter 2002). Realist review approaches are particularly promising in this regard, specifically seeking to document "what works, for whom, and in what contexts" (Jagosh et al. 2011, 2012).

PHR Follows Specific Validity Criteria

PHR incorporates both qualitative and quantitative methods, depending on the type of data required. The methods need to be adapted to the participatory research process which often means a deviation from the methodological standards found in nonparticipatory forms of health research. Important is the adherence to validity criteria specific to participatory research approaches. These include (cf. Greenwood and Levin 2005; Edwards et al. 2008; Roman and Apple 1990; Waterman et al. 2001; Dadds 2008; Sohng 1995; Reason and Bradbury 2008; Lather 1986):

- Participatory validity: the extent to which all stakeholders are able to take an active part in the research process to the full extent possible
- Intersubjective validity: the extent to which the research is viewed as being credible and meaningful by the stakeholders from a variety of perspectives
- Contextual validity: the extent to which the research relates to the local situation
- Catalytic validity: the extent to which the research is useful in terms of presenting new possibilities for social action
- Ethical validity: the extent to which the research outcomes and the changes exerted on people by the research are sound and just
- Empathic validity: the extent to which the research has increased empathy among the participants

PHR Is a Dialectical Process Characterized by Messiness

The knowledge and the action strategies generated by PHR arise out a facilitated, collective research process. The process is characterized by a dialogue among participants with different perspectives on the subject under study. The dialogue does not necessarily result in a consensual view but may reveal and promote several different views resulting in different ways of addressing the health issue at hand. In any case, the dialogical process intends to promote transformational learning based on a critical examination of the causes behind health and illness.

Transformational learning is made possible through a dialectical process in which participants are challenged to investigate assumptions based on their local (tacit) knowledge. Authentic dialogue makes such an investigation possible. Due to the variety of perspectives and ways of knowing found among the participants, a strict adherence to a research protocol and to methodological standards is not appropriate. The rigor in PHR lies in the extent to which the research is facilitated so as to make possible new, transformative insights which offer fresh approaches for action. If the dialectical tension is upheld, a "messiness" arises in the process, participants often exhibiting confusion and irritation as their assumptions are questioned (Cook 2009). The occurrence of messiness in this sense is a fundamental characteristic of PHR, where engaging with the mess is characterized as "…a complex process of inquiry, involving a wide range of techniques, where messy is taken to mean difficult, not careless" (Mellor 1999). This results in a research process which is nonlinear and multi-focused and in research outcomes which cannot be characterized prior to the study. This quality makes it difficult for PHR proposals to meet the requirements of typical research calls, given the necessity of defining in advance the phases of the research project, the methods to be used, and the scope and nature of the results.

Conclusion

In spite of the remarkable variety within participatory health research internationally, common characteristics can be identified which are shared by many. By making explicit this common foundation, participatory researchers can debate and critically reflect on what makes PHR different from other approaches to health research and thus address more effectively issues of quality, credibility, and visibility.

References

ATHENA Network, & Global Coalition on Women and AIDS (GCWA). (2013) Building women's global meaningful participation in the high level meeting on AIDS. http://www.athenanetwork. org/assets/files/HLM/AP_Factsheet.pdf.

Bassey, M. (2001). A solution to the problem of generalisation in educational research: Fuzzy prediction. *Oxford Review of Education, 27*(1), 5–22.

Blackstock, K. L., Kelly, G. J., & Horsey, B. L. (2007). Developing and applying a framework to evaluate participatory research for sustainability. *Ecological Economics, 60*(4), 726–742.

Brandão, C. R. (Org.) (1987). *Repensando a pesquisa participante*. 3 ed. São Paulo: Brasiliense.

Brito, I. (2008). Intervenção de conscientização para prevenção da brucelose em área endémica. Tese de Doutoramento em Ciências de Enfermagem, Instituto de Ciências Biomédicas Abel Salazar ICBAS.

Cargo, M., & Mercer, S. L. (2008). The value and challenges of participatory research: Strengthening its practice. *Annual Review of Public Health, 29*, 325–350.

Conchelos, G., & Kassam, Y. (1981). A brief review of critical opinions and responses on issues facing participatory research. *Convergence, 14*(3), 52.

Cook, T. (2009). The purpose of mess in action research: Building rigour through a messy turn. *Educational Action Research, 17*(2), 277–291.

Cornwall, A. (2008). Unpacking "Participation" models, meanings and practices. *Community Development Journal, 43*(3), 269–283.

Cropper, S., Porter, A., Williams, G., Carlisle, S., Moore, R., O'Neill, M., Roberts, C., & Snooks, H. (2010). *Community health and wellbeing. Action research on inequalities*. Bristol: Policy Press.

Dadds, M. (2008). Empathetic validity in practitioner research. *Educational Action Research, 16*(2), 279–290.

Denzin, N. K., & Lincoln, Y. S. (Eds.). (2011). *The Sage handbook of qualitative research*. London: Sage.

Department of Health (DoH). (1999). *Patient and public involvement in the NHS*. London: Department of Health.

Department of Health (DoH). (2006). *Best research for best health: A new national health research strategy*. London: DH Publications.

Edwards, K., Lund, C., & Gibson, N. (2008). Validity: Expecting the unexpected in community-based research. *Pimatisiwin A Journal of Aboriginal and Indigenous Community Health, 6*(3), 17–29.

Fals-Borda, O., & Rahman, M. (Eds.). (1991). *Action and knowledge. Breaking the monopoly with participatory action research*. New York: Apex.

Freire, P. (1970). *Pedagogy of the oppressed*. New York: Herder & Herder.

Goldberger, N. R., Tanile, J. M., Clinchy, B. M., & Belenky, M. F. (Eds.). (1996). *Knowledge, difference and power: Essays inspired by women's ways of knowing*. New York: Basic Books.

Greenwood, D. J., & Levin, M. (2005). Reform of the social sciences and of universities through action research. In N. K. Denzin & Y. S. Lincoln (Eds.), *The Sage handbook of qualitative research* (3rd ed., pp. 43–64). Thousand Oaks: Sage.

Guba, E. G., & Lincoln, Y. S. (2005). Paradigmatic controversies, contradictions, and emerging confluences. In N. K. Denzin & Y. S. Lincoln (Eds.), *Sage handbook of qualitative research* (pp. 191–215). London: Sage Publications.

Hart, E., & Bond, M. (1995). *Action research for health & social care*. London: Open University.

Institute of Medicine (IOM). (2009). *Initial national priorities for comparative effectiveness research*. Washington, DC: The National Academy Press.

International Collaboration for Participatory Health Research (ICPHR). (2013). *Position paper 1: What is participatory health research? Version: May 2013*. Berlin: International Collaboration for Participatory Health Research.

International Planned Parenthood Federation (IPPF), The Joint United Nations Programme on HIV/AIDS (UNAIDS), Global Network of People living with HIV/AIDS (GNP+), International Community of Women living with HIV/AIDS (ICW). (2013). The people living with HIV stigma index. http://www.stigmaindex.org/.

Ismail, S. (2009). *Participatory health research. international observatory on health research systems*. Cambridge: RAND Europe.

Israel, B. A., Schulz, A. J., Parker, E. A., & Becker, A. B. (1998). Review of community-based research: Assessing partnership approaches to improve public health. *Annual Review of Public Health, 19*(1), 173–202.

Israel, B. A., Schulz, A. J., Parker, E. A., Becker, A. B., Allen, A. J., & Guzman, J. R. (2003). Critical issues in developing and following community-based participatory research principles. In M. Minkler & N. Wallerstein (Eds.), *Community-based participatory research for health* (pp. 56–73). San Francisco: Jossey-Bass.

Jagosh, J., Pluye, P., Macaulay, A. C., Salsberg, J., Henderson, J., Sirett, E., Bush, P. L., Seller, R., Wong, G., Greenhalgh, T., Cargo, M., Herbert, C. P., Seifer, S. D., & Green, L. W. (2011). Assessing the outcomes of participatory research: Protocol for identifying, selecting, appraising and synthesizing the literature for realist review. *Implementation Science, 6*(1), 24.

Jagosh, J., Macaulay, A. C., Pluye, P., Salsberg, J., Bush, P. L., Henderson, J., Sirett, E., Wong, G., Cargo, M., Herbert, C. P., Seifer, S. D., Green, L. W., & Greenhalgh, T. (2012). Uncovering the benefits of participatory research: Implications of a realist review for health research and practice. *The Milbank Quarterly, 90*(2), 311–346.

Johansson, A. W., & Lindhult, E. (2008). Emancipation or workability? Critical versus pragmatic scientific orientation in action research. *Action Research, 6*(1), 95–115.

Kuhn, T. S. (2012). *The structure of scientific revolutions*. Chicago: University of Chicago press.

Lather, P. (1986). Research as practice. *Harvard Educational Review, 55*(3), 290–300.

Ledwith, M., & Springett, J. (2010). *Participatory practice. Community-based action for transformative change*. Bristol: The Policy Press.

Lukesch, H., & Zecha, G. (1978). Neue Handlungsforschung? Programm und Praxis gesellschaftskritischer Sozialforschung. *Soziale Welt, 29*, 26–43.

Macaulay, A., Commanda, L., Freeman, W. L., Gibson, N., McCabe, M., Robbins, C., & Twohig, P. (1999). Responsible research with communities: Participatory research in primary care. *British Medical Journal, 319*, 774–778.

Macaulay, A. C., Jagosh, J., Seller, R., Henderson, J., Cargo, M., Greenhalgh, T., Wong, G., Salsberg, J., Green, L. W., Herbert, C. P., & Pluye, P. (2011). Assessing the benefits of participatory research: A rationale for a realist review. *Global Health Promotion, 18*(2), 45–48.

Mellor, N. (1999). *From exploring practice to exploring inquiry: A practitioner researcher's experience*. PhD thesis. Newcastle: University of Northumbria.

Mercer, G. (2002). Emancipatory disability research. In C. Barnes, M. Oliver, & L. Barton (Eds.), *Disability studies today* (pp. 228–249). Cambridge: Blackwells.

Mezirow, J., et al. (1990). *Fostering critical reflection in adulthood. A guide to transformational and emancipatory learning.* San Francisco: Jossey-Bass.

Minkler, M., & Wallerstein, N. (2008). *Community-based participatory research for health: From process to outcome.* San Francisco: Jossey-Bass.

National Health and Medical Research Council & Consumers' Health Forum of Australia. (2002). *Statement on consumer and community participation in health and medical research.* Canberra: Commonwealth of Australia.

Nutbeam, D (2000) Health Literacy as a Public Health Goal: A Challenge for Contemporary Health Education and Communication Strategies into the 21st Century. Health Promotion International; 15(3): 259–267.

Onwuegbuzie, A. J., Johnson, R. B., & Collins, K. M. (2009). Call for mixed analysis: A philosophical framework for combining qualitative and quantitative approaches. *International Journal of Multiple Research Approaches, 3*(2), 114–139.

Reason, P., & Bradbury, H. (2001). *Handbook of action research: Participative inquiry and practice.* London: Sage.

Reason, P., & Bradbury, H. (Eds.). (2008). *Handbook of action research* (2nd ed.). Thousand Oaks: Sage.

Rifkin, S. B. (1996). Paradigms lost: Toward a new understanding of community participation in health programmes. *Acta Tropica, 61*(2), 79–92.

Roman, L. G., & Apple, M. W. (1990). Is naturalism a move away from positivism? Materialist and feminist approaches to subjectivity in ethnographic research. In E. W. Eisner & A. Peshkin (Eds.), *Qualitative inquiry in education* (pp. 38–73). New York: Teachers' College Press.

Schön, D. (1983). *The reflective practitioner. How professionals think in action.* London: Maurice Temple Smith Ltd.

Smithies, J., & Webster, G. (1998). *Community involvement in health. From passive recipients to active participants.* Aldershot: Ashgate.

Sohng, S. S. L. (1995). *Participatory research and community organizing.* Working paper presented at the New Social Movement and Community Organizing Conference, University of Washington, Seattle, WA. November 1–3, 1995.

Stoecker, R. (2013). *Research methods for community change: A project-based approach.* Thousand Oaks: Sage.

von Unger, H., Block, M., & Wright, M. T. (2007). *Aktionsforschung im deutschsprachigen Raum. Zur Geschichte und Aktualität eines kontroversen Ansatzes aus Public Health Sicht, der Reihe 'Discussion Papers'.* Berlin: Wissenschaftszentrum Berlin für Sozialforschung Berlin.

Viswanathan, M., Ammerman, A., Eng, E., Gartlehner, G., Lohr, K. N., Griffith, D., Rhodes, S., Samuel-Hodge, C., Maty, S., Lux, L., Webb, L., Sutton, S. F., Swinson, T., Jackman, A., & Whitener, L. (2004). *Community-based participatory research: Assessing the evidence, Summary, Evidence Report/Technology Assessment: Number 99. AHRQ Publication Number 04-E022-1, August 2004.* Rockville: Agency for Healthcare Research and Quality.

Von Unger, H. (2012). Participatory health research with immigrant communities in Germany. *International Journal of Action Research, 8*(3), 266–287.

Waterman, H., Tillen, D., Dickson, R., & de Koning, K. (2001). Action research: A systematic review and guidance for assessment. *Health Technology Assessment, 5*(23), 1–166.

Whitelaw, S., Beattie, A., Balogh, R., & Watson, J. (2003). *A review of the nature of action research.* Cardiff: Welsh Assembly Government.

Winter, R. (2002). Truth or fiction: Problems of validity and authenticity in narratives of action research. *Educational Action Research, 10*(1), 143–154.

Wright, M. T. (Ed.). (2010). *Partizipative Qualitätsentwicklung in der Gesundheitsförderung und Prävention.* Bern: Hans-Huber.

Wright, M. T. (2012). Partizipation in der Praxis: die Herausforderung einer kritisch reflektierten Professionalität. In R. Rosenbrock & S. Hartung (Eds.), *Partizipation und Gesundheit* (pp. 91–101). Bern: Hans-Huber.

Wright, M. T. (2016). Partizipative Gesundheitsforschung. In *Bundeszentrale für gesundheitliche Aufklärung (BZgA), Leitbegriffe der Gesundheitsförderung*. http://www.bzga.de/leitbegriffe/?id=angebote&idx=273.

Wright, M. T., Roche, B., von Unger, H., Block, M., & Gardner, B. (2009). A call for an international collaboration on participatory research for health. *Health Promotion International, 25*(1), 115–122.

Wright, M. T., von Unger, H., & Block, M. (2010a). Lokales Wissen, lokale Theorie und lokale Evidenz für die Prävention und Gesundheitsförderung. In M. T. Wright (Ed।)., (2010) *Partizipative Qualitätsentwicklung in der Gesundheitsförderung und Prävention* (pp. 53–74). Hans-Huber: Bern.

Wright, M. T., Gardner, B., Roche, B., von Unger, H., & Ainlay, C. (2010b). Building an international collaboration on participatory health research. *Progress in Community Health Partnerships: Research, Education, and Action, 4*(1), 31–36.

Wright, M. T., Kilian, H., & Brandes, S. (2013). Praxisbasierte Evidenz in der Prävention und Gesundheitsförderung bei sozial Benachteiligten. *Das Gesundheitswesen*. https://doi.org/10.1007/s00103-012-1628-7.

Chapter 2
Building Consensus, Celebrating Diversity: The International Collaboration for Participatory Health Research

Michael T. Wright, Tina Cook, Jane Springett, and Krystyna Kongats

Introduction

Participatory approaches to health research are increasingly drawing the attention of researchers, decision-makers, funders, civil society, and various social groups and communities worldwide. There is a great diversity among these approaches in terms of intention, theory, process, and outcome (Waterman et al. 2001; Ismail 2009; Whitelaw et al. 2003; Minkler and Wallerstein 2008; Rocha and Aguiar 2003; Rodrigues Brandão 2005). This diversity reflects the large variety of people, places, and issues involved in participatory health research (PHR) in many different countries and under widely varying conditions. PHR is often viewed as being a means for achieving positive transformation in society in the interest of people's health, from bringing citizens together to explore and address local issues to changing the way health professionals are educated, the way healthcare institutions work, and the politics and policies affecting the health of society, including issues of health equity.

The International Collaboration for Participatory Health Research (ICPHR) was created in 2009 as a place to bring together what we are learning internationally about the application of participatory research approaches to address health-related

M. T. Wright (✉)
Catholic University of Applied Sciences, Institute for Social Health, Berlin, Germany
e-mail: michael.wright@khsb-berlin.de

T. Cook
Department of Disability and Education, Liverpool Hope University, Liverpool, UK
e-mail: cookt@hope.ac.uk

J. Springett
School of Public Health, University of Alberta, Edmonton, Alberta, Canada
e-mail: jane.springett@ualberta.ca

K. Kongats
School of Public Health, University of Alberta, Edmonton, Alberta, Canada
e-mail: krystyna.kongats@ualberta.ca

© Springer International Publishing AG, part of Springer Nature 2018
M. T. Wright, K. Kongats (eds.), *Participatory Health Research*,
https://doi.org/10.1007/978-3-319-92177-8_2

17

issues (Wright et al. 2009, 2010). The ICPHR is open to everyone interested in promoting the dissemination and further development of PHR embedded in common values and principles. The ICPHR seeks to strengthen the role of PHR in problem definition, intervention design, and decision-making on health-related issues and thus to provide a means for people most affected by these issues to influence how they are understood and addressed in the society.

A central task of the ICPHR has been clarifying what "participation" means when conducting research. The term is often used in an inflationary and diffuse way to mean a broad range of engagement processes, from serving on a steering committee or acting as a consultant on the content of a questionnaire to the co-creation of research led by and for those whose lives or work would be directly affected by the study (Tritter 2009; Martin 2008). By clarifying what we mean by PHR, we can critically examine research practices and outcomes, distinguishing the various forms and effects of participation.

Goals of the ICPHR

The following goals have guided the work of the ICPHR from its founding:

To define PHR: Although the basic idea of participatory research is found in several countries, there has been no internationally accepted definition of what constitutes this type of research (cf. Reason and Bradbury 2001). The practice of PHR spans a multitude of settings, methods, and theoretical assumptions. The challenge is to define what unites the field, particularly in comparison to more widely accepted approaches to generating particular forms of data or evidence, such as clinical trials or population-based social epidemiology. In a first position paper, ICPHR members have described 11 key characteristics of PHR (see Chap. 1: 'What is Participatory Health Research').

To enhance the quality of PHR: It is common in PHR to reject or modify conventional definitions of scientific rigor so as to accommodate the participatory process of generating knowledge. However, this has not yet resulted in a consensus on what constitutes good PHR. In defining quality criteria, such concepts as scientific rigor, validity, generalizability, evidence, and objectivity need to be clarified (Springett et al. 2011). Quality criteria have been identified by the ICPHR, based on what have been proposed as core characteristics of the approach, emphasizing the importance of participation throughout the research process (Cook n.d.).

To reinforce the impact of PHR on public health research and practice: To date, the bulk of the work describing PHR has focused on relational and procedural aspects of the research (the partnership between academia and community, the nature and impact of community involvement, etc.) (e.g., Israel et al. 2006; Seifer 2006) and less on specifying the forms of knowledge which are generated by PHR as compared to other forms of research. Terms such as local knowledge, local theory, and local evidence are used (e.g., Israel et al. 1998; Yamada et al. 2008) without specifying how these fit into the big picture of building knowledge, more generally, or how they inform decision-making in the health field (Roche 2009). In the UK, INVOLVE invoNET—a network funded by the National Institute for Health Research to promote and build evidence, knowledge, and learning about *patient and public involvement* (PPI) in the National Health Service (NHS), public health, and social care research—has produced a helpful bibliography of references on public involvement in these fields (Staley 2010; INVOLVE 2014). This bibliography identifies papers that allude to the impact of public involvement in health research. The broad use of the term PPI means, however, that it is difficult to identify the forms of participation that have taken place and related impacts.

In participatory research more generally, and particularly in action research traditions, impact is embedded in the research. As part of the research process, rather than a defined outcome, the impact is not always easy to articulate and can be lost in accounts of action research in practice (Cook et al. 2017). This is especially true when the impact is a change in perspective, problem definition, or in getting a fuller account of an issue. In addition, while participatory research is set within a collaborative paradigm, the range of approaches means that community participation and co-laboring (Sumara and Luce-Kapler 1993) sit on a participatory spectrum and do not fall neatly into single categorizations for practice. The form and intensity of participation can also change over the course of a research project.

A focus area of the ICPHR is the evaluation of participatory health research projects (see Chaps. 3 and 6), which includes addressing the issue of impact (see Chap. 5). A core evaluation question of ICPHR members is: Under what conditions do which participatory strategies contribute to what kind of outcomes, recognizing that PHR is often imbedded in already complex intervention designs (ICPHR n.d.). A number of reviews by ICPHR members have started to unravel these connections and build the evidence based on the impacts of PHR (Abma et al. 2017; Pearson et al. 2015; Sandoval et al. 2011; Trickett and Beehler 2017). There are also future plans to build an interactive impact repository (the interactive knowledge base) to both retroactively and prospectively assess and document the impact of specific PHR initiatives around the world (see Chap. 5).

Structure and Membership of the ICPHR

The ICPHR was founded by the Research Group Public Health at the Social Science Research Center Berlin (WZB), the Wellesley Institute (WI) in Toronto, and the Liverpool John Moores University (LJMU).[1] There is a *central office* responsible

---

[1] WI is the only founding institution still serving on the executive committee. The staff at the WZB and LJMU have since changed institution, transferring their activity as consortium members to their new workplaces.

for the day-to-day management of the Collaboration. The ICPHR is governed by an executive committee composed largely of the consortium members. Each consortium member provides leadership on a particular focus area. The current focus areas are theory and PHR, ethics in PHR, training in PHR, impact of PHR, mixed methods and PHR, children and PHR, literature reviews, evaluation of PHR, art and PHR, and communication (ICPHR website and other media). Important results from the work of the focus areas are presented in Chaps. 3, 4, 5, 6, and 7 in this book. In addition, there are several working groups focused on various short- and long-term projects, including joint publications. The ICPHR has more than 200 members from over 20 countries in Europe, North America, Latin America, Asia, Oceania, and Africa. The mailing list has over 400 members. Part II of this volume (Chaps. 8, 9, 10, 11, 12, 13, 14, 15, and 16) reflects the variety of regional perspectives represented in the membership and in the practice of PHR, more generally.

The ICPHR members come together at the annual working meeting to work on common projects and to present work they have conducted in their home countries. The meeting takes place each year in a different country. This is truly a working meeting, not a conference, as it is a place where the co-laboring takes place. The work of the Collaboration is publicized through the internet site and the publications of its members.[2]

There are many reasons for becoming a member of the ICPHR. Madsen (2016) conducted an oral history project with eight ICPHR members from Mexico, the UK, the USA, Canada, Germany, and Sweden to uncover their motivations for joining the ICPHR as related to their personal histories in the field of public health, which may be typical for other members. The interviews revealed that most of the researchers had come from a practice background with strong connections to various communities and that none had a typical, straightforward career path to become an academic or a researcher. The participants were drawn to applying participatory principles to academic research, often without any clear role models or consistent support from their work contexts. Thus they were "making the road while walking." The people who influenced the thinking of these researchers varied considerably, depending on the context in which they worked, ranging from feminism to Paulo Freire, the work of Meredith Minkler and Barbara Israel in the USA, and liberation theology. Those interviewed named several obstacles to their work, including particularly (Madsen 2016, p. 305): "1) a history of action or participatory approaches being linked with community development and devalued as research; 2) questioning the rigour of participatory approaches to research based on positivist criteria; 3) co-opting aspects of participatory research for utilitarian purposes but devaluing the underlying principles and values of this approach to research." By joining the ICPHR, those interviewed have sought to address these and other obstacles together, believing in the power of collective action.

---

[2] www.icphr.org

Issues and Challenges

Several issues and challenges have been encountered in building the Collaboration, including the following:

Identifying the primary goal of the Collaboration: A host of needs and interests which could potentially be served by an international collaboration have been discussed. Achieving a higher degree of legitimacy for PHR has been identified as a common concern and a driving issue for the work of the ICPHR. To have an impact on the hierarchically organized structures of academia and healthcare, the ICPHR has created a platform for greater visibility of PHR so as to claim its place in research and decision-making bodies. The Collaboration needs, therefore, to address issues which can have a direct impact on how research is generated, disseminated, and applied by universities, academic journals and publishers, research funding bodies, and healthcare authorities.

Building on current practice: The Collaboration was not created as a corrective to the current practice of PHR but rather to bring together what we know in a systematic way and to develop and clarify collectively the theoretical premises, scientific standards, and methodology of PHR. The ICPHR is not trying to reinvent PHR but rather to deepen the understanding of what PHR is—in all its diversity—and what it can achieve as compared to other approaches.

What's in a name? Finding the best term: Several well-known publications on PHR have originated from the USA where *community-based participatory research* has become a widely accepted term to designate the approach. In other countries, there is often no direct equivalent to the word "community" in the American sense, which has its origins in a particular history of immigration and civil rights. In Latin America, several traditions are explicitly political and emancipatory, based on the work of such pioneers as Paulo Freire and Orlando Fals Borda (Cordeiro et al. 2015). In the UK, the term "action research" is most commonly used in the health sector (Health Development Agency 2000), although the type of participatory engagement within an action research approach varies widely. In contrast, the term "action research" has been discredited in Germany and Sweden, being associated with particular ideological positions in the 1960s and 1970s (von Unger et al. 2007). For this reason, the terms participatory health research (*Partizipative Gesundheitsforschung*) and interactive research (*interaktiv forskning*) have been adopted in Germany and Sweden, respectively. All the various approaches have in common the core principle that the persons being researched have an influence on the research process itself. For that reason, it was agreed to adopt the more inclusive title International Collaboration for Participatory Health Research.

It was also discussed whether the health focus should be dropped to include all forms of participatory research, based on the observation that many of the issues identified are true for participatory research more generally. The decision to maintain the health focus was based on the argument that participatory research in health contexts is confronted with specific challenges which need to be addressed directly in order to impact policy and research on health disparities. These challenges include a hierarchical healthcare system, the dominance of positivist approaches to science, and the focus on particular forms of evidence in intervention research.

The conflict between a participatory ethic and setting standards: There is an ongoing tension in the discussion between the commitment to inclusion through participatory approaches and the exclusion implied by defining criteria and setting standards. This tension is present at two levels: regarding the process of setting up the Collaboration itself and regarding the question of how to set standards for participatory ways of working. There is general agreement that enhancing the impact and legitimacy of PHR necessitates creating more clarity in terms of definitions and quality criteria. It has been recognized that not everyone interested in PHR necessarily can or wants to be part of such a project that will be focused on advancing PHR in academic and political circles. Nevertheless, the ICPHR has sought to find ways to include a broad range of stakeholders, particularly through participation at the annual working meetings, and to explore ways of defining standards that respect the participatory ethic of PHR.

The relationship between theory and results: Addressing questions of scientific legitimacy necessarily involves discussions of theoretical assumptions (epistemology and ontology) and methodological questions. Participatory researchers in the health field are often not explicit about the nature, purpose, and potential of the participatory approach (Cook et al. 2017). There is a danger that such a discussion will become removed from the central goal of PHR—namely, creating social change to improve the health of disadvantaged communities. The theorization, standards, and methodological consistency which the ICPHR proposes will need to be congruent with this goal as a defining characteristic of PHR.

Avoiding the dominance of one language, country, or region: The ICPHR is committed to the participation of PHR practitioners from all parts of the world. The challenge of language and cultural barriers is enormous, particularly when considering that much PHR activity is not implemented in traditional academic contexts. The reporting of PHR takes place predominantly in local languages as part of the "gray literature." The English language and thus the role of English-speaking countries has become dominant in the international scientific discourse, overshadowing the existence of long-standing participatory research traditions in other parts of the world such as Latin America, Scandinavia, or South Asia. Several measures have been taken to expand the membership to more countries, to provide multilingual access to information, to gather information on various traditions, and to share decision-making power among members from various countries. This book is one way to highlight the variety of approaches, traditions, and cultures in the ICPHR.

Conclusion

PHR has emerged as an important approach to health research. The International Collaboration for Participatory Health Research is working to consolidate what is known about PHR and its impact in order to secure its place as a source of knowledge and action to address the world's health problems, particularly the problems of those most disadvantaged in society. The ICPHR is seeking to define more clearly the unique contribution of PHR to promoting the public's health and to bring together the power of what we know to create a different world in which everyone has the same opportunity to live a healthy and fulfilling life.

References

Abma, T. A., Cook, T., Rämgård, M., Kleba, E., Harris, J., & Wallerstein, N. (2017). Social impact of participatory health research: Collaborative non-linear processes of knowledge mobilization. *Educational Action Research, 25*(4) 1–17.

Cook, T. (n.d.). *Ensuring quality: Indicative characteristics of participatory (health) research.* Berlin: International Collaboration for Participatory Health Research Retrieved from: http://www.icphr.org/uploads/2/0/3/9/20399575/qualtiy_criteria_for_participatory_health_research_-_cook_-_version_15_08_21__1_.pdf.

Cook, T., Boote, J., Buckley, N., Vougioukalou, S., & Wright, M. (2017). Accessing participatory research impact and legacy: Developing the evidence base for participatory approaches in health research. *Educational Action Research, 25*(4), 473–488.

Cordeiro, L., Rittenmeyer, L., & Soares, C. B. (2015). Action research methodology in the health care field: A scoping review protocol. *JBI Database of Systematic Reviews and Implementation Reports, 13*(8), 70–78.

Health Development Agency. (2000). *Participatory approaches in health promotion and health planning: A literature review, Summary Bulletin.* London: Health Development Agency http://www.nice.org.uk/nicemedia/documents/participatory.pdf.

ICPHR. (n.d.). Evaluation of participatory health research. Retrieved from: http://www.icphr.org/evaluation-of-participatory-health-research.html.

INVOLVE. (2014). *Evidence bibliography 5.* Eastleigh: INVOLVE Coordinating Centre http://www.invo.org.uk/wp-content/uploads/2014/11/Bibliography5FinalComplete.pdf.

Ismail, S. (2009). *Participatory health research. International observatory on health research systems.* Cambridge: RAND Europe.

Israel, B. A., Schulz, A. J., Parker, E. A., & Becker, A. B. (1998). Review of community-based research: Assessing partnership approaches to improve public health. *Annual Review of Public Health, 19*, 173–202.

Israel, B. A., Krieger, J., Vlahov, D., Ciske, S., Foley, M., Fortin, P., et al. (2006). Challenges and facilitating factors in sustaining community-based participatory research partnerships: Lessons learned from Detroit, New York City and Seattle urban research centers. *Journal of Urban Health, 83*, 1022–1040.

Madsen, W. (2016). 'There and back again': International Collaboration for Participatory Health Researchers' journeys to evidence based practice and practice based evidence. *International Journal of Action Research, 12*(3), 294–314.

Martin, G. P. (2008). 'Ordinary people only': Knowledge, representativeness, and the publics of public participation in healthcare. *Sociology of Health & Illness, 30*(1), 35–54.

Minkler, M., & Wallerstein, N. (Eds.). (2008). *Community-based participatory research for health*. San Francisco: Jossey-Bass.

Pearson, C. R., Duran, B., Oetzel, J., Margarati, M., Villegas, M., Lucero, J., & Wallerstein, N. (2015). Research for improved health: Variability and impact of structural characteristics in federally funded community engaged research. *Progress in Community Health Partnerships: Research, Education, and Action, 9*(1), 17–29.

Reason, P., & Bradbury, H. (2001). *Handbook of action research: Participative inquiry and practice*. London: Sage.

Rocha, M., & Aguiar, K. (2003). Pesquisa-intervenção e a produção de novas análises. [Versão eletrônica]. *Psicologia, Ciência e Profissão, 23*(4), 64–73.

Roche, B. (2009). *New directions in community-based research*. Toronto: Wellesley Institute.

Rodrigues Brandão, C. (2005). Participatory research and participation in research: A look between times and spaces from Latin America. *International Journal of Action Research, 1*(1), 43–68.

Sandoval, J. A., Lucero, J., Oetzel, J., Avila, M., Belone, L., Mau, M., Pearson, C., Tafoya, G., Duran, B., Iglesias Rios, L., & Wallerstein, N. (2011). Process and outcome constructs for evaluating community-based participatory research projects: A matrix of existing measures. *Health Education Research, 27*(4), 680–690.

Seifer, S. D. (2006). Building and sustaining community-institutional partnerships for prevention research: Findings from a national collaborative. *Journal of Urban Health: Bulletin of the New York Academy of Medicine, 83*, 989–1003.

Springett, J., Wright, M. T., & Roche, B. (2011). *Developing quality criteria for participatory health research. An agenda for action, Discussion Paper*. Berlin: Wissenschaftszentrum Berlin für Sozialforschung.

Staley, K. (2010). *Exploring impact: Public involvement in NHS, public health and social care research*. Eastleigh: INVOLVE.

Sumara, D. J., & Luce-Kapler, R. (1993). Action research as a writerly text: Locating co-labouring in collaboration. *Education Action Research, 1*(3), 387–396.

Trickett, E. J., & Beehler, S. (2017). Participatory action research and impact: An ecological ripples perspective. *Educational Action Research, 25*, 1–16.

Tritter, J. (2009). Revolution or evolution: The challenges of conceptualizing patient and public involvement in a consumerist world. *Health Expectations, 12*(3), 275–287.

von Unger, H., Block, M., & Wright, M. T. (2007). *Aktionsforschung im deutschsprachigen Raum. Zur Geschichte und Aktualität eines kontroversen Ansatzes aus Public Health Sicht, der Reihe 'Discussion Papers'*. Berlin: Wissenschaftszentrum Berlin für Sozialforschung, Berlin.

Waterman, H., Tillen, D., Dickson, R., & de Koning, K. (2001). Action research: A systematic review and guidance for assessment. *Health Technology Assessment, 5*(23), iii-157 http://doi.org/10.3310/hta5230.

Whitelaw, S., Beattie, A., Balogh, R., & Watson, J. (2003). *A review of the nature of action research*. Cardiff: Welsh Assembly Government.

Wright, M. T., Roche, B., von Unger, H., Block, M., & Gardner, B. (2009). A call for an international collaboration on participatory research for health. *Health Promotion International, 25*(1), 115–122.

Wright, M. T., Gardner, B., Roche, B., von Unger, H., & Ainlay, C. (2010). Building an international collaboration on participatory health research. *Progress in Community Health Partnerships: Research, Education, and Action, 4*(1), 31–36.

Yamada, S., Slingsby, B. T., Inada, M. K., & Derauf, D. (2008). Evidence-based public health: A critical perspective. *Journal of Public Health, 16*, 169–172.

Chapter 3
Evaluating Participatory Health Research

John G. Oetzel, Jane Springett, Nina Wallerstein, Laura Parajon, Irene Sia, Mark Wieland, Abigail Reese, and Rangimahora Reddy

Introduction

With the growth of participatory health research (PHR) internationally in the recent decades, it becomes increasingly important to document and evaluate this approach. Evaluation of PHR, however, presents unique challenges as it represents distinct values and methods which differ from the dominant positivist worldview of bio-medical research, which seeks to control context within randomized control trials (Whitelaw 2012) or to control interventions across time and space without incorporating dynamic meanings and interpretations assigned by stakeholders (Bell et al. 2012; Shoveller et al. 2016). Unlike biomedical research, PHR is a practice that is epistemologically complex and interdisciplinary, involving multiple participants

J. G. Oetzel (✉)
University of Waikato, Hamilton, New Zealand
e-mail: john.oetzel@waikato.ac.nz

J. Springett
University of Alberta, Edmonton, Canada
e-mail: jane.springett@ualberta.ca

N. Wallerstein · A. Reese
University of New Mexico, Albuquerque, NM, USA
e-mail: nwallerstein@salud.unm.edus

L. Parajon
AMOS Health and Hope, Managua, Nicaragua and Potomac, Potomac, MD, USA
e-mail: lauraparajon@amoshealth.org

I. Sia · M. Wieland
Mayo Clinic College of Medicine, Rochester, MN, USA
e-mail: ia.irene@mayo.edu

R. Reddy
Rauawaawa Kaumātua Charitable Trust, Hamilton, New Zealand
e-mail: ceo@rauawaawa.co.nz

from a range of non-scientific backgrounds. It emphasizes process and learning; has a strong focus on action; is inherently relational, embedded, and connected to context; and has the participation of those affected by the research at its core. Evaluation therefore must be responsive and congruent to these features and the particular questions and values that are promoted (Greene 1994).

The purpose of this chapter is to introduce the key issues and challenges in evaluating PHR and discuss the use of the community-based participatory research (CBPR) conceptual model as one way to address these evaluation challenges. The CBPR conceptual model is a well-tested logic model developed in the context of the USA where PHR is commonly called CBPR. CBPR has a longstanding tradition within public health research where it emerged as a result of the development of formal partnerships between universities and wider society. In recent years, CBPR partnerships have also joined a wider array of community engagement in the USA called community-engaged scholarship (Bowen and Graham 2013). This chapter is organized in the following sections: (a) the key issues/challenges of evaluating PHR are identified; (b) the CPBR conceptual model is introduced; (c) three case studies are discussed to illustrate the model's usefulness; and (d) a conclusion is offered to illustrate how the CBPR model can address the key issues in evaluating PHR.

What Is the Current Status and Key Issues of Evaluating Participatory Health Research?

A first key issue is that the knowledge and information generated from PHR projects and activities can vary widely, dependent on the context in which the research takes place, the participatory research methods used, who participates, the attitudes and abilities of the participants, and the nature of the research question itself (Mantoura and Potvin 2013; Wallerstein et al. 2018). Different social factors can influence the results including the initial capacity of the community in terms of social capital and the capacity of academic researchers to collaborate authentically in equal relationships with all stakeholders (Wallerstein et al. 2018). External contextual factors may also enable or constrain participation, together with historical and contemporary social relationships and power dynamics (Shoveller et al. 2016). Evaluation questions can thus range from issues internal to the partnership, such as quality and level of participation, effectiveness of tools and methods used, and group dynamics, as well as external impact, such as goals of policy change, social transformation, or ability to respond to changing community needs. Much depends as to whether the evaluation is formative or summative, developmental, or outcome-driven, which may also change over time. Given this variety it is impossible to be prescriptive as to the evaluation design; however, participatory approaches will ensure commensurability.

A second key issue relates to differing and often conflicting epistemologies. Recent years have seen the growth internationally of multiple frameworks for evaluating research, as research quality and, more particularly, research impact have become issues of social accountability and governance, with government-funded research monies shrinking under neoliberal economic policies (Guthrie et al. 2013). This has generated a minefield for conflicting epistemologies and values as disciplines compete with one another to demonstrate their worth. While some countries have articulated new frameworks for evaluating research quality, many still rely on bibliometrics and peer review (Turato 2005; Pinto and de Andrade 1999). In some cases, particularly in less developed countries, certain frameworks are imposed by international agencies which distort local systems of thought to meet (usually) "western" models (de Sousa Santos 2014; Devia et al. 2017; Wallerstein and Duran 2006; Coimbra 1999). Yet even within "western" models, there are substantial differences between, for example, the Anglo-American pragmatic utilitarian approach and the European model of the primacy of knowledge and philosophy for its own sake (House 2015; Springett et al. 2011; Trickett 2011). Nevertheless, the trend towards seeking standardization through common frameworks for evaluating research quality provides an opportunity and a challenge for PHR to articulate criteria by which it should be judged and evaluated.

Relatedly, it is important to understand the purpose and perspective of the particular PHR approach in order to guide the evaluation. In the varieties of PHR internationally, there is a wide spectrum of approaches (Trickett 2011). At one end of the spectrum is the pragmatic or utilitarian approach to PHR whereby participation is seen as a way of increasing the relevance of research to local people in terms of health improvement or healthcare. At the other end of spectrum lies transformative or emancipatory PHR which often has a specific aim of social transformation or empowerment, contributing to what has been called knowledge democracy (Johansson and Lindhult 2008; Wallerstein and Duran 2006; Hall et al. 2015; de Sousa Santos 2014). These types of PHR can be large research projects or small-scale projects strongly embedded in marginalized communities, wherein the "expert" researcher, who is not necessarily an academic, builds a community of co-researchers (e.g. group of unemployed youth) and works to create a space for radical inclusivity. Evaluation here might take the form of self-reflection in journals and sharing through poems and art as the main tools (Cahill 2007). The emphasis is on empowerment and learning rather proving added value. These two stereotypes of PHR are, of course, not mutually exclusive; PHR can be both functional and transformative.

A third key issue is recognizing the central role of values and principles in PHR, thus making evaluation of PHR projects more than simply an issue of methods and outcomes (Israel et al. 2018). This includes identifying whose values and principles are meant ("whose reality counts") and how far one is prepared to compromise one's principles to conform to others' expectations (de Sousa Santos 2014; Wallerstein et al. 2018). Developing and advocating the use of appropriate tools and evaluation approaches are therefore not simply about health outcomes or methodological standards but must address how the values of those involved influence the participatory process itself and how the interplay of values and process shapes research methods and intervention development (Oetzel et al. 2015b; Wallerstein et al. 2018).

Unfortunately, in the age of the evaluative state, evaluation is often tied up with political priorities in funding rather than increasing local knowledge about what works and why or contributing to learning and development for transformation (House 2015). There remains a tension between top-down bureaucratic requirements of standardization and control and local-level demands for diversity, complexity, and local direction (Chambers 1998). A further tension is between evaluation to prove and evaluation to *im*prove. When placed in an arena of positivist health science research which emphasizes the notion of linear cause and effect, where social change for health is a matter of strictly formulated "interventions" devoid of context and social relationships and where generalizability is the mission, PHR gets pushed to defend itself against this worldview.

Finally, a fourth challenge is the extensive debate within PHR evaluation on the issue of quality. The ICPHR has put forwards some criteria on quality and a discussion paper that has spurned some debate (Springett et al. 2011). More recently Bradbury-Huang (2014), in the context of action research, challenges us to reimagine our view of quality, away from the mechanistic to the relational. Quality is about relationships, actionability, reflexivity, and acknowledging the self as local change agent and one who can support the flourishing of other persons, communities, and the wider ecology. A key pivotal decision in regard to quality concerns the purpose of the evaluation, whether it is for advocacy, accountability, and allocation of funds or for understanding why or how PHR is effective. In the health field, some funders are concerned as to the added value of participation, while others are more concerned whether there is impact on health status, healthcare, or health equity (Israel et al. 2018; Wallerstein and Duran 2006). With the purpose of any evaluation being pivotal for shaping all other decisions, evaluation design requires being clear on what is actually being evaluated.

A generally recognized primary component of PHR evaluation is to create clarity through generating a logic model which specifies inputs including resources, activities/processes, outputs, intermediate outcomes, and impacts or distal outcomes (Renger et al. 2011; Wallerstein et al. 2008, 2018). The logic model can then be used to generate priorities in indicator development as well as timelines for data collection. It can also elucidate local explanatory models, including what stakeholders' theories of change are, in other words why and how they think the activities being undertaken will lead to change, the role of context that can ameliorate or prevent change, as well as underlying assumptions held by key actors.

While their use is highly regarded, logic models have come under some criticism for their inability to elucidate dynamic interrelationships and multiple perspectives, since consensus is required (Hummelbrunner 2010). There is also concern about the way they have been used often instrumentally and inflexibly by funding agencies. Others have argued that, as long as the processes of development are participatory, some of the criticisms can be overcome (Renger et al. 2011). In participatory evaluation, evaluation from a dynamic perspective is undertaken through workshops and dialogue between all stakeholders. The process of bringing together different ways of knowing not only generates appropriate indicators but also can focus a group of stakeholders as to what will be the priority for the evaluation, as well as understanding different perspectives on what constitutes PHR in that context.

In sum, the key issues around evaluating PHR include the following: (1) the need to integrate context into evaluation, (2) the need to reflect different and local ways of knowing (i.e. conflicting epistemologies in the evaluation), (3) the need to reflect the underlying principles of PHR and local knowledge creation rather than solely focusing on methods and health outcomes, and (4) the need to include high-quality evaluation that reflects dynamic relationships and perspectives in PHR. The next section introduces the CPBR conceptual model and three case studies that illustrate its use. Then, a discussion of how the CBPR conceptual model addresses these key issues concludes this chapter.

CBPR Conceptual Model

The CBPR conceptual model was constructed to identify the added value of community and other stakeholder participation in research and to assess the potential pathways of how promising partnership practices contribute to intermediate system and capacity changes, long-term community transformation, and the improvement of health and health equity. The model identifies mechanisms and theories of change in four domains and associated pathways. It was developed in consultation with a national advisory board of CBPR community and academic experts in the USA, a systematic review of the North American literature, and a survey of American CBPR community and academic experts (Wallerstein et al. 2008). It has also been continuously updated based on consultations with CBPR experts, empirical data from the CBPR literature, the US-based Research for Improved Health (RIH) mixed-methods study of 200 CBPR projects on various health issues among diverse communities (Hicks et al. 2012; Lucero et al. 2018), and the current US National Institutes of Health "Engage for Equity" study of another 192 partnerships to further validate the model (Kastelic et al. 2018; Oetzel et al. 2018). The most recent version of this model is presented in Fig. 3.1.

The model identifies four domains of CBPR characteristics: contexts; participatory processes; intervention and research; and outcomes. *Contexts* are the background features that shape the nature of the research and include five broad elements: social/structural, policy, health importance, capacity and readiness, and historical trust and mistrust among research institutions and communities. The social/structural element encompasses such issues as socio-economic status, the physical environment, and institutional racism. Policy relates to the local and national issues around funding and governing PHR. Health importance is the local perception of the importance of a specific health issue (i.e. should we address this or other issues?). Capacity and readiness includes the academic/research and community capacities to undertake the research and also the readiness to collaborate effectively. Finally, historical trust addresses the nature of the prior relationship among the academic/research institution and the community; it also may include the general trust a community has for research institutions.

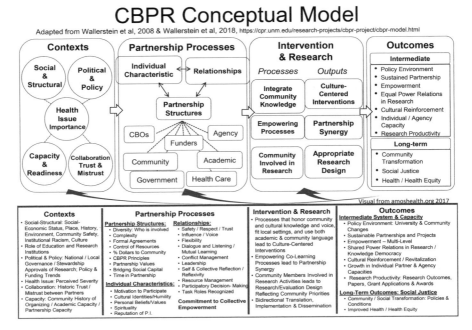

CBPR Conceptual Model

Adapted from Wallerstein et al, 2008 & Wallerstein et al, 2018, https://cpr.unm.edu/research-projects/cbpr-project/cbpr-model.html

Fig. 3.1 CBPR conceptual model. (Adapted from Wallerstein et al. 2008 and Wallerstein and Duran 2010, https://cpr.unm.edu/research-projects/cbpr-project/cbpr-model.html)

Contexts influence the nature of the *partnership processes* which includes three elements: individual characteristics, relationships, and partnership structures. Individual characteristics are qualities of the people involved that allow creation of a strong partnership such as flexibility and cultural humility. Relationships centre on the interactional dynamics of the partnership, including shared decision-making and conflict management. Partnership structures are the structures and values that guide the various agencies and organizations involved in the research, such as formal agreements, advisory boards, sharing of resources, and shared principles. Collectively, these three elements of the partnership processes influence the science or the choice of *interventions and research* methods of the partnership.

Intervention/research includes three interdependent processes and outputs of the research. Integrating community knowledge in the research process increases the likelihood that a culture-centred intervention or research project is created (Wallerstein et al. under review). Empowering processes involving mutual learning leads to partnership synergy or facilitating the group accomplishing more than what they could than individual partners on their own (Khodyakov et al. 2011). Community involvement in multiple phases of research results in an appropriate research design that fits the local contexts and yields strong, valid data.

The choice of intervention and research design affects the outcomes of the partnership project. Intermediate outcomes shape the community and larger environment including policy environment change, sustained partnerships, shared power relations in research, cultural reinforcement, and growth of individual partner and agency capacity. These intermediate outcomes then influence long-term outcomes such as community transformation, social justice, and improved health and health equity.

This model is well-suited to guide evaluation of participatory health research for several reasons. First, the RIH study provided strong empirical research to support the theoretical elements of change and the conceptualization and measurement of many of the constructs in the domains (Oetzel et al. 2015a, b; Pearson et al. 2015). This empirical research provides a set of metrics, tools, and measures (both quantitative and qualitative) that can be used to guide evaluation (Center for Participatory Research A n.d.). Second, the model is flexible to allow individual partnerships to assess elements of the model that matter to them. A new visioning guide for using the CBPR model as a planning and evaluation tool supports partnerships to choose the relevant characteristics in the model and to adapt the model to their own context and evaluation purpose (Center for Participatory Research B n.d.). A beginning partnership could use the model as a planning tool to develop their evaluation indicators. Third, the empirical data in support of the model (Duran et al. under review; Oetzel et al. 2018; Wallerstein et al. under review) can also be used as a targeted approach to evaluation. A partnership can choose the most relevant outcomes for their project and then select the contexts, partnership processes, and intervention characteristics that are significantly associated with those outcomes. Fourth, the model has shown resilience across partnerships, both in the USA (Devia et al. 2017; Lucero et al. 2018) and in the developing world with translations that exist in Portuguese and Spanish.

Case Studies Using the CBPR Conceptual Model

The following cases illustrate evaluation of PHR framed by the CBPR conceptual model. Two of the cases directly used the model to guide evaluation, and one of the cases did not use it directly but did organize evaluation around the four domains. Despite not directly using the conceptual model, this case is included because it illustrates how the model and domains are useful as intuitive frameworks that resonate with efforts to evaluate PHR even when applied in a post hoc manner.

Rochester Healthy Community Partnership, Minnesota

The Rochester Healthy Community Partnership (RHCP) was established in 2004 as a result of a successful project undertaken by community organizations and health researchers in Rochester, Minnesota, to address tuberculosis. The partnership discovered that a CBPR approach had the potential to successfully engage the knowledge and concerns of community members, along with the expertise of clinician-researchers, among Rochester's diverse immigrant communities (Wieland et al. 2012). To leverage this success, RHCP was formed to apply CBPR to multiple other health concerns identified by community partners. In 2014, following a productive decade of CBPR collaboration, RHCP undertook a participatory evaluation process to assess the "health" of our partnership, define future steps, and plan for sustainability. The partnership elected to use the model as the framework for a four-step evaluation process.

The first step of the evaluation was to create a historical timeline identifying key moments in the partnership (Sanchez-Youngman and Wallerstein 2018). This was done through a collaborative process in which partners identified the point at which they joined RHCP and important events, grounding them in their origins and 10-year trajectory.

The partnership then adapted the model to reflect the history and priorities of RHCP. The partners discussed and validated each domain of the model and determined which aspects resonated most strongly with their partners. The focused, adapted model retains many original constructs but also includes new elements from experience (e.g. *deep complexity*, *group process*, and *building community*) reflecting RHCP language and values.

Following this foundational work, the partners collected qualitative and quantitative data from current and former partners. The partners used the adapted model to customize an interview guide and survey instrument developed and validated by the Center for Participatory Research at the University of New Mexico to assure the tools would elicit responses reflective of the extent of their capacity to promote core values of RHCP. The partners conducted 13 interviews of key partnership members and 36 surveys of a wider group.

The fourth step was participatory data analysis by the new RHCP Evaluation Workgroup, a subset of partners who volunteered, examined, and reflected on the aggregated data reports of the large amount of rich data. The findings about partnering practices, their impact on research projects, and outcomes led to both appreciating the long-term commitment to equitable involvement and to outlining challenges. The Workgroup prepared an executive summary of findings in each domain, further revised the adapted model (Rochester Healthy Community Partnership n.d.), and developed key questions to help guide full-partnership discussion of action steps.

This experience indicates that participatory processes are as essential to evaluation as they are to core partnership activities, leading to a level of resonance and utility that would not have been obtained from a traditional programme evaluation. The CBPR conceptual model is a flexible tool that was used to generate an evaluation plan grounded in the partnerships' specific priorities. A key finding of the evaluation was that partnership processes inform outcomes, and the development of authentic participation is one of RHCP's most important contributions.

CBPR and Participatory Evaluation Process at AMOS

This case study describes the use of the CBPR conceptual model for participatory evaluation by a community-based non-profit public health organization based in Nicaragua called AMOS Health and Hope.[1] Nicaragua is the second poorest country in Latin America, characterized by extreme disparities in wealth and health. AMOS was founded in 2006 to reduce health inequities by blending evidence-based global health interventions with CBPR principles, community empowerment strategies, and participatory evaluation for greater impact. AMOS currently works in 26 communities and 5 departments, serving a population of 30,000 people.

AMOS uses an assets-based strategy of community-based primary healthcare (CBPHC), developing community trust, understanding geographic boundaries, and inventorying community strengths. CBPHC is built on a three-way partnership: the *community* identifying their key community priorities and issues, the *government* providing top-down policies and epidemiological priorities, and *non-governmental partners* such as AMOS facilitating participatory processes and evaluation (Taylor 2010). An initial step is the census, which registers every person in the catchment area. With AMOS staff support, the local health council, community health workers (CHWs), and community volunteers conduct the census and analyse and interpret the data with a health equity focus to identify the most vulnerable people (primarily pregnant women and children under 2 years old). These steps are done iteratively each year to prioritize issues, implement a community health plan, and evaluate impact together.

In 2014, AMOS began utilizing the model as a participatory planning and evaluation tool. On a semi-annual basis, staff members, working on projects such as childhood malnutrition, WASH (Water, Sanitation, and Hygiene), Essential Care for Every Baby (ECEB), and service learning, evaluate their work using the four domains. Led by the AMOS monitoring and evaluation team, the participatory evaluation action cycle engages all staff to reflect and dialogue about successes and areas of improvement. The data gathered from the four domains is visualized on a large poster board with the staff and CHWs for interpretation, analysis, and prioritization to develop action plans. Recently, the use of the model helped AMOS improve CBPR efficacy by prioritizing partnerships across all programmes. This led to an organizational action plan to assign one staff member to facilitate long-term partnership processes between communities and the Nicaraguan Ministry of Health to strengthen the three-way partnership for higher sustainability.

While the use of the CBPR conceptual model as a participatory evaluation tool does not require new resources or funding, it does require an organizational commitment to CBPR principles as well as basic staff training. This training is available online (Center for Participatory Research C n.d.) to help other organizations adapt the model for their use. The use of the CBPR model at AMOS has resulted in greater collective efficacy by staff and CHWs to adhere to CBPR principles and to take

---

[1] amoshealth.org

action to influence change. In the words of one of the field staff, "The CBPR framework is an empowering way to help us understand how we can better partner for social justice".[2]

CBRP in New Zealand

In 2011–2012, a community organization that serves Māori *kaumātua* (elders 55+), Rauawaawa Kaumātua Charitable Trust (Rauawaawa), partnered with researchers from several universities to identify why *kaumātua* underutilize palliative care services using a multidimensional health literacy perspective (Zarcadoolas et al. 2005). They captured the voices of *kaumātua*, *whānau* (extended family), and healthcare workers to understand what makes effective communication during the palliative care process.

The evaluation was guided by these goals of understanding health services and reflects the domains of the model, although they only loosely used the model to guide the evaluation. The evaluation was process-focussed to ensure the following of Māori *tikanga* (cultural values and protocols) and participatory principles. The partners were cognizant of the New Zealand history, especially the Treaty of Waitangi. The Treaty was signed in 1840 between the British crown and 500 Māori chiefs, making the land a British colony and providing equal rights to Māori as British citizens (Orange 1987). There were discrepancies about the Treaty due to different languages; to reconcile the differences, the New Zealand government issued a set of principles for interpreting the Treaty—partnership, participation, and protection which emphasized Māori self-determination (Orange 1987; Simpson and Ake 2010).

To address these key contextual issues (*tikanga* and the principles of the treaty), the partnership began with training about PHR (including introduction of the conceptual model and the four key domains) and *kaupapa Māori*. *Kaupapa Māori* is a culturally appropriate methodology to research in the local context as it emphasizes Māori worldviews/practices (Kennedy and Cram 2010). These trainings helped to ensure partners had shared goals and processes for evaluating our work. Further, the project was guided by an advisory board composed of Rauawaawa board members; they stewarded the work and had monthly checks to ensure the project was moving towards the stated goals.

The evaluation of partnership processes consisted of using monthly "check-ins". The partners assessed the structure of meetings and research and found that meetings were collegial and that all parties were willing to express concerns about the research, demonstrating shared power and influence. The structure of the partnership was deemed appropriate, as the community partners led the project and there were memoranda of understanding (MOUs) and shared resources. The board approved the partnership structure and received updates about group dynamics.

---

[2] Acuna, S. AMOS field programme coordinator and former CHW. 2016.

The research included interviews/focus groups with 80+ participants. The original proposal included conventional interview guides of direct and open-ended questions. In one evaluation session, a community partner noted that this approach would not be appropriate. This partner suggested an unstructured approach with probes for *kaumātua* to tell their stories. The data collection included bringing a small group of five to ten participants together and start with *karakia* (prayer) and then *whakawhānaungatanga* (sharing backgrounds). Then there was an individual interview followed by bringing the participants back together to have shared *kai* (food) and *whakawhitiwhiti whakaaro* (collective debrief). Without the process evaluation, this approach would not have been used and the data quality would have suffered.

Finally, the outcomes of the evaluation focused on intermediate outcomes of dissemination of research findings and agency capacity-building. The findings were shared at academic and practitioner conferences, and the evaluation consisted of estimating the dissemination efforts. The other intermediate outcome was whether the Rauawaawa and the University had strong capacity for future PHR, evidenced by continued work and receipt of funding.

Conclusions About Cases

These cases illustrate the conceptual clarity offered by the CBPR conceptual model to address important domains of PHR evaluation. They demonstrate how partnerships can adapt the model to their own histories, experiences, values, and priorities; use their own adapted versions of the model for planning purposes; and engage in step-by-step participatory processes of evaluation of their own participatory research processes. More specifically, the Rochester case illustrates how the model was adapted by the partners to help them evaluate their own 10-year history of partnering and to strengthen their collaboration for improving community health outcomes. The AMOS case demonstrates how the model helped them identify specific content areas for evaluation of distinct projects within a global rural health setting. It, too, illustrated how they adapted the four domains of the model to analyse local community indicators and to reprioritize their own organizational self-capacity-building. The New Zealand case provides support for the validity of the CPBR conceptual model as a general guiding framework for evaluating processes and outcomes of partnerships. The four domains were introduced at the beginning of the project although the specific elements beyond the domains were not invoked in the evaluation. Nonetheless, post hoc analysis reveals that the evaluation fits the CBPR conceptual model.

Conclusion

We presented a CBPR conceptual model, which reflects one interpretation of PHR and provides a useful framework for identifying four broad domains and some shared constructs that might be of interest in any evaluation of PHR. There are other conceptual frameworks (e.g. Schulz et al. 2003 in the USA, Green et al. 1995 or Cargo and Mercer 2008 in Canada; Staley 2009 in the UK), although none have been tested to such a degree. Those generated outside an Anglo-American perspective remain sparse in the health context. There are, however, a range of frameworks developed in the field of education, environmental science, natural resource management, agriculture, and development studies for participatory action research (e.g. Daigneault and Jacob 2009; Wiek et al. 2014).

Most importantly, the CBPR conceptual model provides a useful framework that addresses the four key issues/challenges noted earlier in this chapter. Firstly, the model emphasizes context in PHR and in evaluation. Context is one of the key domains of the model, and tools have been developed to help partners explore their own histories and use the information to shape and improve their practice. All three case studies illustrate how the specific context was used to shape the evaluation process and to strengthen the partnership.

Secondly, the conceptual model recognizes differing epistemologies and integrates these perspectives into processes and intervention/research design. Wallerstein et al. (2008, 2018) argue that partnership outcomes are enhanced when local epistemologies are integrated into the research process and when community members participate in all steps of the research process. The AMOS and New Zealand cases, in particular, introduced different epistemologies to the evaluation process (e.g. *kaupapa Māori*), and all three cases ensured that local perspectives were included in the evaluation process. All three cases also demonstrate the importance of ensuring that the evaluation of PHR is itself participatory to ensure shared power in the production of knowledge.

Thirdly, the CBPR conceptual model includes a variety of intermediate and distal outcomes that reflect various purposes. All three cases have utilitarian elements such as improved health outcomes or understanding of health service utilization. However, they also seek elements of transformative potential such as rebalancing of power in research towards community empowerment and social justice. The model is flexible enough for partnerships to identify their specific purposes and link evaluation to those purposes.

Finally, the conceptual model has strong emphasis on quality and dynamic evaluation. A large amount of empirical evidence (both quantitative and qualitative) has been compiled about measures and tools for evaluating constructs within the four domains. The Rochester and AMOS cases noted that one benefit of the model is that there are valid and proven techniques for evaluating PHR based on the conceptual model. These cases also illustrate the importance of dynamic input from the partners in reshaping and adapting the model to fit their local context and epistemological perspectives.

To move the debate forwards and the evaluation of PHR in general, what is required is that those undertaking PHR should ensure that they take some time for evaluating not just how processes contribute to outcomes but also to specifically document the processes and their broader contribution, as, for example, has been done in the area of agricultural science (Campilan and Prain 2000; Home and Rump 2015). Attention should be paid to those elements that make PHR distinct: the level of participation, what action took place as the result of the research, the degree of capacity-building and empowerment, and the particular influence of context on those dimensions so we can build an evidence base that is acceptable and credible in different cultural contexts.

There are differences between cultures and between countries in the varieties of PHR, reflecting the context in which it was historically developed as well as philosophical traditions (ICPHR 2013). This creates a challenge when developing a common model for evaluating PHR internationally, although the CBPR conceptual model is a promising example in need of further testing and application. In sum, evaluation of PHR is about simple questions of "who participates?", "how?", "who has the power to decide?", and "who benefits?" Defining an ecology of practice for participatory knowledge production in PHR that is truly about participatory power sharing would involve paying equal attention to the general exigencies of both quality and utility. Quality involves the quest for truth and objectivity, usually the concerns of researchers. Utility involves eliciting interest that goes beyond intellectual curiosity, to be actionable for practitioners (Mantoura and Potvin 2013). Both require acceptance and understanding of different ways of knowing, respect for cultural differences, and flexibility and openness to change and ambiguity, all core requirements of PHR itself.

Acknowledgements The following authors are associated with the cases: (a) New Zealand, John Oetzel and Rangimahora Reddy; (b) Rochester, Mark Wieland, Irene Sia, and Abigail Reese; and (c) Nicaragua, Laura Parajon. We also thank our many community partners and colleagues with whom we have collaborated and learnt from over the years. The CBPR model was originally developed and tested with US National Institutes of Health NARCH funding (U261HS300293; U261IHS0036-04-00) and revised under "Engage for Equity" National Institute of Nursing Research funding (1R01NR015241-01A1).

References

Bell, S., Morse, S., & Shah, R. A. (2012). Understanding stakeholder participation in research as part of sustainable development. *Journal of Environmental Management, 101*, 13–22.

Bowen, S. J., & Graham, I. D. (2013). From knowledge translation to engaged scholarship: Promoting research relevance and utilization. *Archives of Physical Medicine and Rehabilitation, 94*, S3–S8.

Bradbury-Huang, H. (2014). Quality in action research. In M. Brydon-Miller, D. Coghlan, & P. Gaya (Eds.), *Encyclopedia of action research*. London: Sage.

Cahill, C. (2007). The personal is political: Developing new subjectivities through participatory action research. *Gend Place Culture, 14*, 267–292.

Campilan, D., & Prain, G. (2000). Self-assessment as an approach to evaluating participatory research: An Asian experience. In N. Lilja & L. Sperling (Eds.), *Assessing the impact of participatory research and gender analysis* (pp. p172–p182). Cali: CGIAR SWP-PRGA.

Cargo, M., & Mercer, S. L. (2008). The value and challenges of participatory research: Strengthening its practice. *Annual Review of Public Health, 29*, 325–350.

Center for Participatory Research A (n.d.). CBPR project: Research for improvement health 2009–2013. Available via https://cpr.unm.edu/research-projects/cbpr-project/research-for-improved-health.html. Accessed: 2 Nov 2017.

Center for Participatory Research B (n.d.). CBPR model visioning guide for planning and evaluation. Available via https://cpr.unm.edu/research-projects/cbpr-project/index.html. Accessed: 2 Nov 2017.

Center for Participatory Research C (n.d.). Empowerment curriculum. Available via http://cpr.unm.edu/curricula--classes/empowerment-curriculum.html. Accessed: 2 Nov 2017.

Coimbra, C. E. A., Jr. (1999). Scientific production in public health and international bibliographic bases. *Caderno Saúde Pública, 5*, 883–888.

Chambers, R. (1998). Foreword. In J. Holland and J. Blackburn (eds.). Whose voice? Participatory research and policy change. London. Immediate Technology Publications.

de Sousa Santos, B. (2014). *Epistemologies of the south: Justice against epistemicide.* Boulder: Paradigm Publishers.

Daigneault, P.-M., & Jacob, S. (2009). Toward accurate measurement of participation rethinking the conceptualization and operationalization of participatory evaluation. *American Journal of Evaluation, 30*, 330–348.

Devia, C., Baker, E., Sanchez-Youngman, S., et al. (2017). CBPR to advance social and racial equity: Urban and rural partnerships in black and Latino communities. *International Journal for Equity in Health, 16*, 17.

Duran, B., Oetzel, J.G., Pearson, C., et al. (under review). Promising practices in community-based participatory research: Evidence from a national study.

Green, L. W., George, M. A., Daniel, M., et al. (1995). *Study of participatory research in health promotion: Review and recommendations for development of participatory research in health promotion in Canada.* Ottawa: The Royal Society of Canada.

Greene, J. C. (1994). Qualitative program evaluation practices and promise. In N. K. Denzin & Y. S. Lincoln (Eds.), *Handbook of qualitative research* (pp. 530–544). London: Sage Publications., London.

Guthrie, S., Wamae, W., Diepeveen, S., et al. (2013). *Measuring research: A guide to research evaluation frameworks and tools.* Europe: RAND.

Hall, B., Tandon, R., & Tremblay, C. (2015). *Strengthening community university research partnerships: Global perspectives.* Victoria: University of Victoria.

Hicks, S., Duran, B., Wallerstein, N., et al. (2012). Evaluating community-based participatory research (CBPR) to improve community-partnered science and community health. *Progress in Community Health Partnerships, 6*, 289–299.

Home, R., & Rump, N. (2015). Evaluation of a multi-case participatory action research project: The case of SOLINSA. *The Journal of Agricultural Education and Extension, 21*, 73–89.

House, E. R. (2015). *Evaluating: Values, biases, and practical wisdom.* Charlotte: IAP.

Hummelbrunner, R. (2010). Beyond logframe: Critique, variations and alternatives. In N. Fujita (Ed.), *Beyond logframe: Using systems concepts in evaluation.* Tokyo: Foundation for Advanced Studies on International Development.

International Collaboration for Participatory Health Research (ICPHR). (2013). *Position paper 1: What is participatory Health Research?* Berlin: International Collaboration for Participatory Health Research.

Israel, B. A., Schulz, A. J., Parker, E. A., et al. (2018). Critical issues in developing and following CBPR principles. In N. Wallerstein, B. Duran, J. G. Oetzel, & M. Minkler (Eds.), *Community-based participatory research for health* (3rd ed., pp. 31–44). San Francisco: Jossey-Bass.

Johansson, A. W., & Lindhult, E. (2008). Emancipation or workability?: Critical versus pragmatic scientific orientation in action research. *Action Research, 6*, 95–115.

Kastelic, S., Wallerstein, N., Duran, B., et al. (2018). Socio-ecologic framework for CBPR: Development and testing of a model. In N. Wallerstein, B. Duran, J. G. Oetzel, & M. Minkler (Eds.), *Community-based participatory research for health* (3rd ed., pp. 77–94). San Francisco: Jossey-Bass.

Kennedy, V., & Cram, F. (2010). Ethics of researching with Whānau collectives. *MAI Review, 2010*(3), 1–8.

Khodyakov, D., Stockdale, S., Jones, F., et al. (2011). An exploration of the effect of community engagement in research on perceived outcomes of partnered mental health services projects. *Social Mental Health, 1*, 185–199.

Lucero, J., Wallerstein, N., Duran, B., Alegria, M., Greene-Moton, E., Israel, B., Kastelic, S., Magarati, M., Oetzel, J., Pearson, C., Schulz, A., Villegas, M., & White Hat, E. (2018). Development of a mixed methods investigation of process and outcomes of community-based participatory research. Journal of Mixed Methods Research, 12, 55–74.

Mantoura, P., & Potvin, L. (2013). A realist–constructionist perspective on participatory research in health promotion. *Health Promotion International, 28*, 61–72.

Oetzel, J. G., Villegas, M., Zenone, H., et al. (2015a). Enhancing stewardship of community-engaged research through governance. *American Journal of Public Health, 105*, 1161–1167.

Oetzel, J. G., Zhou, C., Duran, B., et al. (2015b). Establishing the psychometric properties of constructs in a community-based participatory research conceptual model. *American Journal of Health Promotion, 29*, e188–e202.

Oetzel, J. G., Duran, B., Sussman, A., et al. (2018). Evaluation of CBPR partnerships and outcomes: Lessons and tools from the Research for Improved Health study. In N. Wallerstein, B. Duran, J. G. Oetzel, & M. Minkler (Eds.), *Community-based participatory research for health* (3rd ed., pp. 237–250). San Francisco: Jossey-Bass.

Oetzel, J.G., Wallerstein, N., Duran, B., et al. (in press). Community-engaged research for health: A test of the CBPR conceptual model. *BioMed Research International.*

Orange, C. (1987). *The story of a treaty*. Wellington: Allen & Unwin.

Oetzel, J. G., Wallerstein, N., Duran, B., Villegas, M., Sanchez-Youngman, S., Nguyen, T., Woo, K., Wang, J., Schulz, A., Kaholokula, Israel, B., & Alegria, M. (2018). Community-engaged research for health: A test of the CBPR conceptual model. BioMed Research International. 2018, Article ID: 7281405

Pearson, C. R., Duran, B., Oetzel, J., et al. (2015). Research for improved health: Variability and impact of structural characteristics in federally- funded community engaged research. *Progress in Community Health Partnerships, 9*, 17–29.

Pinto, A. C., & de Andrade, J. B. (1999). Factor of impact in scientific journals: What is the meaning of this parameter? *Química Nova, 22*, 448–453.

Renger, R., Wood, S., Williamson, S., et al. (2011). Systemic evaluation, impact, evaluation and logic models. *Evaluation Journal of Australasia, 11*, 24–30.

Rochester Healthy Community Partnership (n.d.). Our research model. Available via https://rochesterhealthy.org/our-research-model; Accessed on 2 Nov 2017.

Sanchez-Youngman, S., & Wallerstein, N. (2018). Appendix 7: Partnership river of life: Creating an historical timeline. In N. Wallerstein, B. Duran, J. G. Oetzel, & M. Minkler (Eds.), *Community-based participatory research for health* (3rd ed., pp. 375–378). San Francisco: Jossey-Bass.

Schulz, A., Israel, B. A., & Lantz, P. (2003). Instrument for evaluating dimensions of group dynamic within community-based participatory research partnerships. *Evaluation Program Planning, 26*, 249–262.

Shoveller, J., Viehbeck, S., Di Ruggiero, E., et al. (2016). A critical examination of representations of context within research on population health interventions. *Critical Public Health, 26*, 487–500.

Simpson, M., & Ake, T. (2010). Whitiwhiti korero: Exploring the researchers' relationship in cross-cultural research. *Journal of Intercultural Communication Research, 39*, 185–205.

Springett, J., Wright, M. T., & Roche, B. (2011). *Developing quality criteria for participatory health research. An agenda for action, WZB Discussion Paper*. Berlin: Wissenschaftszentrum Berlin für Sozialforschung.

Staley, K. (2009). *Exploring impact: Public involvement in NHS, public health and social care research*. Eastleigh: INVOLVE.

Taylor, C. (2010). What would Jim Grant say now? *Lancet, 375*, 1236–1237.

Trickett, E. J. (2011). Community-based participatory research as worldview or instrumental strategy: Is it lost in translation(al) research? *American Journal of Public Health, 101*, 1353–1355.

Turato, E. R. (2005). Qualitative and quantitative methods in the health care field: Definitions, differences and the objects of research. *Revista Saúde Pública, 39*, 507–514.

Wallerstein, N., & Duran, B. (2006). Using community based participatory research to address health disparities. *Health Promotion Practice, 7*, 312–323.

Wallerstein, N., & Duran, B. (2010). Community-based participatory research contributions to intervention research: The intersection of science and practice to improve health equity. *American Journal of Public Health, 100*, S40–S46.

Wallerstein, N., Oetzel, J., Duran, B., et al. (2008). CBPR: What predicts outcomes? In M. Minkler & N. Wallerstein (Eds.), *Community-based participatory research for health: From process to outcomes* (2nd ed., pp. 371–392). San Francisco: Jossey-Bass.

Wallerstein, N., Oetzel, J. G., Duran, B., et al. (under review). Cultural-centeredness in community-based participatory research: Culture as power and agency.

Whitelaw, S. (2012). The emergence of a 'dose–response' analogy in the health improvement domain of public health: A critical review. *Crit Public Health, 22*, 427–440.

Wiek, A., Talwar, S., O'Shea, M., & Robinson, J. (2014). Toward a methodological scheme for capturing societal effects of participatory sustainability research. *Research Evaluation, 23*, 117–132.

Wieland, M. L., Weis, J. A., Yawn, B. P., et al. (2012). Perceptions of tuberculosis among immigrants and refugees at an adult education center: A community-based participatory research approach. *Journal of Immigrant and Minority Health/Center for Minority Public Health, 14*, 14–22.

Zarcadoolas, C., Pleasant, A., & Greer, D. S. (2005). Understanding health literacy: An expanded model. *Health Promotion International, 20*, 195–203.

Chapter 4
Participatory Health Research in the Education of Health and Social Work Professionals

Irma Brito

> *Participatory Health Research is a need to health care. All over the world politicians, stakeholders and citizens stated that more professional health workers are needed. It is also clear that those efforts to scale up health professionals' education and training must not only increase the quantity of health workers, but should address issues of quality and relevance in order to address community and population health needs and engage people on searching for healthy settings and lifestyle.* (WHO 2006, 2013)

Participatory Health Research is a need to Health Care

New approaches in health professionals' education aim to transform health-care systems, moving away from the traditional focus on person-centered care to initiatives that foster community engagement. But in academia, the education of researchers remains traditionally separated from disciplines whose focus is social intervention or community development. In most community health and social work graduate programs, there is a strong distinction between courses on research and those on practice methods. The research courses emphasize a particular understanding of generating evidence by means of empiricism, whereas the practice courses emphasize what can be called practice-based evidence (Schaffer et al. 2013; Drisko 2014; Bal 2017). This may lead to a dichotomy between research and intervention, contributing to weaknesses in the design and evaluation in community-based interventions because of different understandings of what constitutes good practice.

This tension between community involvement and research raises questions about the goals of community health and social work education and therefore about the institutions in which future professionals are educated. Participatory health research (PHR) can be one way to address the perspectives of both community involvement and research. This means teaching PHR in research courses and

I. Brito (✉)
Nursing School of Coimbra, Coimbra, Portugal
e-mail: irmabrito@esenfc.pt

increasing the engagement of graduate and postgraduate students and professionals in PHR projects. PHR results in a co-creation of multiple forms of knowledge that go beyond the usual forms of academic knowledge. And community health and social work professionals benefit personally and professionally from learning how to design and implement intervention projects focused and anchored in targeted communities.

Participatory Health Research Impact Beyond Academic Knowledge Production

Participatory health research (PHR) aims to maximize the participation of people whose life or work is the subject of research at all stages of the research process. The key aspect of PHR is its explicit intention to bring about social change, with an impact beyond the production of academic knowledge (ICPHR 2013a). Thus, it can lead to a reform both in professional education and in the practice of action research because PHR investigates explicitly for the purpose of change, involving various people and communities.

Most often PHR is focused on a health problem which those most affected by the problem and/or professionals wish to change for the better. It should be noted PHR can also focus on the experience of something that works well and which those involved wish to reproduce or expand, adapting it to other local contexts. Although in theory there is a difference between the elements "participation," "action," and "research," this difference can be resolved in practice by way of numerous cycles of reflection on the participatory action. These cycles generate learning about the action, resulting in new practices that are the subject of further reflection. So the change does not happen at the end of a PHR project but rather throughout the process. According to Kneebone and Wadsworth (1998), the main feature of a true participatory action-research process is that it can change shape and focus over time (and sometimes unexpectedly) with participants reorienting their understanding of what is really happening and what is really important to them. This is the feature that makes reporting PHR process complex and sometimes "chaotic" as stated in the first ICPHR position paper: "PHR is a dialectical process characterized by messiness… The occurrence of messiness in this sense is a fundamental characteristic of PHR" (2013a: 20).

Starting from the intention of improving practice for the purpose of social change, the teaching of practice and research methods cannot be considered separate entities. There must be experiential and shared social learning (learning together and with each other) because a fundamental dimension of the PHR process is the continuous cycle of "looking, reflecting, acting" that underpins the dynamics of the connected knowledge. It also means trying to understand the other person or idea through dialogue, through relationships of trust and empathy (Goleman 2006; Boyatzis 2008; Goleman and Boyatzis 2011). Thus, all participants in a PHR project learn to be coinvestigators in varying degrees. Ideally, the process should involve participants in transformative learning, i.e., changes in the way they see the world and themselves (Freire 1980; Mezirow 1990; Kolb 2014) which is the result of interactive processes that address both the personal and the collective. In turn, these processes support the intention to be able to act based on the results of the research, thus having a greater impact than can be achieved by the usual academic research. PHR is pragmatic due to its emphasis on the usefulness of the research to promote positive change in practice; and it is emancipatory to the degree which it is focused on collectively transforming the way people think and act in their world (Jagosh et al. 2015).

In an extensive review of the impact of public involvement in health and social welfare research, Staley (2009) identified various forms of impact at five different levels: the public involved, researchers, research participants, the community at large, and community organizations. Public involvement was associated positively with the acquisition of new skills and knowledge, personal development, support and friendship, pleasure and satisfaction, and financial rewards. Negative aspects of involvement included emotional overload, more work, exposure through the media, and frustration with the limitations to the degree of involvement. At the level of the research participants, there were benefits such as helping people feel more comfortable with the issue under study, providing emotional support, providing access to information and services, and giving inspiration/hope. For the wider community, the benefits included reinforcing and building trust and acceptance of research, keeping projects anchored and focused on community benefits, and improving relationships between communities and practitioners. At the level of community organizations, the following benefits were identified: gaining knowledge, gaining more visibility, partnering with other community members/organizations, and contributing positively to community development. Negative effects included financial costs and an increased demand for a service that is difficult to provide. For researchers, the benefits of engaging the public were better knowledge and understanding of the community, pleasure and satisfaction, career benefits, and challenges to beliefs and attitudes. The negative aspects identified were greater demands on resources and a slower speed of research, loss of power, forced changes in work practice, and questioning the values and assumptions of the researchers.

Taking into account the above and the author's experience as a higher education teacher and a teacher in PHR (Brito and Mendes 2015), we consider that, from the academy's point of view, training community health professionals and social workers in PHR can have benefits for:

1. The academic institution. Both practice-based and scientific knowledge can be generated; PHR projects can promote the public visibility of the institution; partnerships with community organizations are made possible; and the institution can contribute positively to community development.
2. Future professionals in community health and social work. New skills and knowledge can be gained; the usual professional stance can be challenged in relation to beliefs and attitudes; personal development can be promoted at various levels; support and friendship can be obtained by working with the various partners; pleasure and satisfaction as a result of the cooperative relationships can

be reached; better knowledge and understanding of the community can be obtained; direct benefits for the future career can be achieved, for example, through networking and learning a unique set of skills; the future professionals can attain a new level of trust and acceptance of research; the student projects can be better anchored and focused on benefits to the community; and a better relationship with communities can be built which goes beyond the usual relationship between communities and professionals.
3. The community. The members can be actively involved in the production of knowledge and can take responsibility for the dissemination of the same among peers.

There are already some curricula for community-based participatory research (CBPR), a form of PHR found in North American, that aim to increase knowledge and understanding of particular forms of PHR practice and to integrate that knowledge with interventions and social/political changes to improve the health and quality of life of members from targeted communities. These courses are recommended for academic researchers in various fields such as public health, education, nursing, medicine, social work, and urban planning. The resources serve primarily as an introduction to CBPR for the initial phases of planning (Green 2006; Lantz et al. 2006; Wallerstein and Duran 2010; Sheikhattari and Kamangar 2010).

Assuming that PHR is an approach with specific requirements for teaching and learning, the participants in PHR training should have the opportunity to reflect on its various dimensions for the purpose of conducting their own projects. Since there are still few opportunities for shared learning on participatory research in the fields of health and social welfare, four institutions affiliated to the ICPHR have developed an international course (presented in English, German, and Portuguese). The purpose is to disseminate the use of participatory research while working together to define the core competencies. The international course (ICPHR 2017) aims to enable participants to develop new skills in the design and implementation of participatory research projects. Considering that each training group is unique and that the teaching culture in the countries involved varies, a standardization of training is not possible. PHR courses should be designed to address the interests, motivations and level of knowledge of the participants, as well as the interests of the organization that sponsors the training. However, such training has specific general teaching and learning requirements that are reflected in its structure and implementation strategies.

Participatory Health Research Education Requires Specific Forms of Learning and Teaching

The question regarding the purpose of PHR training for health and social work professionals requires attention to an overall concept for teaching and learning focused on the notions of problematizing the current order and contextualizing the research practice. This concept should be based on experiential learning as a powerful and proven approach to teaching and learning: people learn better through experience (Kolb 2014). The pedagogy of freedom (Freire 2014) offers an additional basis for teaching PHR, requiring a broad approach focused on the subject (person or group). The problematizing and liberating nature of education proposed by Freire breaks with the verticality of traditional teaching practices, in which the teacher "deposits" the knowledge in the student. For Freire, educator and educated need to establish a dialogue in order to perceive the reality of the world in which they live as a basis for reflection and action. The perception of reality happens in the first contact and in the dialogue between the teacher/facilitator and the group of participants: what Freire calls "generating themes," which carry a world view, language, and thoughts of a well-defined historical-social context. This includes identifying the "limiting situations" which still exist, those barriers to understanding the reality lived by the subjects and the obstacles for their liberation. This dialogical way of working seeks to establish a dialectical relationship between the participants and the world in which they live by emphasizing historical aspects of their situation and discussing the contradictions present in the current reality. The result is "a praxis which, being reflection and action truly transforming into reality, is a source of reflective knowledge and creation" (Freire 2014: 108). Thus, the training in PHR should start from the presentation and reflection on the ideas/projects of the participants as they see them in their lived reality.

Freire proposed a thematic approach involving three interrelated aspects: coding, problematizing, and decoding. The "coding and decoding" is a process of understanding the place of the subject in the construction of knowledge. Freire establishes a dialectical relation between the person and world by way of a reading of reality which is shared by a collective subject, but not separated from him or her. It is the understanding of what can be understood as *praxis*, real-time reality, historically and socially situated, that enables the investigation of the performance of this subject in this reality. And from this dialectical relationship arises the problematization. Problematizing for Freire goes beyond the idea of using a problem to introduce preselected concepts by the teacher. But rather, it is a process in which the learner is confronted with situations in his or her praxis, destabilizing his or her previous knowledge and creating a gap that makes him or her feel a lack of knowledge about the current reality. The critical reflection of the distance between the knowledge of the subject and the knowledge of the reality she or he seeks to change is characterized by an exploration of the contradictions and the limits of that knowledge, resulting in the learner realizing the importance of knowing more and seeking this knowledge. This process can be hampered by distortions in meaning: epistemic, sociocultural, and psychic (Mezirow 1990). The social representations of phenomena are often constructed in the consensual sphere, rather than in the scientific sphere. Although not completely watertight, both have different purposes and are effective and indispensable for human life. So if we consider that science does not happen inside a bubble, isolated from society, we can see how the framework that surrounds it also affects its production of scientific knowledge. PHR brings new conceptual tools to analyze the angles of reality put on the agenda, combining new views coming from the struggles of social movements, creativity, and questions in the field of science. In terms of PHR training, the participant's research project is the starting point for this process of exploration, promoting the participant to move from a level of "real effective consciousness" (*coding*: a realization of what the current situation is) to the level of "maximum possible consciousness" (*decoding*: discovering the possibilities for liberation) (Freire 1980: 126). The conceptions and representations which arise during the training are the product of wrestling with the values, customs, and needs of the community in which the trainee is inserted. The problematizing happens in several dimensions: the level of participation of research subjects in the research, the purpose of the research and the way it was outlined (usually by professionals or academics), the process of collecting and analyzing data for research, as well as the ownership of research and cooperation between researchers and the way knowledge is disseminated.

But decoding in this sense may not happen; that is, the trainee doesn't move from his or her starting point and fails to connect the abstract principles of PHR with the concrete situation in which the research is being conducted. In these cases, we find that both the trainee and the others participating in the PHR project are involved in the construction of knowledge but that the vision for what is possible is limited. The understanding of reality in the sense which Freire describes requires the trainee to transcend the usual boundaries of academic knowledge which also means going beyond the usual physical space in which the trainee usually works. This requires the trainee to examine his or her predisposition to change in his or her praxis, to move from abstraction to a new reality, and thereby to dare to dream about possibilities. We note that for many academic researchers, this transformation is complex and difficult because it differs markedly from the usual research practice. But for many health and social welfare professionals, such a transformation is necessary, providing an opportunity to review and improve their practice and thus to better promote community development.

The process of experiential and shared learning in PHR training supports directly this process of transformation. It questions the assumptions of authority in the process of learning, challenging orthodoxy and the assumption that the position of "teacher" engenders knowledge. It offers possibilities to learn by reflecting on and making personal and collective sense of the experience of the various trainees trying to conduct PHR. So the benefits of experiential learning come from its connection with the social and political aspects of work and with the dilemmas and problems that make up the experience of working with and in communities. The training also enables the creation of connections between projects of the trainees, enhancing networking and, consequently, professionalism as an ongoing process of learning and learning to learn. In PHR training, the message is transported that, in order to successfully implement PHR projects, action is not enough and praxis is completed and consolidated by ongoing reflection; if action is seen as the ultimate goal of the process, there is a risk of not changing reality, but only producing more activism which only appears to change the status quo. Martins and Brito (2013) have repeatedly identified this gap in participatory research: working with the community has generated action proposals for change that never went beyond proposals. Such an outcome may discredit the research and prevent future projects with the community in question, which raises an ethical dimension generally not considered in participatory research (ICPHR 2013b).

A Participatory Health Research Curriculum

In the discussion thus far, we have sought to provide a better understanding of some of the pedagogical presuppositions that anchor PHR training as proposed by the ICPHR, especially the elements of contextualization and the need for a consistent problematizing. Based on the framework that led to the creation of the international PHR course, we will describe how a PHR course can be structured both inside and outside institutions of higher education. It is not the author's intention to present this curriculum as developed by the ICPHR as the only possibility for PHR training but rather to point to elements to consider when teaching PHR to community health professionals and social workers.

A curriculum structures knowledge and is itself a social construction that helps to discipline the emotions, the intellect, and the behavior of the individuals. Academic disciplines (and other ways of organizing knowledge) exert a power of normalization through modes of teaching and learning. An International Course for Participatory Researchers is thus to be understood broadly, relying on pedagogy as a science of education and on didactics, a discipline that deals with teaching and learning methods, processes, and techniques (Brydon-Miller and Maguire 2009; Shaw and Lunt 2012; Agnello 2016).

In a more traditional approach to curriculum development, which can be seen in some CBPR training programs, the curriculum design follows a logic of efficiency which results in the training being carried out by specialists who are in charge of determining the skills to be developed by the trainees, the training methods, and the measurement/evaluation of the skills obtained. The teacher takes into account the interests of the trainees and seeks to provide an appropriate atmosphere for experiential learning, with the support of his/her institution. The focus is on practical solutions to problems in participatory research projects by means of deliberation. The underlying pragmatism depends heavily on a humanist discourse and a liberal organization while emphasizing rational decision-making on the part of the trainee who coordinates the research.

The PHR curriculum as developed by the ICPHR presupposes a participatory approach to and sharing and generating various forms of knowledge, based on the experience of the trainees. Aligned with Habermas's critical theory of society (Habermas 2002), we advocate for a praxis that makes sense to the trainees, based on the paradigm shift from an *instrumental rationality* to a *communicative rationality*. This approach seeks to overcome the usual fragmentation and overspecialization of knowledge and the separation of theory and practice. PHR is thus taught not as a specific skill set or procedure but rather as a process which the trainees experience over the course of their projects. The learning is comprised of making sense out of that experience.

Making sense of the PHR experience means making it meaningful through interpretation. It is in the process of interpretation of decision-making or action where learning occurs. The interpretation is guided by a stance characterized by critical reflection which requires the training not only to question his or her actions but also the assumptions and beliefs which underlie those actions (Mezirow 1990). This means especially empowering the trainees working with communities to question how goals of democracy and social justice can be met. According to Sousa-Santos (1999): 9), this means "an epistemological concern with the nature and validity of scientific knowledge, an interdisciplinary vocation, a refusal to use scientific knowledge at the service of political and economic power... a society that privileges the identification of conflicts and interests (...), an ethical commitment that links universal values to the processes of social transformation".

Strategies to implement the teaching of PHR. The PHR course of the ICPHR includes strategies to implement the teaching of PHR so as to promote transformative learning within the context of developing and implementing the concrete projects of the trainees. Considering the needs of health professionals and social workers, the course takes into account the following: (1) sessions comprised largely of dialogue; (2) a design which follows the steps in the process of conducting PHR, thus directly related to the experience of the trainees; and (3) a continual and dynamic process of adaptation to the situation of the trainees, supported by ongoing evaluation. This involves didactic choices that are meaningful to the trainees so as to promote critical discussion and knowledge sharing. The educator-educated approach becomes essential in the pedagogical proposal of thematic research. Freire describes several aspects as being essential to the process which we can apply to PHR teachings: deepening local PHR practices, comprehension of the contradictions inherent in the projects, identification of central themes arising in the work, examining the themes systematically and from various perspectives, reducing the themes to their essential qualities, examining modes of communication regarding the identified themes, applying appropriate didactic material to address the themes, constantly returning to the subject focus (the perspective and experience of the trainees), and then presenting the program tailored to participants' needs. The teacher can add themes that have not emerged from the work of the trainees but that are fundamental for a reflection on action, what we call *hinge themes*. These themes are hinges in that they enable connections between the themes raised by the trainees. These include the principles of PHR, ethics in PHR, health advocacy, and formal and informal ways of disseminating findings. It is expected that the knowledge gained will be mobilized for the local PHR projects – that is, beyond the training space – which requires set times for an alternating rhythm of action and collective reflection, as found in the course plan (see Table 4.1).

In both curricula, the trainees have the opportunity to share knowledge in the classroom (6 to 8 sessions) over the course of 8–12 months. Both courses are designed as continuing education courses, not as courses within degree programs. There is a sufficient interval between sessions for work in the local research teams which is then discussed in the classroom, for example, sharing innovate approaches

Table 4.1 The plan of two courses from Germany and Portugal

Participatory social research (http://www.khsb-berlin.de/weiterbildung/zertifikatskurse/partizipative-sozialforschung/)	International course on participatory health research (http://www.esenfc.pt/event/3cipapes)
Module 1. Background and Introduction	Module I. = 40H (28H in class+12H virtual)
• Origins and Theoretical Basis	1. Introduction and Presentation of Training Objectives
• Definitions	2. Background to Participatory Health Research
• Forming a Research Team	• Historical background and theoretical foundations
	• Fundamentals, concepts and definitions of participatory research
Between modules 1 and 2: Trainees organize a local research team	3. How to Organize a Research Group
	4. Ethics and Peer research in the Development of Participatory Research
Module 2. Ethics, Roles, Developing a Research Design	• Ethical and leadership issues in participatory research
• Ethical Questions	• Defining functions: "peer research"
• Clarification of Roles	5. Building Dialogic Communities
• Developing a Research Design (Part 1)	6. Development of a Participatory Research Project
	• Formulation of a research project
	• Research design
Between modules 2 and 3: Trainees develop their projects together with the local research teams	7. Data Collection and Analysis in Participatory Research
Module 3. Developing a Research Design (Part 2)	
	• Practical issues of each project
	• Reproduction, transformation and impact of participatory research
	• Reproducibility and transferability of knowledge
Between modules 3 and 4: Trainees develop a research design with their local teams	8. Project Stories: Discussion and Problem-Solving
Module 4. Data Collection and Analysis	• Presentation of projects
• Developing a Strategy for Data Collection and Analysis	• Problem-solving and/or alternatives suggested by participants
	• Dissemination of participatory research and mass media use
Between modules 4 and 5: Data collection and analysis with the local research teams	• Reflections on the links between national and international projects and the sustainability of participatory research
Module 5. Consultation	

(continued)

Table 4.1 (continued)

Participatory social research (http://www.khsb-berlin.de/weiterbildung/zertifikatskurse/partizipative-sozialforschung/)	International course on participatory health research (http://www.esenfc.pt/event/3cipapes)
• Discussion of the Local Research Processes	MODULE II = 60H (22H in class +38H virtual)
• Developing Problem-Solving Strategies	9. Discussion and Presentation of the Results of Participatory Research Projects
	• Development and presentation of projects in seminar
	• Development of links between national and international projects and preparation of funding applications
Between modules 5 und 6: The research projects are brought to a close and the presentation of the projects is planned	10. Dissemination of PHR projects
Module 6. Presentation of the Project Results	
• Project Presentations	• Writing scientific articles and doing news for media
• Sustainability in Participatory Research	

as well as doubts and stories of success as well as failure. It should be emphasized that the training contexts of the country and the institution greatly influence the curriculum and didactics. For example, the course offered by the Center for Professional Development at Central Queensland University is made available by distance learning mode, given the large geographic dispersion of potential participants and the desire to reach English speakers in other countries. In Portugal and Germany all meetings are in-person at the host institution with participants from various parts of the country.

There is a didactic challenge in streamlining classroom sessions based on dialogue. As argued above, this dialogue is, however, central to the process of teaching PHR. Dialogue among professionals from various settings is key to increasing knowledge about real needs and thus enhances their projects. Dialogue is supported through interactive methodologies which bring to light the perspectives of the different actors involved in the projects and how these perspectives affect PHR.

Examining the two curricula in light of the previous discussion, four points of convergence emerge:

1. The thematic approach based on elements of the research process and the associated didactic materials
2. The interdisciplinary perspective of pedagogical work in the training of community health professionals and social workers
3. The role of the teacher/facilitator in the process of teaching and learning
4. The accreditation of training for academic and professional advancement

Making PHR curricula explicit and public provides an opportunity for improving the training of community health and social work professionals. The curricula developed by the ICPHR provides a pedagogical basis consistent with the mission of these professionals, addressing the social, political, and economic issues inherent in the field of health promotion and community development.

Strategies for Implementing Participatory Health Research in Health and Social Welfare Higher Education

Boaventura Sousa Santos states that among the characteristics that mark the crisis of the public university, the contradiction between the (traditional) rigidity of university education and the volatility of the qualifications demanded by the market has led to the commercialization of education and the "transition of university knowledge to pluriversity" (Sousa-Santos 2008: 16). This means that in the last decades, a model has emerged that opposes the scientific knowledge produced in universities (or similar institutions) which is predominantly disciplinary and often with some "social irresponsibility" for not being cautious of the results from the application of the knowledge produced (p. 16). In the so-called pluriversity model, the production of knowledge is contextual, insofar as the organizing principle of its production is how it should be applied. And as the application takes place outside the university, it is necessary to identify criteria of relevance based on a partnership between academic researchers and knowledge users. The research enterprise is transformed into one of transdisciplinary knowledge that requires dialogue and confrontation with other forms of knowledge, thus evolving toward a more open and less hierarchical organization of universities.

In order to overcome these conflicting demands, it has been sought to create nonuniversity systems of modular training, as a result of pressures both to shorten periods of university education and to make training more flexible and transdisciplinary, with a focus on supporting lifelong learning. Including PHR training in community health and social work education – both at undergraduate and advanced levels – may be another way to address the transformation of higher learning. As we have described here, the PHR curriculum for community health and social workers provides a theoretical and practical basis for transformative learning, emphasizing issues of communication, emancipation, and reflexivity.

We take, for example, the experience of a transdisciplinary approach to training nurses in curriculum of the University of Cape Verde. Several workshops for undergraduates and postgraduates on PHR have been conducted, as well as the PHR course of the ICPHR. The goal of the degree programs is to train students to adequately diagnose problem situations and to design social intervention strategies in a community context. In the first year, the students learn concepts of community development, health promotion, and participatory health research. Together with a local community, they identify problem situations, negotiate solutions, and reflect on them. During the following years, the students begin with an identified problem situation, and then they develop an innovative idea to address that situation.

By way of workshops with undergraduate or graduate students in Angola, Brazil, and Portugal, we have built capacity to increase the participation of those who are the subject of research. The analysis of the activities developed shows that introducing the PHR approach in an undergraduate and postgraduate course allowed not only the development of cultural competency in researchers but also a view of caring for people beyond the scope of health-care institutions. This work was piloted using the PHR course designed by the ICPHR and the structures of the PEER project – Peer-education Engagement and Evaluation Research, a PHR network coordinated by the author (Brito 2009, 2014). These pilots showed that it is possible to support social change by delivering person-centered services, improving responsiveness, and promoting inclusion in health care. We concluded that PHR education fits both with the mission of health-care teaching institutions and in two of the pillars of health services: continuing education and research.

Using PHR approaches can also lead to better care practices on the part of those who have health problems by supporting participation and knowledge transfer. PHR works best when it is designed and implemented through multisector activities (including all relevant public and private sector stakeholders and policy makers); it is rooted in the socioeconomic and developmental context of communities/populations; it meets the health needs and expectations of the population served; and it is adapted to the evolution of epidemiological profiles and burden of disease. Teaching community health professionals and social workers to use PHR is an asset, but it requires the investment of the training institutions, which includes providing resources, accessibility to training courses, and educational credits. It is also important that the institutions provide for the involvement of community-based organizations to engage in participatory action-research partnerships. Trainers/facilitators have a demanding role in ensuring an atmosphere which promotes critical reflection and emancipation through co-creation of various forms of knowledge.

By continuing to gather and share experience in conducting PHR training in several countries, we hope to be able to collect concrete information on the impact of such trainings. By bringing together data of this sort, we can continue to advance PHR as an integral part of professional education in the fields of health and social work.

References

Agnello, M. F. (2016). 'Finding Foucault': Contextualising power in the curriculum through reflections on students' dialoguing about foucauldian discourses. In V. Perselli (Ed.), *Education, theory and pedagogies of change in a global landscape: 110–126*. London: Palgrave Macmillan. https://doi.org/10.1057/9781137549235_6.

Bal, R. (2017). Evidence-based policy as reflexive practice. What can we learn from evidence-based medicine? *Journal of Health Services Research & Policy, 22*(2), 113–119. https://doi.org/10.1177/1355819616670680.

Boyatzis, R. (2008). Competencies in the 21st century. *Journal of Management Development, 27,* 5–12.

Brito, I. (2009) PEER – Peer education engagement and evaluation research. In Escola Superior de Enfermagem de Coimbra. ESEnfC. Available via ESEnfC/UICISA-E http://web.esenfc.pt/public/index.php?module=ui&target=outreach-projects&id_projecto=54&id_linha_investigacao=1&tipo=UI Accessed 03 Jan 2017.

Brito, I. (2014). Um modelo de planeamento da promoção da saúde: Modelo PRECEDE-PROCEED. In R. Pedroso, & I. Brito (Eds.), Saúde dos estudantes do ensino superior de enfermagem: Estudo de contexto na Escola Superior de Enfermagem de Coimbra: Unidade de Investigação em Ciências da Saúde: Enfermagem, Escola Superior de Enfermagem de Coimbra (pp. 17–31).

Brito, I., & Mendes, F. (2015). Curso Internacional de Pesquisa-ação Participativa em Saúde em português (CIPaPS). Escola Superior de Enfermagem de Coimbra. ESEnfC. Available via ESEnfC/UICISA-E. http://www.esenfc.pt/event/3cipapes. Accessed 03 Jan 2017.

Brydon-Miller, M., & Maguire, P. (2009). Participatory action research: Contributions to the development of practitioner inquiry in education. *Educational Action Research, 17*(1), 79–93.

Drisko, J. (2014). Research evidence and social work practice: The place of evidence-based practice. *Clinical Social Work Journal, 42*(2), 123–133. https://doi.org/10.1007/s10615-013-0459-9.

Freire, P. (1980). *Conscientização* (3rd ed.). São Paulo: Moraes.

Freire, P. (2014). *Pedagogy of hope: Reliving pedagogy of the oppressed.* New York: Bloomsbury Publishing.

Goleman, D. (2006). *Inteligencia social (5).* Barcelona: Kairós.

Goleman, D., & Boyatzis, R. (2011). Inteligência social e a biologia da liderança. Available via Harvard Business Review Brasil http://hbrbr.uol.com.br/inteligencia-social-e-a-biologia-da-lideranca/. Accessed 03 Jan 2017.

Green, L. W. (2006). Public Health Asks of Systems Science: To Advance Our Evidence-Based Practice, Can You Help Us Get More Practice-Based Evidence?. *American Journal of Public Health, 96*(3):406–409 https://doi.org/10.2105/AJPH.2005.066035

Habermas, J. (2002). *On the pragmatics of social interaction: Preliminary studies in the theory of communicative action.* Cambridge: MIT Press.

ICPHR. (2013a). What is participatory health research? Position paper 1. Available via International Collaboration for Participatory Health Research: http://www.icphr.org/position-papers/position-paper-no-1. Accessed 03 Jan 2017.

ICPHR. (2013b). Participatory health research: A guide to ethical principles and practice. Position Paper 2. Available via International Collaboration for Participatory Health Research: http://www.icphr.org/uploads/2/0/3/9/20399575/ichpr_position_paper_2_ethics_-_version_october_2013.pdf. Accessed 03 Jan 2017.

ICPHR. (2017). An international course for participatory researchers. Available via International Collaboration for Participatory Health Research: http://www.icphr.org/international-course.html. Accessed 03 Jan 2017.

Jagosh, J., Bush, P. L., Salsberg, J., et al. (2015). A realist evaluation of community-based participatory research: Partnership synergy, trust building and related ripple effects. *BMC Public Health, 15*(1), 725.

Kneebone, S., & Wadsworth, Y. (1998) What is participatory action research? In Action Research International online journal. Research for real. Available via http://www.research-for-real.co.uk/resources. Asp. Accessed 03 Jan 2017.

Kolb, D. (2014) Experiential learning: Experience as the source of learning and development. Prentice Hall, New Jersey

Lantz, P.M., Israel, B., Schulz, A.J., Reyes, A. (2006) Community-based participatory research: Rationale and relevance for social epidemiology. In Oakes, JM & Kaufman, JS (Edits) *Methods in social epidemiology*, Jossey-Bass, San Francisco (pp. 239–266)

Lawrence W. Green, (2006) Public Health Asks of Systems Science: To Advance Our Evidence-Based Practice, Can You Help Us Get More Practice-Based Evidence?. *American Journal of Public Health, 96*(3):406–409.

Martins, E., & Brito, I. (2013). Investigação-acção participativa em saúde: revisão integrativa da literatura em língua portuguesa. In Escola Superior de Enfermagem de Coimbra. ESEnfC. Available via http://repositorio.esenfc.pt/private/index.php?process=download&id=27076&code=480 Accessed 03 Jan 2017.

Mezirow, J. (1990). How critical reflection triggers transformative learning. *Fostering Critical Reflection Adulthood, 1*, 20.

Schaffer, M. A., Sandau, K. E., & Diedrick, L. (2013). Evidence-based practice models for organizational change: Overview and practical applications. *Journal of Advanced Nursing, 69*(5), 1197–1209. https://doi.org/10.1111/j.1365-2648.2012.06122.x.

Shaw, I., & Lunt, N. (2012). Constructing practitioner research. *Social Work Research, 36*(3), 197–208. https://doi.org/10.1093/swr/svs013.

Sheikhattari, P., & Kamangar, F. (2010). How can primary health care system and community-based participatory research be complementary? *International Journal of Preventive Medicine, 1*(1), 1.

Sousa-Santos, B. (1999). Porque é tão difícil construir uma teoria crítica? *Revista Crítica de Ciências Sociais, 54*, 197–215.

Sousa-Santos, B. (2008) A Universidade no século XXI: Para uma universidade democrática e emancipadora. In N. Almeida, & B. Sousa-Santos (Eds.) *A Universidade no século XXI, para uma Universidade Nova* (pp. 15–78). Almedina Coimbra.

Staley, K. (2009). Exploring impact: Public involvement in NHS. Public health and social care research. Available via INVOLVE http://www.invo.org.uk/posttypepublication/exploring-impact-public-involvement-in-nhs-public-health-and-social-care-research/. Accessed 03 Jan 2017.

Wallerstein, N., & Duran, B. (2010). Community-based participatory research contributions to intervention research: The intersection of science and practice to improve health equity. *American Journal of Public Health, 100*(SUPPL. 1), 1:S40-46. https://doi.org/10.2105/AJPH.2009.184036.

WHO. (2013). Good practices in nursing and midwifery: From expert to expert. Available via http://www.euro.who.int/__data/assets/pdf_file/0007/234952/Good-practices-in-nursing-and-midwifery.pdf. Accessed 03 Jan 2017.

World Health Organization. (2006). STOP the global epidemic of chronic disease: A practical guide to successful advocacy. Available via http://www.who.int/chp/advocacy/chp.manual.EN-webfinal.pdf?ua=1. Accessed 03 Jan 2017.

Chapter 5
Demonstrating Impact in Participatory Health Research

Krystyna Kongats, Jane Springett, Michael T. Wright, and Tina Cook

The Focus on Impact

Internationally, there is increasing pressure to demonstrate research impact through improvements in policy, practice, and health outcomes in order to substantiate research value to funding organisations and the wider community (Penfield et al. 2014; Milat et al. 2015; Cook et al. 2017). On the flip side, there is also an expectation that policy and practice developments are evidence-based and informed by research (Banks et al. 2017). Traditionally, impact in academic contexts has been assessed by counting the number of papers produced, publishing in high-impact journals, and counting the number of citations on a publication (Milat et al. 2015). However, there is an increasing push for academics to define research impact beyond the academy. For example, in the UK, research impact is commonly defined as "an effect on, change or benefit to the economy, society, culture, public policy or services, health, the environment or quality of life, beyond academia" (Higher Education Funding Council for England n.d.). In Canada, research impact in a health context is defined as including "outputs and outcomes, and may also include additional contributions to the health sector or to society... [and] effects that may not have been part of the research objectives such as contributions to a knowledge based society or to economic growth" (Panel on Return on Investment in Health

K. Kongats (✉) · J. Springett
School of Public Health, University of Alberta, Edmonton, Alberta, Canada
e-mail: krystyna.kongats@ualberta.ca; jane.springett@ualberta.ca

M. T. Wright
Catholic University of Applied Sciences, Institute for Social Health, Berlin, Germany
e-mail: Michael.Wright@KHSB-Berlin.de

T. Cook
Department of Disability and Education, Liverpool Hope University, Liverpool, UK
e-mail: cookt@hope.ac.uk

© Springer International Publishing AG, part of Springer Nature 2018
M. T. Wright, K. Kongats (eds.), *Participatory Health Research*,
https://doi.org/10.1007/978-3-319-92177-8_5

Research 2009, pp. A-311). While these definitions are relatively broad, they do highlight a shift in seeing research as predominately a tool for *knowledge collection* to seeing it as an opportunity to bridge *what is known* with *action* (i.e. research into practice) (Springett 2017).

Despite increasing demands to exhibit research impact, the issue of *what is research impact* in the first place is not a benign matter. The worldview or paradigms we explicitly or implicitly subscribe to ultimately shape what we count as relevant impact and the meanings we attribute to these respective impacts (Kuhn 1996). Further, we also have a tendency to *measure what can be easily counted* rather than assess *what counts* in regard to more meaningful impacts, which further limits how we conceptualise impact in research (Milat et al. 2015). On the whole, how we define research impact depends on the lens we use (Trickett and Beehler 2017). From this premise, we argue that impact in participatory health research (PHR) needs to reflect the participatory worldview and the related values, principles, and processes (International Collaboration for Participatory Health Research (ICPHR) 2018). In this chapter, we define PHR as research done with people whose life or work is the focus of the research in an active and meaningful way across all phases of the research process (International Collaboration for Participatory Health Research 2013). In Chap. 1, *What Is Participatory Health Research*, a more complete discussion of the principles and values of PHR is presented.

In this chapter, we present three essential dimensions in conceptualising impact in PHR. We then begin to unravel the challenge of accessing and assessing the impact of PHR in the health context (e.g. the dominance of the evidence-based medicine or EBM worldview). We argue that a key factor contributing to this challenge is the different epistemological and ontological principles and assumptions that underpin PHR. Last, we share a few examples from practice on how to assess impact in PHR including an internationally led initiative called the interactive knowledge base (iKB) which aims to assess the legacy of impact in PHR.

Impact in PHR: Three Essential Dimensions

The three essential dimensions of impact in PHR are *co-impact, social impact,* and *embedded and ecological impact*. These dimensions are a reflection of recent discussions among members of the International Collaboration for Participatory Health Research (ICPHR) on the impact of PHR that were first initiated at an International Scientific Meeting on this same topic in Bielefeld, Germany, in Spring 2015 (Wright 2015). Subsequently, these discussions have been further articulated in a special themed issue on the conceptualisation and articulation of impact in PHR (Cook and Roche 2017). Discussions of what impact in PHR *is* and what impact in PHR *is not* are still in the early phases. The essential dimensions presented in this chapter are a starting point for articulating the core dimensions of impact in PHR that we hope will continue with the development of a systematic and dynamic evidence base on impact in PHR (i.e. the interactive knowledge base that will be presented later on in this chapter).

Co-impact

Co-impact, sometimes also referred to as *co-creation* or *co-production*, is an umbrella term defined as "the generation of change as a result of individuals, groups and organisations working together" (Banks et al. 2017, p. 542). Banks et al. (2017) have outlined three different types of co-impact in PHR:

- *Participatory impact:* relates to "changes in the thinking, emotions and practice of researchers and core partner organisations, which happen as a result of their involvement in conducting [PHR]" (Banks et al. 2017, p. 543). For example, these types of participatory impacts may be reported as developing confidence, becoming passionate about an issue, or feeling more empowered to take action (Banks et al. 2017; Cook et al. 2017). While these types of impacts may occur in other forms of research, the unique emphasis of co-impact in PHR is that the focus is on the project process and the learning that happens together (Banks et al. 2017).
- *Collaborative impact:* refers to "the take-up and use of the findings of collaborative research by individuals and organisations to change practice and policy, and influence attitudes and culture" (Banks et al. 2017, p. 543). This type of approach to co-impact is more utilitarian and findings-based. However, it is collaborative in that it is a result of people working together.
- *Collective impact:* is "a deliberate strategy on the part of the research partners (and sometimes others) to achieve a specific, targeted change in practice and/or policy based on issues highlighted via the research" (Banks et al. 2017, p. 543). This type of approach to co-impact is particularly important for groups working to address *wicked problems* and contribute to social change (Banks et al. 2017).

While Banks et al. (2017) have conceptually differentiated these three different types of co-impact in PHR, in reality there is significant overlap. The *Debt on Teesside* project – an action research project that aimed to research, alleviate, and advocate on the high levels of debt caused by predatory tactics of some credit card companies – illustrates a detailed case study on how these three forms of co-impact interact in practice at micro- and macro-levels (Banks et al. 2017). Further, these three types of co-impact provide a useful framework for evaluating impact in PHR projects (Banks et al. 2017).

Co-impact is a fundamental aspect of impact in PHR; however it remains an under-assessed and under-reported domain in the field. The under-reporting of co-impact is, in part, a reflection and consequence of the dominance of more traditional (i.e. linear) guidelines for how research is carried out and disseminated. As the impact of co-creation is not pertinent in such forms of research, space is not afforded for either considering or reporting this element that is fundamental to PHR. When participatory researchers have to report to funders, or indeed write in traditional academic journals, the impact of co-creation is thus omitted. The lack of documentation of co-impact by PHR researchers may, however, also be because participation is so central to the heart of PHR that its value and role in impact are taken for granted. For example, a UK-based study, led by co-author Tina Cook, found that participatory researchers tended to underemphasise both the breadth and depth of the engagement processes that took place in their reporting of the project (Cook et al. 2017). In a later section of this chapter, we provide some examples from practice to assist PHR researchers in accessing and articulating co-impact within their projects.

Social Impact

What differentiates impact in PHR from impact in more conventional health science fields is the explicit commitment to enabling action, with a focus on contributing to social impact, through developing human agency (Baum et al. 2006; International Collaboration for Participatory Health Research 2013). While there is no single definition of social impact, this concept is commonly defined as "the net effect of an activity on a community and well-being of individuals and families" (Centre for Social Impact n.d.). For example, these social impacts in PHR can range from improvements in the health of a specific group of people to addressing the social determinants of health by improving living standards or addressing the political determinants of health by changing repressive or restrictive policies.

While other forms of health research may strive for similar social impacts, what differentiates this type of impact from a PHR perspective is the consideration for the role of empowerment (i.e. developing human agency) as part of the change or action process (International Collaboration for Participatory Health Research 2013). Developing human agency is an important aspect of assessing social impact in PHR for a number of reasons. First, from a participatory worldview, it is assumed that people are better motivated to take action on an issue (a) when they have been involved in systematically learning more about the issue and (b) when they have become empowered to take action on that knowledge (International Collaboration for Participatory Health Research 2013). Therefore, in assessing the social impact of PHR, it is also important to assess the role of developing human agency and empowerment in the change process.

Embedded and Ecological Impact

The third essential dimension of impact in PHR is that impact is ecological and embedded in the PHR process [i.e. a result of interdependent processes and relationships nested in particular contexts (McLaren and Hawe 2005)]. To illustrate, the impacts that occur in PHR do not only occur at the end after data collection, analysis, and dissemination are complete; rather, impact is embedded throughout the entire PHR process. For example, in PHR there are many iterative cycles of knowledge co-creation, action, and reflection (Ledwith and Springett 2010). It is during these cycles, and through dialogue among project members, that many of the embedded participatory impacts previously discussed can occur (e.g. changes in thinking, becoming passionate about an issue, or feeling empowered to take action).

Being aware of these embedded impacts in PHR has a number of implications for researchers looking to better articulate and assess impact in PHR. First, impact in PHR is not something that can be *caught* at the end, but needs to be carefully considered throughout the lifecycle of the project, as it can be a challenge to retrospectively reflect on certain turning points in the project that contributed to certain impacts. In a later section of this chapter, we provide an example of how to approach assessing embedded impact across the project.

Impact in PHR should also be considered from an ecological or holistic/systems lens in order to articulate a more interconnected and holistic understanding of impacts in PHR (Trickett and Beehler 2017). As John D. Sterman in Trickett and Beehler (2017) states, "there are no side effects – just effects. Those we expected or that prove beneficial we call the main effects and claim credit. Those that undercut our policies and cause harm we claim to be side effects, hoping to excuse the failure of our intervention" (p. 528). From this ecological perspective, action in one part of the system will subsequently create a ripple effect in another part of that same system. Assessing impact from an ecological approach prepares PHR researchers to keep an open eye and ear for emergent impacts across different settings (i.e. individual, community, institutional) or different groups of people. As impact in PHR is co-produced and involves many different stakeholders, it is valuable to assess impact across these various settings and groups as well as the relationships between them (see the example from practice below).

While these essential dimensions of impact in PHR are presented as separate entities, in reality they are interconnected and build on each other in telling the *impact story* in PHR. The nature of these dimensions presents unique challenges to PHR researchers in unravelling the impact of their PHR projects; these challenges will be further discussed in the following sections.

Unravelling the Challenges of Assessing Impact in Participatory Health Research

Participatory health researchers experience unique challenges in assessing and articulating the impact of participatory health research. These include the dominance of the linear nature of assessing impact in the health sciences field (Springett 2017), the wide and imprecise use of the term *participatory* (Cook et al. 2017), and the perceived lack of appropriate existing outcome indicators to assess impact specific to PHR projects (Sandoval et al. 2012). While these challenges exist across the disciplines in which participatory research approaches are practised, they are further exacerbated in the context of the health sciences.

The Health Sciences Context

One of the underlying challenges in assessing the impact of PHR in the health sciences context is the strong dominance of the evidence-based medicine (EBM) paradigm. EBM is commonly defined as "the conscientious, explicit, and judicious use of current best evidence in making decisions about the care of individual patients" (Sackett et al. 1996, p. 71). It is argued that evidence-based practices "maintain an antiquated understanding of evidence as 'facts' about the world in the assumption that scientific beliefs stand or fall in light of the evidence" (Goldenberg 2006, p. 2622). The appeal of this positivist approach to evidence is that it claims to explain complex social processes (Goldenberg 2006). Our issue, like Holmes et al. (2006), is that EBM has come to be considered a *regime of truth* in the health sciences, disregarding other important forms of evidence (and impact) such as social efficacy (Rod et al. 2013), unanticipated outcomes, intuitive knowledge (Ledwith and Springett 2010), and interactions between intervention and context (Rychetnik et al. 2002; Goldenberg 2006). Within the EBM paradigm, evidence is most commonly perceived as quantifiable data. While qualitative evidence has made progress in gaining credibility in public health, stories as evidence are still marginalised. Such forms of knowledge have traditionally been characterised within the dominant EBM paradigm as subjective and unreliable (Baum et al. 2006). While, as Greenhalgh and Fahy (2015) suggest, in the UK the understanding of quality in EBM has been misappropriated and distorted by vested interests, they also argue that EBM is maturing from its early focus on epidemiology to embrace a wider range of disciplines and methodologies. Further, "the unenhanced 'logic model' of impact, comprising inputs (research funding)→activities (research)→outputs (e.g. papers, guidelines)→outcomes (e.g. changed clinician behaviour, new service models)→impacts (e.g. reduced mortality), is increasingly viewed as over simplistic" (Greenhalgh et al., 2015, p. 3). They go on to argue, however, that there remain a number of potential biases in EBM, including the low value given to knowledge through experience, that contributes to devaluing what they term *the patient and carer agenda* (Greenhalgh et al. 2015).

For PHR researchers, the dominance of forms of research in EBM that rely on distance as a key element of rigour creates a climate where participatory approaches are still seen as subservient. This means trying to demonstrate scientific merit and impact against quality guidelines and impact frameworks informed by the positivist ontology of EBM (South 2013). The consequence here is that many of the different forms of impact in PHR (e.g. relational impacts) are not valued under EBM's hierarchy of evidence and hence end up unarticulated and missing from the evidence base on impact. This contextual challenge is also faced by qualitative researchers, of course, but its effect is particularly acute for participatory researchers working in the health field because of the primacy given to *practical* and *living* knowledge (Heron and Reason 1997).

Three Unique Challenges to Assessing the Impact of Participatory Health Research

While there are a number of unique challenges that participatory health researchers may experience in assessing and articulating the impact of PHR, here we unravel what we believe are three central challenges. The first challenge is that traditional (i.e. more linear) approaches to reporting research impact within the health sciences are not compatible with the processes in PHR initiatives (Springett 2017). Current approaches to assessing impact in the health field tend to follow a linear pathway beginning with developing the research question, collecting data, disseminating findings, and concluding with the generation of impact (Banks et al. 2017). Similarly, the guidelines for reporting research in many health sciences journals also mirror this linear pathway of impact. This linear pathway does not reflect the emergent and iterative cycles of reflection, learning, action, and impact that occur repeatedly throughout the lifecycle of a PHR initiative.

Many PHR researchers can attest that trying to fit *what actually happens* in the PHR process into these linear guidelines is like trying to fit a square into a circle: much of what happens does not fit and ends up being left out of reporting and subsequently the wider evidence base on impact (Cook et al. 2017). This dissonance between what actually happens (e.g. the unanticipated actions and detours, where perspectives are challenged, and where unlearning and new learning take place) and how it is reported brushes over the *mess* that is commonly experienced by PHR researchers (Cook 2009). The *messiness* of the PHR process should not be seen as *noise*, but as a critical component that contributes to the rigour and impact of PHR (Cook 2009; Trickett et al. 2014). The exclusion of mess in the PHR process has brushed over the unique purpose of PHR and subsequently made it "difficult for future researchers to understand how outcomes were achieved and how they might build on those outcomes" (Cook 2009, p. 289).

While there are journals in the field of community psychology (Trickett et al. 2014) and research and practice in educational settings (Cook and Roche 2017) that have demonstrated support in publishing on issues of impact in PHR, part of addressing this challenge moving forward will be to advocate for reporting frameworks that allow the PHR story to be told with all the essential *messy* components. In 2017, the ICPHR developed a working group to draft criteria for writing up and appraising PHR from an international perspective, to begin to address this challenge (International Collaboration for Participatory Health Research 2018). Although still in the early phases, the key elements include outlining transparent criteria for describing types of participation, criteria on validity and credibility specific to the participatory worldview, as well as opportunities to demonstrate outcomes and impact beyond written text (i.e. multimedia dissemination).

The second major challenge in assessing impact in PHR is the broad use of the term *participatory*. The resulting breadth of research falling under this label makes assessing expected impacts from this approach very difficult (Cook et al. 2017). So much so that the concept of participation has been described as "infinitely mallea-

Table 5.1 Dimensions for participation matrix example

Place an '✓' in the appropriate column to indicate the type of participation across the various phases of the research project.

Project publication reference: Cook and Inglis (2012). Participatory research with men with learning disability: informed consent. *Tizard Learning Disability Review*, 17(2), 92–101.

Type	Deciding on research focus	Designing research methodology	Data generation	Data analysis	Report writing	Dissemination	Action	Other
Co-option								N/A
Compliance	✓							
Consultation		✓		✓	✓			
Co-operation		✓	✓	✓	✓	✓	✓	
Co-learning		✓	✓	✓		✓	✓	
Collective action							✓	

Adapted from Cook et al. (2017)

ble...[and] can be used to evoke- and to signify- almost anything that involves people" (Cornwall 2008, p. 269). There are a number of different models outlining various levels of participation including Arnstein's ladder of participation and Cornwall's (1996) typology of participation (see Table 5.1). Articulating the type of participation in a PHR project using one of these frameworks can help develop a more transparent understanding of the types of impacts that result or can be expected.

The third challenge with assessing impacts in PHR is the lack of reported indicators and strategies to capture the link between participatory processes and participatory impacts. For example, a literature review by Sandoval et al. (2012) identified 46 different instruments and 224 measures that related to four components of PHR (in this case the review focused specifically on community-based participatory research (CBPR)): (1) context, (2) group dynamics, (3) the extent of the community role in intervention and/or research design, and (4) the impact of these participatory processes on system change and health outcomes. Interestingly, of the 224 different measures of CBPR characteristics identified in the literature, there were relatively few measures specific to assessing outcomes ($n = 34$) (Sandoval et al. 2012). The outcome measures that were identified primarily focused on empowerment and community capacity, changes in practice or policy, unintended consequences, and health outcomes (Sandoval et al. 2012). However, there were no measures identified in the review that explored changes in power relations, culturally based effectiveness, or cultural revitalisation and renewal (Sandoval et al. 2012), all key aspects of PHR that are subsequently missing from the impact evidence base. While the aim in PHR should not be to mandate a set of standardised indicators to assess impact, PHR researchers may find it useful to draw on a library of different strategies and indicators to assess impact depending on how a PHR project emerges within its respective context.

It is timely then that the ICPHR has developed a participatory epidemiology working group to continue to explore and identify strategies to assess impact from a quantitative lens (International Collaboration for Participatory Health Research 2018). However, quantitative measures are only one approach to assessing impact and, alone, cannot holistically capture the different outcomes and impacts of PHR projects. In the following section, we present different qualitative approaches that have been used to capture PHR impacts from a systems and ecological perspective that is attuned to the participatory and relational dimensions of PHR. Ultimately, a systems approach to capturing impact drawing on both qualitative and quantitative disciplines will be essential, as attributing impact or change to any single effort may be unrealistic given the complex and dynamic natural environments in which PHR projects are situated (Trickett and Beehler 2013; Sandoval et al. 2012).

Tangible Approaches to Building the Impact Evidence Base

In this section, we share different tangible approaches to assessing and documenting impact in PHR that align with the essential dimensions of impact in PHR previously presented (i.e. co-impact, social impact, and embedded and ecological impact). The examples below mainly draw from a qualitative lens and nicely complement the quantitative instruments and measures previously identified (Sandoval et al. 2012).

Community asset mapping and ripples and social network analysis are two methods suggested by Trickett and Beehler (2017) to help PHR researchers assess ripple effects and ecological impacts. Community asset mapping is defined as "a process of documenting the tangible and intangible resources of a community by viewing the community as a place with strengths or assets that need to be preserved and enhanced, not deficits to be remedied" (Kerka 2003, p. 3). There are a variety of toolkits available online that PHR researchers may find useful as a starting point, including the *Community Capacity Inventory* and the *Questions to Ask While Community Mapping* tools hosted on the Community Toolbox website.[1] These methods could be used at varying time points over the life of a PHR initiative and even beyond to assess changes in assets. However, Trickett and Beehler (2017) suggest that mapping assets on its own is not enough from an ecological participatory perspective, as it misses out on key impacts including the relationships between the assets. Therefore, from a PHR lens, it is important to also map "the interdependence of such assets and their history of working together (or not)" to provide a more dynamic picture of PHR ripple impacts (Trickett and Beehler 2017, p. 533).

Social network analysis is another method recommended by Trickett and Beehler (2017) to assess the relational dimension of PHR that contributes to co-impact (an essential dimension of impact in PHR). One of the anticipated outcomes of PHR is that relationships are expected to change as a result of participatory involvement and may include increased (and potentially decreased) connections among project members. The value of strengthening these relationships among project members is that it can support groups to better support the goals they wish to collectively

---

[1] https://ctb.ku.edu/en

achieve. Therefore, assessing how social networks change over time is a useful method in capturing impact in PHR from a relational lens. A social network is "the articulation of a social relationship, ascribed or achieved, among individuals, families, households, villages, communities, regions, and so on" (Bandyopadhyay et al. 2011, p. 1). Social network analysis then is the analysis of "various characteristics of the pattern of distribution of relational ties… drawing inferences about the network as a whole or about those belonging to it considered individually or in groups" (Bandyopadhyay et al. 2011, p. 4). The unique value of social network analysis for exploring impact in PHR is that it can also be used as an approach to assess changes in power in research relationships over time (Neal and Neal 2011; Trickett and Beehler 2017). Understanding this power element is important to capture, as the dialogical processes at the centre of PHR are only successful to the extent that power dynamics are acknowledged and better understood (International Collaboration for Participatory Health Research 2013). There are many different tools and software available to assist in conducting a social network analysis, a sample of which is summarised on the Knowledge Sharing Toolkit webpage.[2]

Alongside community asset mapping and ripples, and social network analysis, the ICPHR is developing a framework to help PHR researchers assess the link between participation and impact across different phases of the research lifecycle building on the work of the APRIL (Accessing Participatory Research Impact and Legacy) project in the UK led by co-author Tina Cook (Cook et al. 2017). The *Dimensions for Participation Matrix* example (Table 5.1) can help researchers to categorise the depth of participation across the various phases of the research, informed by Cornwall's (1996) levels of participation. In the APRIL project, use of this matrix helped researchers to be more precise and explicit about the breadth and depth of participation that occurred in the research (Cook et al. 2017). Working through this matrix can help to stimulate further discussion and reflection on types of participation and impact, as was the case in the APRIL project (Cook et al. 2017), on aspects such as:

- What was the impact across various stakeholders and where did it occur?
- Were there any perceived links between participation and the quality of the research design?
- Who benefited most from the participation in the study, what did that benefit look like, and when did it occur? (p. 481)

The *Impact in Participatory Health Research* grid (Table 5.2) helps researchers to categorise what impact they think the project will have (to assist with prospective mapping) or to reflect back and assess the impact the project has had (a retrospective analysis) across the different phases. Together, these two draft frameworks can assist PHR researchers in linking the specific types of participation to the different forms of impact that have occurred, resulting in a more transparent articulation of the impact and value of participation in research. These frameworks are currently being piloted by members of the ICPHR and, when revised, will form the basis for

---

[2] http://www.kstoolkit.org/

Table 5.2 Impact in participatory health research (*Place an 'x' in the appropriate column*)

Degree of impact: scale where 1 is lowest						Category
1	2	3	4	5	N/A	
						On research agenda
						Initiating this research topic
						Identifying different research questions
						Influencing funding decisions
						On research design
						Amending the focus of this research
						Shaping the question (s) for this research
						Designing data collection/generation approach
						Designing approach to data analysis
						Designing approaches to trustworthiness and rigour
						Quality of the data
						On research process
						Supporting recruitment
						Collecting/generating data
						Analysing data
						Writing up
						Dissemination
						On participatory researchers
						Knowledge of research
						Self esteem
						Confidence
						Other
						On academic/community-based researchers
						Affected perceptions
						Affected engagement with communities of practice
						Affected access to data
						Affected understandings of topic area
						Affected dissemination strategy
						On services
						Affected health outcomes
						Affected patient care
						Affected costs
						Provided new products
						Improved educational dimension
						Changed service provision
						Changed organisational processes
						Changed organisational behaviours
						On policy
						Influenced debate
						Influenced policy making (legislation, guidelines, etc.)
						Other: Please specify

a newly proposed interactive knowledge base to bring together and share the various impacts of PHR projects in a dynamic and systematic manner.

These three examples of possible strategies highlight different tangible methods to assist researchers in documenting the impact of their PHR projects. These methods emphasise different elements of conceptualising impact in PHR: co-impact (relational), social (collective) impact, and ecological (embedded ripple effects) impact. There is no single method or tool to capture all the different elements; PHR researchers will be required to experiment with different methods in an additive fashion to holistically capture impact in PHR. For PHR researchers, it will also be important to capture impact in a systematic yet dynamic way to begin building an international evidence base on the unique contributions and impact of PHR.

Moving Forward on the Issue of Impact: The Interactive Knowledge Base (IKB)

The interactive knowledge base (iKB) is an expansion of the earlier APRIL project (Cook et al. 2017) and aims to unravel and systematically capture the dynamic impacts of participatory health research. The next steps in the development of the iKB are being led by members of the ICPHR in Canada and the UK (International Collaboration for Participatory Health Research n.d.). The aim of the iKB in the long term is to map the relationship between participation and impact, the scope of impacts that can be expected, and how these impacts manifest in different contexts of health research (i.e. different issues, locations, people involved, etc.). The iKB will be a gathering point for different types of data such as traditional scholarly articles, web archives, and visual data including videos, photographs, and stories.

The pilot framework to retrospectively assess and document impact will focus on (1) how impact manifested in the research project; (2) what types of impact can be rationally expected from participatory health research; (3) how impact can be observed, demonstrated, and documented; (4) what indicators would be most useful in assessing genuine participation and impact; and (5) what the connection between impact and participation is. The aim is to seek clarity through informed descriptions of past implementation of the research process to help make explicit the acquisition, transformation, and dissemination of impact during and after the participatory process.

Inspired by the Cochrane Library (Cochran Community n.d.), practitioners of PHR (academic and non-academic) will be given the opportunity to register their projects online and be given web space to upload academic scholarship as well as other materials into an online database. It is intended that the multimedia format will allow all types of stakeholder groups (e.g. academic, clinical, community) to participate. In contrast to the Cochrane Library, however, the interactive knowledge base will have advanced features whereby registrants have discussion space to reflect on their experience of doing PHR and stakeholders can read about and connect with other PHR groups and add their own reflections after project completion.

This aspect of the interactive knowledge base is important because, as had been confirmed in the APRIL project, many of the extended benefits of PHR remain undocumented (i.e. outside the scope of academic publication) and require the involvement of practitioners and stakeholders in dialogic and self-reflective processes (Cook et al. 2017). Thus, the iKB will engage PHR participants directly in a social learning process and thereby increase their understanding of impact and its articulation.

The iKB will help to inform a clearly articulated conceptualisation and mapping of impact in PHR that will be translated into a usable internationally accepted framework that in turn can inform future PHR projects while being sensitive to different local cultural contexts and health conditions. Furthermore, the proposed iKB will help PHR stakeholders (academic and non-academic) identify how their research fits with currently recognised dimensions of participation (hence addressing the challenge of poor articulations of participation) and impact and to further develop them where appropriate. The participatory and dynamic features of the iKB provide a space for PHR researchers to tell the whole story without being limited by a linear reporting framework and, in essence, make what actually happens a heuristic for PHR impact theory (Trickett 1991).

Conclusion

In this chapter, we have outlined why conceptualising impact in PHR needs to reflect the values, principles, processes and overall worldview of a participatory lens. The three essential dimensions of impact in PHR that we have presented in this chapter – co-impact, social impact, and ecological impact – represent a jumping off point for further formulating the core dimensions of impact in PHR. While PHR researchers experience a number of challenges in demonstrating impact in the health sciences context, it is our hope that the development of the new interactive knowledge base will advance the science of PHR by providing a common nomenclature about how participation and its impacts should be described and operationalised. This will in turn provide much needed empirical evidence to help PHR contribute more effectively to the improvement of people's health and to the development of health services and policies internationally.

References

Bandyopadhyay, S., Rao, A., & Sinha, B. (2011). *Models for social networks with statistical applications*. Thousand Oaks: SAGE Publications. Available at: http://methods.sagepub.com/book/models-for-social-networks-with-statistical-applications

Banks, S., Herrington, T., & Carter, K. (2017). Pathways to co-impact: Action research and community organising. *Educational Action Research, 25*, 541–559. https://doi.org/10.1080/09650792.2017.1331859.

Baum, F., MacDougall, C., & Smith, D. (2006). Participatory action research. *Journal of Epidemiology and Community Health, 60*(10), 854–857. https://doi.org/10.1136/jech.2004.028662.

Centre for Social Impact. (n.d.). About social impact. http://www.csi.edu.au/about-social/. Accessed Feb 2018.

Cochran Community. (n.d.). Proposing and registering new Cochrane Reviews. http://community.cochrane.org/review-production/production-resources/proposing-and-registering-new-cochrane-reviews. Accessed Feb 2018.

Cook, T. (2009). The purpose of mess in action research: Building rigour though a messy turn. *Educational Action Research, 17*(2), 277–291. https://doi.org/10.1080/09650790902914241.

Cook, T., & Inglis, P. (2012). Participatory research with men with learning disability: Informed consent. *Tizard Learning Disability Review, 17*(2), 92–101. https://doi.org/10.1108/13595471211218875.

Cook, T., & Roche, B. (2017). Editorial. *Educational Action Research, 25*(4), 467–472. https://doi.org/10.1080/09650792.2017.1358516.

Cook, T., Boote, J., Buckley, N., Vougioukalou, S., & Wright, M. (2017). Accessing participatory research impact and legacy: Developing the evidence base for participatory approaches in health research. *Educational Action Research, 25*(4), 473–488. https://doi.org/10.1080/09650792.2017.1326964.

Cornwall, A. (1996). Towards participatory practice: Participatory rural appraisal (PRA) and the participatory process. In K. De Koning & M. Martin (Eds.), *Participatory research in health: Issues and experiences*. London: Zed Press.

Cornwall, A. (2008). Unpacking 'participation': Models, meanings and practices. *Community Development Journal, 43*(3), 269–283. https://doi.org/10.1093/cdj/bsn010.

Goldenberg, M. J. (2006). On evidence and evidence-based medicine: Lessons from the philosophy of science. *Social Science & Medicine, 62*(11), 2621–2632. https://doi.org/10.1016/j.socscimed.2005.11.031.

Greenhalgh, T., & Fahy, N. (2015). Research impact in the community-based health sciences: An analysis of 162 case studies from the 2014 UK Research Excellence Framework. *BMC Medicine, 13*(1), 232. https://doi.org/10.1186/s12916-015-0467-4.

Greenhalgh, T., Snow, R., Ryan, S., Rees, S., & Salisbury, H. (2015). Six 'biases' against patients and carers in evidence-based medicine. *BMC Medicine, 13*(1), 200. https://doi.org/10.1186/s12916-015-0437-x.

Heron, J., & Reason, P. (1997). A participatory inquiry paradigm. *Qualitative Inquiry, 3*(3), 274–294. https://doi.org/10.1177/107780049700300302.

Higher Education Funding Council for England. (n.d.). REF impact. http://www.hefce.ac.uk/rsrch/REFimpact/. Accessed Feb 2018.

Holmes, D., Murray, S. J., Perron, A., & Rail, G. (2006). Deconstructing the evidence-based discourse in health sciences: Truth, power and fascism. *International Journal of Evidence-Based Healthcare, 4*(3), 180–186. https://doi.org/10.1111/j.1479-6988.2006.00041.x.

International Collaboration for Participatory Health Research. (2018). Projects. http://www.icphr.org/projects.html. Accessed Feb 2018.

International Collaboration for Participatory Health Research. (n.d.). Focus areas. http://www.icphr.org/focus-areas-overview.html. Accessed Feb 2018.

International Collaboration for Participatory Health Research (ICPHR). (2018). *Position paper 3: What is impact in participatory health research?* Berlin: International Collaboration for Participatory Health Research.

International Collaboration for Participatory Health Research May 2013. (2013). *Position paper 1: What is participatory health research?* Berlin: International Collaboration for Participatory Health Research Report Available at: http://www.icphr.org/uploads/2/0/3/9/20399575/ichpr_position_paper_1_defintion_-_version_may_2013.pdf.

Kerka, S. (2003). *Community asset mapping: Trends and issues alert (no. 47)*. Columbus: ERIC clearinghouse on adult, career, and vocational education.

Kuhn, T. S. (1996). *The structure of scientific revolutions*. Chicago: University of Chicago Press.

Ledwith, M., & Springett, J. (2010). *Participatory practice*. Bristol: The Policy Press.

McLaren, L., & Hawe, P. (2005). Ecological perspectives in health research. *Journal of Epidemiology & Community Health, 59*(1), 6–14. https://doi.org/10.1136/jech.2003.018044.

Milat, A. J., Bauman, A. E., & Redman, S. (2015). A narrative review of research impact assessment models and methods. *Health Research Policy and Systems, 13*(1), 18. https://doi.org/10.1186/s12961-015-0003-1.

Neal, J. W., & Neal, Z. P. (2011). Power as a structural phenomenon. *American Journal of Community Psychology, 48*(3–4), 157–167. https://doi.org/10.1007/s10464-010-9356-3.

Panel on Return on Investment in Health Research. (2009). *Making an impact: A preferred framework and indicators to measure returns on investment in health research*. Ottawa: Canadian Academy of Health.

Penfield, T., Baker, M. J., Scoble, R., & Wykes, M. C. (2014). Assessment, evaluations, and definitions of research impact: A review. *Research Evaluation, 23*(1), 21–32. https://doi.org/10.1093/reseval/rvt021.

Rod, M. H., Ingholt, L., Bang Sørensen, B., & Tjørnhøj-Thomsen, T. (2013). The spirit of the intervention: Reflections on social effectiveness in public health intervention research. *Critical Public Health, 24*(3), 296–307. https://doi.org/10.1080/09581596.2013.841313.

Rychetnik, L., Frommer, M., Hawe, P., & Shiell, A. (2002). Criteria for evaluating evidence on public health interventions. *Journal of Epidemiology and Community Health, 56*(2), 119–127. https://doi.org/10.1136/jech.56.2.119.

Sackett, D. L., Rosenberg, W. M., Gray, J. M., Haynes, R. B., & Richardson, W. S. (1996). Evidence based medicine: What it is and what it isn't. *BMJ, 312*(7023), 71–72. https://doi.org/10.1136/bmj.312.7023.71.

Sandoval, J. A., Lucero, J., Oetzel, J., Avila, M., Belone, L., Mau, M., et al. (2012). Process and outcome constructs for evaluating community-based participatory research projects: A matrix of existing measures. *Health Education Research, 27*(4), 680–690. https://doi.org/10.1093/her/cyr087.

South, J. (2013). *People centred public health*. Bristol: The Policy Press.

Springett, J. (2017). Impact in participatory health research: What can we learn from research on participatory evaluation? *Educational Action Research, 25*(4), 560–574. https://doi.org/10.1080/09650792.2017.1342554.

Trickett, E. J. (1991). Paradigms and the research report: Making what actually happens a heuristic for theory. *American Journal of Community Psychology, 19*(3), 365–370.

Trickett, E. J., & Beehler, S. (2013). The ecology of multilevel interventions to reduce social inequalities in health. *American Behavioral Scientist*, 1227–1246. https://doi.org/10.1177/0002764213487342.

Trickett, E. J., & Beehler, S. (2017). Participatory action research and impact: An ecological ripples perspective. *Educational Action Research*, 525–540. https://doi.org/10.1080/09650792.2017.1299025.

Trickett, E. J., Trimble, J. E., & Allen, J. (2014). Most of the story is missing: Advocating for a more complete intervention story. *American Journal of Community Psychology*, 180–186. https://doi.org/10.1007/s10464-014-9645-3.

Wright, M. T. (2015). International scientific meeting on the impact of participatory health research. *ZiF Mitteilungen* (pp. 43–45). Bielefeld: ZiF.

Chapter 6
Reviewing the Effectiveness of Participatory Health Research: Challenges and Possible Solutions

Janet Harris

Introduction

Ageing populations and people with long-term and chronic conditions are creating rising health-care costs and increasing demands on health systems. As a result, there is renewed interest in looking to participation in health research as a possible solution. For example, health systems are concentrating on reducing the expensive hospital services by tasking primary care with keeping people in the community. Primary care in turn is partnering with communities to promote self-care and reduce risk for developing chronic and long-term conditions. Community-based strategies for promoting health and wellbeing have experienced various levels of success, and a number of explanations have been produced for what works. Cultural relevance and appropriateness are seen as key (Liu et al. 2012) as are coalitions and partnership working (Anderson et al. 2012). Partnership working proposes that forming good relationships across community, government and academia can encourage active participation in addressing the conditions that affect health, producing interventions that integrate community knowledge with research (Oetzel and Minkler 2017).

Several systematic reviews examining the impact of community engagement and participation in health research (Roussos and Fawcett 2000; Viswanathan et al. 2004; O'Mara-Eves et al. 2015; Rifkin 2014) have found that collaborative partnerships can engage communities, and use of a participatory health research (PHR) paradigm can mobilise communities to take action on upstream circumstances relating to health (Roussos and Fawcett 2000). The most recent systematic review has found solid evidence that community engagement is positively associated with individuals achieving health outcomes across a range of conditions (O'Mara-Eves et al. 2015), but other reviews have found that outcomes may

J. Harris (✉)
University of Sheffield, School of Health and Related Research (ScHARR), Sheffield, UK
e-mail: janet.harris@sheffield.ac.uk

© Springer International Publishing AG, part of Springer Nature 2018
M. T. Wright, K. Kongats (eds.), *Participatory Health Research*,
https://doi.org/10.1007/978-3-319-92177-8_6

be related to resolving 'non-health' issues such as housing or crime at the level of community empowerment (Milton et al. 2011).

Although the relationships between participation and health have been validated (Oetzel et al. 2015), documenting the effectiveness of participatory health research is difficult. Few health studies analyse relationships between the process of participation and improved health status (Rifkin 2014). Methods for conducting systematic reviews of the effectiveness of participatory health research need to be developed because health care is increasingly being shifted to communities without a corresponding shift in funding. Community-based services will need evidence of effectiveness in order to ensure adequate funding and present strong arguments for their approaches which are for the most part participatory. This chapter outlines the challenges of conducting reviews of participation in health research, which include:

- Assembling an experienced review team
- Defining participation and impact
- Formulating a review question
- Conducting sensitive searches
- Deciding which literature to include
- Extracting meaningful information from studies
- Synthesising findings
- Disseminating to promote use of the review

Solutions for reviewing participation are presented, based on experiences of conducting several reviews.

Assembling a Review Team

Review teams usually include experienced reviewers alongside health researchers with expert knowledge of the health issue or intervention. A wider group of stakeholders may be involved including service providers, users of services, carers and agencies advocating for people with health and social needs, commissioners of services and policymakers. They are typically consulted when framing the questions for the review or checking the findings (Oliver et al. 2015). Reviews that aim to produce explanations, such as realist reviews, may opt for more involvement by convening stakeholders at key stages to produce explanatory accounts of the process and results (Pearson et al. 2015). While stakeholders as consultants can influence aspects of a review, the review team has the power to make decisions about how the contributions are used. This is called *epistemological power* – i.e. power to decide what it actually means to know something or what really counts as evidence (Barreto 2014). The group in control makes the decisions about what to do with stakeholder knowledge, thereby influencing each stage of the knowledge creation process (Van de Ven 2007). When reviewing participatory health research, experts in the PHR approach need to be included, as well as people with experience of doing PHR. Further, these experts and the wider stakeholder group need to be given opportunities to contribute at all stages of the review. It can be argued that periodic stakeholder contact may not produce the dialogue needed to develop understanding of what is being found, risking the exclusion of important perspectives from people who have lived experience of the health issue. Including people with little experience of systematic reviewing challenges academics, who may not have the skills to facilitate co-production with people who have limited research experience. Including stakeholders throughout a review, however, can raise awareness of epistemological bias. Further, when stakeholders with experience of delivering or receiving the intervention are involved across different stages of the review, they can identify missing elements of intervention or context. Co-production contributes to several types of validity that are used in participatory research (ICPHR 2013):

- Participatory validity, e.g. getting stakeholders to actively engage in the review process as much as possible
- Intersubjective validity, e.g. the extent to which the research included in the review is seen as credible from different perspectives
- Contextual validity, e.g. the extent to which the research included in the review is seen as relating to local situations (different ethnic groups and economic, social and geographical settings) of people who will be the end users of the review

We found that a co-production approach was instrumental in producing a credible review of the impact of peer support on reducing health inequalities (Harris et al. 2016, 2015b), and our methods for assembling the team are described in Box 6.1.

Box 6.1 Assembling a Participatory Review Team
We developed an approach that we have called 'participatory systematic reviewing' because it embodies the paradigm of doing research with providers and recipients of interventions, rather than relying on academics to make judgements based solely on the information in the primary studies. We assembled a group of people with lived experience of delivering or receiving peer support using snowballing and networking. We decided to describe this as an Advisory Network. With the exception of writing the proposal, the Network contributed to each stage of the review. They described the intervention and constructed a programme theory explaining how, when and why peer support works. They reviewed the key elements of peer support that had been researched and identified one critical element – instrumental support – that had been dismissed as unimportant in health settings. Their descriptions of instrumental support enabled us to recognise it in the research. The theory produced by the Network was also compared to theories produced in the research. Their role was similar to that of topic experts who belong to a systematic review panel, contributing to shaping and conducting the review as well as reviewing findings.

The Network engaged with academics in a process of collective sense-making (Weick 1995) where interactions produced explanations of the relationship between peer support and health outcomes that were grounded in the experiences of providers and service users. The inclusion of practical knowledge about instrumental peer support was critical to developing the final theory (Harris et al. 2016).

Conceptualising Participation and Impact

A number of authors have noted that there are diverse definitions of participation (Cook 2012; Beresford 2013; Rifkin 2014), so the review team must make decisions on the population, setting and dimensions of participation and impact. The population may be defined by the type of participation, e.g. people who contribute to designing, delivering and evaluating an initiative, people who receive interventions or services or both groups. It can be further refined by age, cultural group and setting. 'Setting' can be problematic, as studies that describe themselves as 'community-based' may have very different definitions of community. For example, in a recent review of diabetes, the notion of community included a neighbourhood served by community agencies and a health centre (Chesla et al. 2013), an urban district of 150,000 (Daivadanam et al. 2013), a Native American tribe of less than 7000 (Macaulay et al. 1997) and African Americans in the Alabama Black Belt, a rural area comprised of 8 counties (Andreae et al. 2012). Decisions need to be made, therefore, on whether to define community as an area bounded by a health service, a geographical region or an ethnic group.

Participation can be conceptualised by level, the timing or the frequency/intensity of the interaction. There are a number of frameworks that can be used to conceptualise levels. One of the most common is based on Sherry Arnstein's classic ladder of participation (1969) and contains six levels (Box 6.2, Cornwall 2008).

Box 6.2 Levels of Participation
1. *Co-option* – where token representatives are chosen but have no real input or power in the research process
2. *Compliance* – where outsiders decide the research agenda and direct the process, with tasks assigned to participants and incentives being provided by the researchers
3. *Consultation* – where local opinions are asked for, but outside researchers conduct the work and decide on a course of action
4. *Co-operation* – where local people work together with outside researchers to determine priorities, with responsibility remaining with outsiders for directing the process
5. *Co-learning* – where local people and outsiders share their knowledge in order to create new understanding and work together to form action plans, with outsiders providing facilitation
6. *Collective action* – where local people set their own agenda and mobilise to carry out research in the absence of outside initiators and facilitators

In our experience, these levels are not usually reported in health research studies, unless a PHR paradigm has been used. Another framework allows data to be extracted from studies by the stage of research at which the participant was involved (Shippee et al. 2015). The stages are characterised as priority setting, proposal writing, intervention design and implementation. The most recent framework (Lucero et al. 2016) allows extraction by the *process* of participation. Although articles will identify the stage at which people participate, they may not describe the process of participation. Key elements of the process therefore need to be included in the definition of participation to help reviewers decide which articles should be included in the review. These models and frameworks are potentially useful for documenting the impact of participation but are very dependent upon what is actually reported in the literature.

The timing of participation may be important because it may be more difficult to engage and to establish equal partnerships when people are brought on board after priorities have been set and funding proposals have been submitted (Andreae et al. 2012). Frequency and intensity of participation have been identified as a possible key factor in enabling people to achieve health outcomes (Cargo et al. 2015).

For our reviews, we defined participation as the agency of a person or a group of people to exert influence on health research, health structures, practices, services or policies that have an effect on their health and wellbeing. This includes the concept of empowerment, defined as a social action process of individuals, organisations and communities to transform life conditions for greater health and equity (Wallerstein 1992).

Our definitions of impact (Box 6.3) are based on Chap. 5, a working paper being developed by the ICPHR (International Collaboration for Participatory Health Research 2018) and the CBPR conceptual model (Lucero et al. 2016; Wallerstein and Duran 2010).

Box 6.3 Definitions of Impact in Participatory Health Research
- Changes in the design or conduct of an intervention or research project, incorporating local experiential knowledge and culture, norms and practices
- Transformative learning, e.g. generation of new knowledge, evidence or theory as a result of learning together
- Building capacity to make decisions about lifestyle, environment, health and wellbeing
- Changing relationships and group dynamics, e.g. changes in traditional hierarchies or historical relationships, formation of new or expanded partnerships, creation of more equitable collaborations and coalitions
- Improving the lives of those involved in the design, conduct, analysis and dissemination of the research and/or evaluation of the research process
- Structural impacts, e.g. changes in traditional structures, practices, cultures, power relations and policies
- Improved health, reduced disparities and increased social justice

Impact can occur at different levels, including the people directly involved in the research; the local organisations, areas or community groups where the research is taking place; and networks that are developed via the research process (local, national, international) and systems (political, economic, social, technological).

Impact level should be selected based on the interests of the audience – those who are commissioning and using the results of the review. The extent of impact can range from single to cumulative to a wider-reaching 'ripple effect' generating unanticipated outcomes. Finally, impact can occur at different points in time – during the project, immediately after the project or over the medium or longer term. Before undertaking a review of long-term impact, the literature needs to be scoped to determine whether there are an adequate number of studies reporting longer-term effects.

These definitions for participation and impact are given to make the point that when conducting a review, the review team needs to craft their definitions to suit the knowledge that is available while satisfying the interests of those commissioning the review.

Formulating a Review Question

Review questions are formulated using a set of mnemonics to focus on a specific population, intervention or outcome, but the element of participation needs to be incorporated into the mnemonic as shown in Box 6.4. While the PICO format is most often used in review of effectiveness, it can only be used if there is research comparing one form of intervention with another. This makes it difficult to use for reviews of participatory health research, because there are no studies yet that compare a participatory approach with other approaches.

Box 6.4 Formats for Questions About Participatory Health Research

PICO (Richardson et al. 1995)

Population: In people with diabetes
Intervention: Do interventions that are codesigned by patients and the wider community
Comparison: When compared with interventions that are not codesigned
Outcome: Produce more appropriate interventions

SPICE (Booth 2006)

Setting – Where? In what context? In North American tribes
Perspective – For whom? People with diabetes who codesign and research diabetes interventions
Intervention (phenomenon of interest) – What? Who? Promote better uptake of the intervention

(continued)

Box 6.4 (continued)

Comparison – What else? Than projects that do not involve people with diabetes in codesign

Evaluation – How well? What result? Improved self-management of diabetes

CHIP (Shaw 2010)

Context: In communities where there are high levels of diabetes and pre-diabetes

How the study was conducted: Does participatory health research

Issues examined: Enable the circumstances leading to diabetes risk to be identified

People involved: By people who are at risk

3WH (Sandelowski et al. 2007)

What topic: Can risks be associated with high levels of diabetes in a community

Who population: Be identified by the people who are at risk, working in partnership with academics and community leaders

When temporal: Before people are hospitalised

How methodological: Using participatory health research

CIMO (Wong et al. 2013)

Context: Do participatory health research projects that use academic-community partnerships

Intervention: To co-produce diabetes education programmes

Mechanisms: Engage people with diabetes and the wider community

Outcomes: In producing relevant and appropriate education that empowers people to take control of diabetes and reduce diabetes-related risk

The SPICE format also requires a comparison. In our current review, we have found that it remains difficult to compare different levels of participation because they are often poorly reported in primary studies (Harris et al. submitted). The CHIP and 3WH mnemonics are more open ended, allowing exploration of the effectiveness of PHR without doing a comparison. The sample question for the CIMO framework shows that in participatory health research, process outcomes are included alongside impact outcomes. This is a critical point to consider, as the process of participation has a direct influence on whether people are able to participate in the intervention and are supported to achieve health outcomes. The types of questions that can be asked in a review, to capture process, are shown in Table 6.1 below.

Review questions can focus on impact within projects or beyond projects. Within projects, the relative contribution of participation at various stages can be the focus

Table 6.1 Questions for reviews of the process of participation

Type of inquiry	Types of review questions
Implementation inquiry: How do participatory approaches contribute to the process for designing and delivering the intervention or programme?	How were people involved in deciding the components of the intervention?
	Were local people consulted or engaged in developing recruitment strategies? Did they do the recruiting? Were there barriers to recruitment that can be attributed to lack of engagement?
	Who participated? How many over time? Did the programme attract the target audience?
	What were the frequency, duration and intensity of the intervention? Did it reflect the levels of participation that the target group would consider realistic or appropriate?
	Did participants actually engage with the intervention? How did participants experience the intervention and did their experiences affect engagement?
	What were provider experiences of delivering the intervention?
	Was the intervention implemented as planned? Why or why not?
Appropriateness inquiry: To what extent does the approach to participation fit (or is it likely to fit) with the cultural, ethical or equity context?	Is the approach appropriate, acceptable and accessible to people within their local context?
	How does the participatory intervention (potentially) impact on equity from both a positive and negative perspective for different population groups?
	Are the desired outcomes the outcomes that are valued by the population?
	Are the desired outcomes consistent with people's priorities and/or beliefs?
	What is the population's perception/experience of negative consequences of the intervention?
Effectiveness inquiry: Do participatory approaches work?	What is the effectiveness of a community-based (intervention) compared to interventions that do not use participatory approaches for the population?
	Do the effects vary in relation to subgroups within the population?
	Do effects vary in relation to the country context and history of using participatory approaches in health?

Adapted from Cargo et al. (2015), Pearson et al. (2005) and Harris et al. (2018)

of the review, or the review question can ask whether participation 'works' in terms of achieving the desired health outcomes. These questions may be combined within a single review. There is also a 'beyond-project' set of review questions, assessing impact in terms of broader and more far-reaching changes, often occurring after the original study has been completed, which have social, economic, environmental and health benefits for individuals, groups, communities and systems (Table 6.2). During the project, it is likely that researchers and local participants will be the main beneficiaries, while policymakers and nonacademics are the main beneficiaries after the study is completed (Phipps et al. 2016).

Table 6.2 Questions for reviews of the impact of participation

Impact questions
Did sharing of local experiential knowledge and culture, norms and practices instigate a change in the design or conduct of the intervention or research project?
Did participation improve the lives of those involved in the design, conduct, analysis, evaluation and/or dissemination of the research?
Did participation change historical relationships, group dynamics and traditional hierarchies? Did it lead to more equitable partnerships and collaborations?
Did participation lead to the formation of new or expanded partnerships, collaborations or coalitions?
Did participation create transformative learning, e.g. generation of new knowledge, evidence or theory as a result of learning together?
Did participation increase capacity on individual and/or collective levels to make decisions about lifestyle, environment, health and wellbeing?
Did participation promote a social action process across individuals, organisations and communities to transform life conditions for greater health and equity?
Did participation have structural impacts, where changes occurred in traditional structures, practices, cultures, power relations and policies?
Did participation lead to improved health and wellbeing, reduced disparities and increased social justice?

Conducting a Scoping Review

A scoping review is useful in deciding the parameters of a review of participation. Scoping reviews are a way of mapping the territory of participation for a particular health topic. They not only serve to develop definitions for participation and impact but also help in making decisions about the boundaries of the review (Joanna Briggs Institute 2015).

The first question to ask of the abstracts that have been retrieved is: Is the article about participation? Our process for excluding articles based on definitions of participation is described in Box 6.5.

> **Box 6.5 Using Definitions of Participation and Impact to Refine the Search**
>
> A preliminary scoping of the literature was conducted, and abstracts including the population and condition of interest were retrieved. For our review, this was all adults with diabetes or at risk for developing diabetes, where relevant keywords are related to the phenomenon of interest, e.g. participatory, engagement and involvement. Because our review aimed to identify effective approaches to involving patients and the wider community in diabetes research, we excluded studies in the first instance that claimed to use participation but that didn't describe one of the levels (co-option through collective

(continued)

Box 6.5 (continued)

action). Over 92% of the abstracts were excluded; 211 articles were retrieved, the full text was read to see if participation was described and a further 154 were excluded. The remaining 57 all described participation at one or more stages of the research (Harris et al. 2015a, b). We included articles with both thin and detailed descriptions of impact, in order to map how impact was defined and assessed.

After restricting the number of articles to those that truly included participation, other questions can be asked to set boundaries for the review, for example:

- What is the context in which participation takes place?
- What is the aim of the participation?
- What is the length of time over which the impact of participation is assessed?

The period of time covered by the project is important because it is related to different types of impact. Whereas 'within-project' impact is created by those who are on the research team, 'beyond-project' impact is created by nonacademic partners such as policymakers and community members who use the learning to inform decisions and programme development.

It is rare to find short-term and longer-term impact in one publication, unless a journal is devoted to reporting a single project (Hasnain-Wynia 2003; Trickett et al. 2014). Journals often require authors to publish methodology and results for intervention studies separately. If included articles are limited to those that report only health outcomes, reviewers will be working with articles where 'years of partnership development and collaboration must be distilled to few words in a small number of journals willing to publish this more descriptive science' (Viswanathan et al. 2004, p. 5). Articles reporting on longer-term impact, as well as those describing process, may not be indexed to the original study because they are seen as separate. This has implications for searching, as a straightforward search on outcomes will rarely produce citations for process or longer-term participation impact.

A method called cluster searching can be used to identify all documents related to a particular project in order to trace pathways to impact (Booth et al. 2013). Cluster searching is an iterative process, where forwards and backwards chaining is done using the relevant article – the index paper – to identify all related materials (Fig. 6.1). Relevant materials are not limited to journal articles – grey literature such as evaluation reports can be included, as can documents describing the process of participation (meeting notes) and the value of participation. The aim is to compile as complete a picture as is possible for the overall process.

An example of an exhaustive search for community engagement (which includes all synonyms for participation) can be found in Chap. 2 of Harris et al. (2015a, b). As more reviews of participation are produced, it is likely that even more efficient search strategies will be developed and reviewers are advised to consult published reviews of participation when constructing the search strategy. It is likely, however, that searches on participation will retrieve much that is not

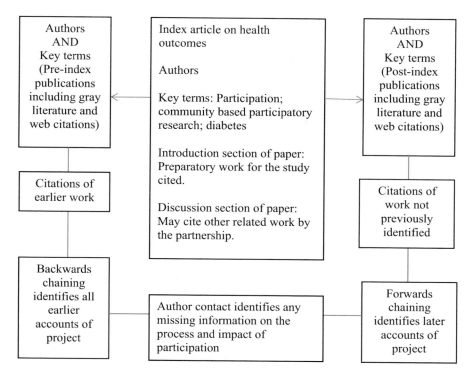

Fig. 6.1 Cluster searching: a worked example

relevant (high specificity) because articles are poorly indexed, making the abstract sift time-consuming as described in Box 6.5.

The scoping review will produce information on the types of studies that have been published on participation, which can be used to decide upon the type of systematic review that can be conducted. As of 2009, 14 different systematic review types had been identified (Grant and Booth 2009), and the number continues to rise. As studies exploring participation in health research are relatively new, it is likely that the most appropriate review types will involve (a) mapping, where an overview is presented and research gaps are identified; (b) qualitative reviewing where constructs and themes are identified illustrating the contribution of participation to health research; or (c) mixed methods reviews that combine learning from both process and outcomes studies to relate participation and intervention.

Deciding Which Studies to Include in Reviews of Participation

When explaining the relative impact of participation, issues of reporting, quality and relevance need to be addressed. Reporting refers to whether the process of participation contains enough detail to enable reviewers to make decisions about impact. Reviewers can construct a list of 'inclusion questions' such as those listed in Box 6.6.

> **Box 6.6 Judging Whether Participation Has Been Adequately Reported**
> - Are the aims of the participatory approach described? How is participation expected to contribute to impact?
> - Is there a description of the types of people that were included (patients, service users, members of health interest groups, other communities of identity or place, health practitioners, other relevant practitioners, managers and policymakers)?
> - Does the paper explain why the participation of these particular stakeholders was considered important?
> - How people were included – how were they invited to take part and what was done to help them feel included?
> - How was a collective process of learning fostered? What enabled people to participate?
> - What did people contribute to the design and conduct of the research?
> - How did their input contribute to the design and implementation of the research? For example, were recruitment methods informed by participant norms for what would be appropriate and acceptable? Were outcomes collaboratively constructed rather than externally driven?
> - How did people collaborate/work together?
> - How were their contributions used to make decisions about the research process?

Decisions about excluding on the basis of thin reporting are difficult, because many primary studies contain little information on process. Review authors have noted that information on the characteristics of partnerships and coalitions is often missing or inadequate, making it difficult to explain underlying mechanisms that promote health (Anderson et al. 2012). Few primary studies describe whether or how space is created for relationship building, deliberation and dialogue and knowledge co-creation although descriptions of the process are key to understanding whether the process fostered inclusivity and involvement. O'Mara-Eves et al. (2013) found that explaining effectiveness was difficult because experimental and process evaluations provided only partial descriptions of structure and process. A conceptual model of PHR developed by Lucero et al. (2016) presents how group dynamics and partnership formation are influenced by and interact with local contexts, which in turn influences development of the intervention and appropriateness of the research. But without information on organisational contexts, political environments and prevailing priorities, it becomes impossible to identify what influences the process and outcomes of interventions and initiatives using participatory approaches.

Because we know that reporting of participation is thin, relevance of information becomes very important. Relevance quite simply means that the information contained in a paper makes an important contribution to answering the review questions. Papers may contain important 'nuggets' of information explaining the effect of participation, identified after much sifting. When these nuggets are located, decisions need to be made about whether to include papers that have relevant information even if the overall study is of poor quality (Heyvaert et al. 2013).

Judgements on the value of 'nuggets' can be made through the use of logic models. A logic model is a graphic representation of the structure and/or the process of an intervention or service (Funnell and Rogers 2011). They can be used to engage stakeholders at an early stage in describing how participation contributes to the design, implementation and effects of health research in theory. The initial searches are then used to further populate the model. When information is lacking, additional searches can be used as well as contact with stakeholders to find relevant information.

Appraisal of quality for different types of studies usually asks whether the research was conducted in an ethical manner and whether it is relevant to practice or policy, the clarity of reporting, the coherence of the findings and the appropriateness and rigour of the methods (Cohen and Crabtree 2008). The appraisal process acts as a filter, supporting decisions to exclude studies of poor methodological quality. Filtering is useful when a large number of studies – perhaps too many for the review – have been identified. Filtering also removes poor-quality studies that may not enable decisions about whether the contribution of PHR to impact was a true effect (Viswanathan et al. 2004).

Issues of thin reporting, relevance and quality may be addressed through the use of cluster searching. Cluster searching is a method where all documents related to a particular project are located in order to trace pathways to impact (Booth et al. 2013). As noted by some reviewers, relationships between participation and health outcomes may be reported separately (Viswanathan et al. 2004); in some cases the relationships are reported long after the original study as they are considered of lesser interest (Adams et al. 2012); and there are few opportunities to report on proximal, intermediate and distal outcomes in a single article because funding is often limited to evaluating short-term outcomes (Roussos and Fawcett 2000). In PHR, a number of articles may be produced as a result of long-term partnerships that continue despite variations in research funding (Jagosh et al. 2015). Cluster searching maximises the opportunities to represent impact from a single initiative or multiple initiatives emerging from the partnership, over time.

Developing a Preliminary Theory for Impact

If it is possible to cluster papers on process, outcomes and impact, a rich picture can be produced tracing the pathway from participation to impact (Harris et al. 2015a, b).

Table 6.3 An a priori theoretical framework for participation in diabetes research

Propositions about involvement by stage of research
Priority setting: getting people to identify the most important issues and participate in setting priorities for research will increase interest in participating in codesign of the intervention. Deciding priorities without involvement leads to questions on the relevance of the research
Proposal writing: involving people in writing proposals for funding increases collective ownership for research projects. Involving people after proposals are written risks less ownership and may make people feel that they are not equal partners in the project
Intervention design: asking people to help with the design of the intervention produces more culturally acceptable interventions, more appropriate approaches to recruitment and more user-friendly information and tools. Excluding people from the design process may lead to project information that is difficult to understand, less cultural acceptance and lower recruitment rates
Implementation: involving people in (a) Recruitment produces high recruitment rates because they are able to help participants understand the relevance and benefits of the research (b) Delivering the intervention may increase trust and communication and foster relationships which lead to high retention rates and good levels of active participation (c) Data collection and analysis may produce additional insight into how and why an intervention works (or doesn't work)
Dissemination: involvement at any stage (a) promotes understanding of the aims and benefits of the research, creates local ownership and likelihood that a local network is created to share what is learned and (b) helps to ensure that findings is relevant and understandable

In both primary studies and systematic reviews, a preliminary conceptual map of how participation works can be developed using existing research and stakeholder experiences. A theoretical or conceptual framework can be developed that proposes general relationships between participation and impact (see, e.g. Khodyakov et al. 2011). Alternatively, a logic model can be developed which illustrates the relationships between participation, research design, implementation and outcomes for specific populations in a given context (Allmark et al. 2013; Anderson et al. 2011; Baxter et al. 2010, 2014). Reviewers can develop their own model or use a pre-existing framework such as the CBPR conceptual model (Lucero et al. 2016; Oetzel and Minkler 2017).

For example, in our review of patient and wider community involvement in diabetes (Harris et al. submitted), we proposed that participation at different stages of the project could enhance the processes of clarifying problems related to diabetes, setting priorities for the research, designing the intervention, recruiting participants, collecting and analysing data and disseminating learning (Table 6.3).

Frameworks and models can be used a priori to ensure that the search strategy explicitly looks for key concepts. They can also be used during the review to iteratively develop explanations for how participation works (Kneale et al. 2015; Rowher et al. 2016).

Judging Quality and Relevance

When deciding which studies ought to be included in a review, concerns related to the quality of the primary research need to be addressed. Appraisal of quality generally asks whether the research was conducted in an ethical manner and whether it is relevant to practice or policy, the clarity of reporting, the coherence of the findings and the appropriateness and rigour of the methods (Cohen and Crabtree 2008). Filtering removes poor-quality studies that may not enable decisions about the effectiveness of participatory research. Reviews that include studies with experimental or quasi-experimental research designs assessing the effectiveness of participation may use critical appraisal tools that are appropriate in the specific study design to assess methodological rigour.

Whereas the review question wants to know how and why something works, however, qualitative studies or studies with descriptive elements may be included on the grounds of relevance because they contribute to developing the explanation. In this instance, the appraisal process is used to make judgements about relevance. Studies containing 'nuggets' of relevant explanation are included, rather than just including studies based on assessment of overall methodological quality (Heyvaert et al. 2013).

Synthesising Information on the Impact of Participation

Synthesis is dependent upon the amount of information available on the process and impact of participation, as well as whether there is a thick description of the process. As a general rule of thumb:

- *If* there is adequate reporting of the process of participation
- *And* local context is detailed enough to assess comparability across studies
- *And* studies have evaluated using similar time periods
- *Then* synthesis could be done to explore impact of participation

Impact can be conceptualised for individuals, groups, organisations, partnerships or systems over different periods of time. Documenting the interaction between participation and health impact remains a major challenge. O'Mara-Eves et al. (2013) found that 'there is no clear evidence of the causal pathway between community engagement, improvements in social capital/cohesion and improvements in health outcomes (mortality, morbidity, health behaviours)' (2013, p. 75). Causal pathways too are difficult to establish because health outcomes are usually conceptualised as the product of a distinct intervention, but interventions need to be conceptualised as social processes in a wider community system (Trickett et al. 2011; Hawe et al. 2009). Changes in processes and relationships should be considered as outcomes in themselves, because they have short-term and intermediate impacts that lead to achieving better health.

As a first step, reviewers need to take the reporting of impact as the compass for deciding how to conduct the synthesis. Data for impact can be organised according to whether it answers the following questions – which are closely related to the elements of impact in our earlier definition:

1. Did participation in setting priorities for research have an impact on the research questions?
2. Were local experiences, knowledge, culture, norms and practices incorporated into the research design and plans for the conduct of the research?
3. Did changes in relationships and group dynamics impact on priority setting, design and/or conduct of the research?

These impact questions link wider processes between researchers and local people to the research that will be conducted. If this process is successful, then a second set of impact questions can be asked, which concern the effect on individuals receiving or delivering the intervention:

4. Did the process have impact on individual capacity to make decisions about lifestyle, environment and wellbeing?
5. Did the process improve the lives of those involved in the design, conduct, analysis, dissemination of the research and/or evaluation of the research process?

Finally, questions can be asked at the systems level, which may focus on whether both participation in research design and conduct and individual impact:

6. Influenced improvement in health, reduced disparities and increased social justice
7. Produced structural changes, traditional structures, practices, cultures, power relations and policies

The questions that can be asked will depend on the information available, but the main point here is to illustrate that impact focuses on drawing relationships between processes of participation at different stages over the short or longer term.

Summary

This chapter has introduced methods that can be used or adapted to synthesise evidence on the impact of participation in health research. As methods continue to be developed, however, it is likely that it will need to be updated or supplemented with methodological articles. For the present, we can conclude based on our experiences that researchers need to consider whether and how participation could affect the research. Ideally, this starts by framing the problem to be researched, but when that is not possible, then participation issues need consideration at the design stage. More description is needed of how the participatory process contributes to the design of studies, their implementation and the process of generating research knowledge. Primary research often contains inadequate descriptions of participation. Researchers could develop a priori logic models or theories that conceptualise how participation may affect the intervention and include evaluation of the process alongside findings. Authors could consider ways to provide more information about context, relationships and participatory processes, by (a) integrating the information within the article, (b) publishing as a separate methods article or (c) providing material supplementary to the publication.

When conducting a review of participatory health research, reviewers should consider:

- Contextual issues (e.g. SES, salience of the health issue to the community, history of collaboration among stakeholders) and how these shape participation, relationships, research design and intervention choices
- The theoretical and conceptual mechanisms through which participation impacts interventions and outcomes, presenting these as a theoretical framework or logic model where possible

Reviews should start with an explicit definition of participation. While this is good practice for all reviews, the definition needs to describe whether:

- Different levels and types of participation will be considered.
- Non-health outcomes will be included.
- Outcomes will include proximal, intermediate and distal outcomes.
- Projects at different stages will be included.
- How different cultural and system contexts will be dealt with.
- How degree of alignment between the intervention and the context will be assessed.
- The length and process of collaboration can be included as a criterion for selecting and extracting data from primary studies.

When deciding what studies to include in the review, reviewers need to ask:

- Does the primary research actually meet the definition for real participation (conceptual security)?
- Is the amount of information on context, development of partnerships and relationships between partnership processes and context adequately reported?
- Can strategies that compensate for thin description be used, such as:
  - Identifying all papers related to a specific project (cluster searching)?
  - Contacting authors and/or conducting interviews with participants?
  - Including participants in the process of systematic review (participatory review)?
- Should primary research, that is, of poor quality, be included when it meets criteria for relevance, e.g. important information contributing to explanations of impact?

Reviewers need to ask whether differences between studies by cultural context, health or political system, partnership processes, type of population, intervention or outcome warrant the analysis of impact by splitting papers into subgroups and conducting subgroup analysis. Further, when considering subgroup analysis, decisions need to be made about whether to split papers by their participatory stance, with the assumption that projects with utilitarian aims may actually represent very different forms of participation than those that have aims of empowerment.

The use of a framework to categorise and judge the quality of participation could be considered, although none of the current frameworks have been used for a systematic review.

Last but not the least, studies need to be viewed using a relational lens, examining processes of participation, how these processes foster relationships and how relationships may lead to positive outcomes that reflect changes in community conditions, policies and services, alongside health outcomes.

References

Adams, A. K., LaRowe, T. L., Cronin, K. A., Prince, R. J., Wubben, D. P., Parker, T., & Jobe, J. B. (2012). The Healthy Children, Strong Families intervention: design and community participation. The journal of primary prevention, 33(4), 175–185.

Allmark, P., Baxter, S., Goyder, E., Guillaume, L., & Crofton-Martin, G. (2013). Assessing the health benefits of advice services: Using research evidence and logic model methods to explore complex pathways. *Health & Social Care in the Community, 21*(1), 59–68.

Anderson, L. M., Petticrew, M., Rehfuess, E., Armstrong, R., Ueffing, E., Baker, P., Francis, D., & Tugwell, P. (2011). Using logic models to capture complexity in systematic reviews. *Research Synthesis Methods, 2*(1), 33–42.

Anderson LM, Adeney KL, Shinn C, Krause LK, Safranek S. (2012). Community coalition-driven interventions to reduce health disparities among racial and ethnic minority populations (Protocol). Cochrane Database of Systematic Reviews. Issue 6. Art. No.: CD009905. https://doi.org/10.1002/14651858.CD009905.

Andreae, S. J., Halanych, J. H., Cherrington, A., & Safford, M. M. (2012). Recruitment of a rural, southern, predominantly African-American population into a diabetes self-management trial. *Contemporary Clinical Trials, 33*(3), 499–506.

Arnstein, S. R. (1969). A ladder of citizen participation. *Journal of the American Institute of Planners, 35*(4), 216–224.

Barreto, J. M. (2014). Epistemologies of the South and human rights: Santos and the quest for global and cognitive justice. *Indiana Journal of Global Legal Studies, 21*(2), 395–422.

Baxter, S., Killoran, A., Kelly, M. P., & Goyder, E. (2010). Synthesizing diverse evidence: The use of primary qualitative data analysis methods and logic models in public health reviews. *Public Health, 124*(2), 99–106.

Baxter, S. K., Blank, L., Woods, H. B., Payne, N., Rimmer, M., & Goyder, E. (2014). Using logic model methods in systematic review synthesis: Describing complex pathways in referral management interventions. *BMC Medical Research Methodology, 14*(1), 62.

Beresford, P. (2013). Theory and practice of user involvement in research: Making the connection with public policy and practice. In Involving service users in health and social care research (pp. 15–26). London: Routledge.

Booth, A., Harris, J., Croot, E., Springett, J., Campbell, F., & Wilkins, E. (2013). Towards a methodology for cluster searching to provide conceptual and contextual "richness" for systematic reviews of complex interventions: Case study (CLUSTER). *BMC Medical Research Methodology, 13*(1), 118.

Booth, A. (2006). Clear and present questions: Formulating questions for evidence based practice. *Library Hi Tech, 24*(3), 355–368.

Cargo, M., Stankov, I., Thomas, J., Saini, M., Rogers, P., Mayo-Wilson, E., & Hannes, K. (2015). Development, inter-rater reliability and feasibility of a checklist to assess implementation (Ch-IMP) in systematic reviews: the case of provider-based prevention and treatment programs targeting children and youth. *BMC medical research methodology, 15*(1), 73.

Chesla, C. A., Chun, K. M., Kwan, C. M., Mullan, J. T., Kwong, Y., Hsu, L., Huang, P., Strycker, L. A., Shum, T., To, D., & Kao, R. (2013). Testing the efficacy of culturally adapted coping skills training for Chinese American immigrants with type 2 diabetes using community-based participatory research. *Research in Nursing & Health, 36*(4), 359–372.

Cook, T. (2012). Where participatory approaches meet pragmatism in funded (health) research: The challenge of finding meaningful spaces. In *Forum Qualitative Sozialforschung/Forum: Qualitative Social Research, 13*(1).

Cohen, D. J., & Crabtree, B. F. (2008). Evaluative criteria for qualitative research in health care: Controversies and recommendations. *The Annals of Family Medicine, 6*(4), 331–339.

Cornwall, A. (2008). Unpacking 'participation': Models, meanings and practices. *Community Development Journal, 43*(3), 269–283.

Daivadanam, M., Wahlstrom, R., Ravindran, T. S., Sarma, P. S., Sivasankaran, S., & Thankappan, K. R. (2013). Design and methodology of a community-based cluster-randomized controlled trial for dietary behaviour change in rural Kerala. *Global Health Action, 6*(1), 20993.

Funnell, S. C., & Rogers, P. J. (2011). *Purposeful program theory: Effective use of theories of change and logic models* (Vol. 31). Hoboken: Wiley.

Grant, M. J., & Booth, A. (2009). A typology of reviews: An analysis of 14 review types and associated methodologies. *Health Information & Libraries Journal, 26*(2), 91–108.

Heyvaert, M., Hannes, K., Maes, B., & Onghena, P. (2013). Critical appraisal of mixed methods studies. *Journal of Mixed Methods Research, 7*(4), 302–327.

Harris, J., Cook, T., Gibbs, L., Oetzel, J., Salsbury, J., & Shinn, C. (2018). Searching for the Impact of Participation in Health and Health Research: Challenges and Methods. BioMed Research International. https://doi.org/10.1155/2018/9427452/.

Harris, J., Croot, L., Thompson, J., & Springett, J. (2016). How stakeholder participation can contribute to systematic reviews of complex interventions. *Journal of Epidemiology and Community Health, 70*(2), 207. https://doi.org/10.1136/jech-2015-205701.

Harris, J., Graue, M., Dunning, T., Haltbakk, J., Austrheim, G., Skille, N., Rokne, B., & Kirkevold, M. (2015a). Involving people with diabetes and the wider community in diabetes research: A realist review protocol. *Systematic Reviews, 4*(1), 146.

Harris, J., Graue, M., Dunning, T., Haltbakk, J., Kirkevold, M., & Austrheim, G (submitted). How patient and community involvement in diabetes research influences health outcomes: A realist review.

Harris, J., Springett, J., Booth, A., Campbell, F., Thompson, J., Goyder, E., Van Cleemput, P., Wilkins, E., & Yang, Y. (2015b). Can community-based peer support promote health literacy and reduce inequalities? A realist review. *Journal of Public Health Research, 3*(3).

Hasnain-Wynia, R. (2003). Overview of the community care network demonstration program and its evaluation. *Medical Care Research and Review, 60*(4_suppl), 5S–16S.

Hawe, P., Shiell, A., & Riley, T. (2009). Theorising interventions as events in systems. *American Journal of Community Psychology, 43*(3–4), 267–276.

International Collaboration for Participatory Health Research (ICPHR). (2018). *Position paper 3: What is impact in participatory health research?* Berlin: International Collaboration for Participatory Health Research.

International Collaboration for Participatory Health Research (ICPHR). (2013). *Position paper 1: What is participatory health research? Version: May 2013*. Berlin: International Collaboration for Participatory Health Research.

Jagosh, J., Bush, P. L., Salsberg, J., Macaulay, A. C., Greenhalgh, T., Wong, G., Cargo, M., Green, L. W., Herbert, C. P., & Pluye, P. (2015). A realist evaluation of community-based participatory research: Partnership synergy, trust building and related ripple effects. *BMC Public Health, 15*(1), 725.

Joanna Briggs Institute. (2015). *Methodology for JBI scoping reviews, Joanna Briggs Institute Reviewers' Manual*. University of Adelaide, Adelaide, Australia.

Khodyakov, D., Stockdale, S., Jones, F., Ohito, E., Jones, A., Lizaola, E., & Mango, J. (2011). An exploration of the effect of community engagement in research on perceived outcomes of partnered mental health services projects. *Society and Mental Health, 1*(3), 185–199.

Kneale, D., Thomas, J., & Harris, K. (2015). Developing and optimising the use of logic models in systematic reviews: Exploring practice and good practice in the use of programme theory in reviews. *PLoS One, 10*(11), e0142187.

Liu, J. J., Davidson, E., Bhopal, R. S., White, M., Johnson, M. R. D., Netto, G., Deverill, M., & Sheikh, A. (2012). Adapting health promotion interventions to meet the needs of ethnic minority groups: Mixed-methods evidence synthesis. *Health Technology Assessment (Winchester, England), 16*(44), 1.

Lucero, J., Wallerstein, N., Duran, B., Alegria, M., Greene-Moton, E., Israel, B., Kastelic, S., Magarati, M., Oetzel, J., Pearson, C., & Schulz, A. (2016). Development of a mixed methods investigation of process and outcomes of community-based participatory research. *Journal of Mixed Methods Research*, 1558689816633309.

Macaulay, A. C., Paradis, G., Potvin, L., Cross, E. J., Saad-Haddad, C., McComber, A., Desrosiers, S., Kirby, R., Montour, L. T., Lamping, D. L., & Leduc, N. (1997). The Kahnawake schools diabetes prevention project: Intervention, evaluation, and baseline results of a diabetes primary prevention program with a native community in Canada. *Preventive Medicine, 26*(6), 779–790.

Milton, B., Attree, P., French, B., Povall, S., Whitehead, M., & Popay, J. (2011). The impact of community engagement on health and social outcomes: A systematic review. *Community Development Journal, 47*(3), 316–334.

Oetzel, J. G., & Minkler, M. (2017). Community-based participatory research for health: advancing social and health equity. John Wiley & Sons.

Oetzel, J. G., Zhou, C., Duran, B., Pearson, C., Magarati, M., Lucero, J., Wallerstein, N., & Villegas, M. (2015). Establishing the psychometric properties of constructs in a community-based participatory research conceptual model. *American Journal of Health Promotion, 29*(5), e188–e202.

Oliver, K., Rees, R., Brady, L. M., Kavanagh, J., Oliver, S., & Thomas, J. (2015). Broadening public participation in systematic reviews: A case example involving young people in two configurative reviews. *Research Synthesis Methods, 6*(2), 206–217.

O'Mara-Eves, A., Brunton, G., McDaid, G., Oliver, S., Kavanagh, J., Jamal, F., ... & Thomas, J. (2013). Community engagement to reduce inequalities in health: a systematic review, meta-analysis and economic analysis. Public Health Research, 1(4).

O'Mara-Eves, A., Brunton, G., Oliver, S., Kavanagh, J., Jamal, F., & Thomas, J. (2015). The effectiveness of community engagement in public health interventions for disadvantaged groups: A meta-analysis. *BMC Public Health, 15*(1), 129.

Pearson, A., Wiechula, R., Court, A., & Lockwood, C. (2005). The JBI model of evidence-based healthcare. *International Journal of Evidence-Based Healthcare, 3*(8), 207–215.

Pearson, M., Brand, S. L., Quinn, C., Shaw, J., Maguire, M., Michie, S., Briscoe, S., Lennox, C., Stirzaker, A., Kirkpatrick, T., & Byng, R. (2015). Using realist review to inform intervention development: Methodological illustration and conceptual platform for collaborative care in offender mental health. *Implementation Science, 10*(1), 134.

Phipps, D., Pepler, D., Craig, W., Cummings, J., & Cardinal, S. (2016). The co-produced pathway to impact describes knowledge mobilization processes. *Journal of Community Engagement and Scholarship, 9*, 31.

Richardson, W. S., Wilson, M. C., Nishikawa, J., & Hayward, R. S. (1995). The well-built clinical question: A key to evidence-based decisions. *ACP Journal Club, 123*(3), A12–A12.

Rifkin, S. B. (2014). Examining the links between community participation and health outcomes: A review of the literature. *Health Policy and Planning, 29*(suppl_2), ii98–ii106.

Roussos, S. T., & Fawcett, S. B. (2000). A review of collaborative partnerships as a strategy for improving community health. *Annual Review of Public Health, 21*(1), 369–402.

Rowher, A., Booth, A., Pfadenhauer, L., Brereton, L., Gerdhardus, J., Mozygemba, K., Oortwijn, W., Tummers, M., van der Wilt, G. J., & Rehfuess, E. (2016). Guidance on the use of logic models in health technology assessments of complex interventions. *International Journal of Technology Assessment in Health Care.*

Sandelowski, M., Barroso, J., & Voils, C. I. (2007). Using qualitative metasummary to synthesize qualitative and quantitative descriptive findings. *Research in Nursing & Health, 30*(1), 99–111.

Shaw, R.L. (2010). Conducting literature reviews. In M. Forrester (Ed.) Doing qualitative research in psychology: A practical guide (pp.39–52). London: Sage.

Shippee, N. D., Domecq Garces, J. P., Prutsky Lopez, G. J., Wang, Z., Elraiyah, T. A., Nabhan, M., Brito, J. P., Boehmer, K., Hasan, R., Firwana, B., & Erwin, P. J. (2015). Patient and service user engagement in research: A systematic review and synthesized framework. *Health Expectations, 18*(5), 1151–1166.

Trickett, E. J., Beehler, S., Deutsch, C., Green, L. W., Hawe, P., McLeroy, K., Miller, R. L., Rapkin, B. D., Schensul, J. J., Schulz, A. J., & Trimble, J. E. (2011). Advancing the science of community-level interventions. *American Journal of Public Health, 101*(8), 1410–1419.

Trickett, E. J., Trimble, J. E., & Allen, J. (2014). Most of the story is missing: Advocating for a more complete intervention story. American journal of community psychology, 54(1–2), 180–186.

Van de Ven, A. H. (2007). *Engaged scholarship: A guide for organizational and social research.* Oxford: Oxford University Press on Demand.

Viswanathan, M., Ammerman, A., Eng, E., Gartlehner, G., Lohr, K. N., Griffth, D., et al. (2004). *Community-based participatory research: Assessing the evidence, Evidence Report/Technology Assessment No. 99; Prepared by RTI International-University of North Carolina.* Rockville: Agency for Healthcare Research and Quality.

Wallerstein, N. (1992). Powerlessness, empowerment, and health: Implications for health promotion programs. *American Journal of Health Promotion, 6*(3), 197–205.

Wallerstein, N., & Duran, B. (2010). CBPR contributions to intervention research: The interaction of science and practice to improve health equity. *American Journal Public Health S1, 100,* 540–546.

Weick, K. E. (1995). *Sensemaking in organizations.* Thousand Oaks: Sage.

Wong, G., Greenhalgh, T., Westhorp, G., Buckingham, J., & Pawson, R. (2013). RAMESES publication standards: Realist syntheses. *BMC Medicine, 11*(1), 21.

Chapter 7
Kids in Action: Participatory Health Research with Children

Lisa Gibbs, Katitza Marinkovic, Alison L. Black, Brenda Gladstone, Christine Dedding, Ann Dadich, Siobhan O'Higgins, Tineke Abma, Marilyn Casley, Jennifer Cartmel, and Lalatendu Acharya

Fig. 7.1 Kids in Action logo

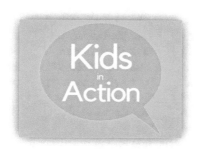

L. Gibbs (✉) · K. Marinkovic
University of Melbourne, Melbourne, Australia
e-mail: lgibbs@unimelb.edu.au; katitza.marinkovic@unimelb.edu.au

A. L. Black
University of the Sunshine Coast, Sippy Downs, Australia
e-mail: ablack1@usc.edu.au

B. Gladstone
University of Toronto, Toronto, Canada
e-mail: brenda.gladstone@utoronta.ca

C. Dedding · T. Abma
VU University Medical Centre, Amsterdam, The Netherlands
e-mail: c.dedding@vu.nl; t.abma@vumc.nl

A. Dadich
Western Sydney University, Parramatta, Australia
e-mail: A.Dadich@uwesternsydney.edu.au

S. O'Higgins
National University of Ireland, Galway, Ireland
e-mail: Siobhan.ohiggins@nuigalway.ie

M. Casley · J. Cartmel
Griffith University, Logan, Australia
e-mail: m.casley@griffith.edu.au; j.cartmel@griffith.edu.au

L. Acharya
Purdue University, West Lafayette, IN, USA

© Springer International Publishing AG, part of Springer Nature 2018
M. T. Wright, K. Kongats (eds.), *Participatory Health Research*,
https://doi.org/10.1007/978-3-319-92177-8_7

Introduction

Participatory health research (PHR) is a particularly useful way to understand the health and well-being of children. It does this by providing children with opportunities to show their unique point of view and competencies and to use their perspectives and experiences to shape research topics and methods, and the interpretation and reporting of findings. This chapter presents some of the principles, processes, and ethical debates about PHR with children to promote discussion and encourage good practice. Photos, examples, and quotes from the authors as PHR adult researchers and from child researchers are embedded throughout to illuminate the issues. A cartoon image is used to signify child quotes (Fig. 7.2).

PHR as an approach has been defined earlier in this book (see Chap. 1). Despite the reported value of PHR, much of the literature describes its use with adult consumers, neglecting its use with children (Veale 2005; van Staa et al. 2010; Salmon et al. 2010; Ramsden et al. 2015). In some cases, reports of PHR aiming to improve children's health appear to involve advocates for and representatives of children, rather than the children themselves (Israel et al. 2005). This bias toward adult participants is problematic for at least two reasons. First, it suggests that PHR with children might be less relevant, less important, difficult, or inappropriate; second, it offers limited guidance to those with an interest in involving children in research to address child and youth health issues.

The limited literature on PHR with children reports positive benefits for the children involved, including empowerment, healthy development and well-being, social skills, self-esteem, and citizenship (Cargo et al. 2004; Foster-Fishman et al. 2005; Wong et al. 2010; Wallerstein et al. 2002). PHR with children can also be a positive experience for the adults involved and for the social and community context of the research (Kellett 2010b). Although there is guidance on good practice in PHR with children, some of which is explored in this chapter, it is an anomaly that in seeking to define and promote child participation in research, we inevitably place it within an adult-centric structure (Malone and Hartung 2010). In this sense, authors like

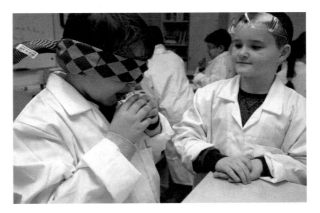

Fig. 7.2 The KLIK project in the Netherlands (see Case Study 2), where the children researched differences in taste between cooked and raw and warm and cold foods

Lesley-Anne Gallacher and Michael Gallagher (2008) warned that "the very notion of having an agenda to which everyone would adhere… is itself a participatory norm based on (adult) democratic ideals" (p. 507). This would mean that children's participation in the setting is still defined and understood from an adult perspective, and what does not fit into those categories might be labeled as subversive behavior (Gallacher and Gallagher 2008).

In response to current gaps in the literature, the Kids in Action Network was established in 2016 to increase the profile of PHR with children under the age of 14 years, offer projects increased support and credibility through membership in an international collaboration, and provide a platform for shared learning and the development of PHR methods with children (http://www.icphr.org/kids-in-action.html). Members meet regularly by teleconference to share strategies and useful references and co-generate publications and resources to promote good practice in PHR with children. Additionally, members have individually established strategic alliances and collaborations with organizations that can help to achieve this aim, such as television networks, educational organizations, and health services. In doing this, the aim of the Kids in Action Network is to promote and uphold children's right to speak out and be heard and to have their views considered in decision-making, particularly in the context of research relating to their health and well-being.

What Do We Mean by "Children"?

The definitions of childhood are diverse and are influenced by many factors including cultural, historical, economic, and legal aspects. This diversity means we should not refer to one universal "childhood," but rather, multiple childhoods. In this sense, PHR aims to give voice to children, particularly those who are marginalized due to ethnicity, socioeconomic status, gender, culture, disability, mental health issues, drug use, and other reasons:

> Power-sharing requires a view that children – despite age, ability, mental health, and levels of maturity and understanding – have something important to teach adults and that children should be allowed to express themselves according to their needs, age, ability, mental health, and levels of maturity and understanding. (Liegghio et al. 2010)

Terminology for older children, including youth, adolescents, young people, students, and juveniles, is also contested. These terms can be problematic for different reasons – they are imprecise; they can be politically laden; and they might also be unpopular among and rejected by the individuals they refer to. In this chapter, the term "children" represents an inclusive term to refer to people 18 years of age and under, as per the United Nations Convention on the Rights of the Child (1989). In response to the challenges presented by use of any specific terminology, the Kids in Action Network has agreed that, rather than having a set of universal terms, the terminology will be negotiated in each future study with the child researchers involved.

Why Do PHR with Children?

PHR with children is a rights-based approach, consistent with the United Nations Convention on the Rights of the Child (Lundy and McEvoy 2012a). PHR provides safe spaces for children's expression and participation. It accommodates different levels of communication skills and acknowledges children as capable social actors who have their own views and agency. It creates conditions for children's empowerment, encouraging their contributions to issues that are relevant to them and their community (Kellett 2010a). In this sense, PHR with children can impact children's lives at personal, familial, communal, and institutional levels and can influence global issues (Hart et al. 2004). Plan International, a development and humanitarian organization that advances children's rights, has demonstrated children's capacity to contribute in post-disaster contexts. After landslides in the Philippines, Plan International involved children and young people in risk-mapping and risk-reduction activities (Ray 2010). One of the child contributors noted:

> Being a student survivor, I have my responsibility to get involved with this. We lost our loved ones and we have to honour and treasure the memories.

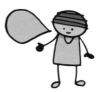

Case study 1 provides an example of a participatory research study that introduced children to local industry. Although not specific to health, it demonstrates how participatory research can provide children with opportunities to present their research to an adult audience and, in doing so, have an impact beyond the individual participants.

Case Study 1
A research project in the mining town of Gladstone in Queensland, Australia, focused on listening to children's views of place and industries in their local environment. The children's representations of Gladstone were publicly displayed in a local gallery alongside the work of a local artist, Margaret Worthington. Margaret had worked as an artist in residence with the children. The children's creative works were displayed with Margaret's work as part of an interactive installation where visitors could engage with children's ideas. It furthered community thinking about children's competencies as meaning makers.

Observing the project and standing among the activity of it – engagement and multiple interactions and conversations – the adult researchers and other stakeholders were encouraged to examine their own responses and taken-for-

(continued)

Case Study 1   (continued)

granted "ways of seeing" children. Initially, they had different perspectives about children and their capabilities. When considering options for the art gallery and the installation, art gallery staff were hesitant about having interactive activities for young children in the same space as "artists' art." During the project, their doubts about children's capabilities and engagement gradually subsided, and they became open to new ideas. In the end, the gallery staff chose to display some of the documentation of the research process in the exhibition. When children's representations and voices were made visible and shared with others, a profound respect for children as knowledgeable experiencers of their world was generated, and their positioning shifted. The public's response was so positive that gallery staff intend to create interactive spaces for children alongside upcoming and future exhibitions.

Many of the child researchers attended the gallery on the night of the exhibition. They moved throughout the gallery, viewing the exhibition and interacting with people. We observed these children stopping and talking to Margaret as a fellow artist. One of the children, Mitchell, was heard saying, "I like working with Margaret. She is a real artist." Mitchell highlights for us the importance of authentic relationships. The children knew that Margaret was a real artist who created paintings and sculpture, and because their ideas were privileged in the same way that Margaret's were, they positioned themselves as fellow artists who also created paintings and sculpture to represent their ideas and understandings.

Study conducted by co-author Ali Black, School of Education, University of the Sunshine Coast, Australia, with colleagues Black, Gillian Busch and Marion Hayes (2015).

Researching with children can offer rich opportunities for collaborative knowledge production and deepen understandings of their lifeworld (Sinclair 2004; Tizard and Hughes 2002). Having their perspectives and research valued by adults can increase their sense of empowerment and self-esteem. As reported by co-author Tineke Abma, one child researcher at a presentation for the KLIK project in the Netherlands (see Case study 2) said:

Wow, are we famous or something?
Are all these people here for us?

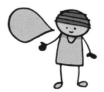

Deeper insights into children's views and experiences can also provide adults with a better understanding of current childhoods, rather than ideas tempered by their own memories of what it was like to be a child (O'Higgins and Nic Gabhainn 2010).

How Is PHR with Children Different from PHR with Adults?

The core principles of PHR, and indeed many of the techniques, are the same regardless of whether adults or children are involved. PHR recognizes participants as co-researchers, not just informants, and requires a shift in research strategies to achieve this. Models of PHR with children address the additional power imbalance between adults and children (Alderson 2001; Arnstein 1969; Charles and DeMaio 1993; Feingold 1976; Hart et al. 2008; Shier 2001; Treseder 1997; Wong et al. 2010; Woodhead 2010). Notions of participation that are hierarchical and that set an ideal of no adult involvement have been critiqued (Shier 2001). In practice, different types and levels of participation are usually observed, even within the same study, depending on the topic and situation (Wong et al. 2010). This includes varying levels of child contribution to decision-making throughout the research process – from study design to problem definition, data collection, analysis, dissemination, and completing related action steps. A new participatory analytical tool developed by Harry Shier helps adult researchers to plan, define, and report these multistage arrangements (Shier forthcoming).

Instead of expecting children to function as adults, research methods that are fun and interesting for children are likely to facilitate creative, meaningful, and enjoyable participation. Accordingly, research methods should be adapted to children instead of the other way around. Multiple methods are likely to accommodate different preferences for communication and expression (Darbyshire et al. 2005). Using play as a research tool is a shift from adult-directed to child-directed research, by accepting play as an important part of children's everyday experiences. When play is recognized as the norm, children are empowered by having some control over the space they occupy with adults (Moss and Petrie 2002). Therefore, when adults' knowledge and acceptance of play is used in research with children, it becomes a means of building relationships and learning together, creating a sense of cohesion (Moss and Petrie 2002; Boddy 2011; Cameron 2013; Lester and Russell 2008).

Case Study 2

In the Netherlands, project KLIK (an acronym which translates into Children Learn Inventive Power) started in July 2015. In KLIK, photos help children to explore their lifestyle and their neighborhood. KLIK therefore stands for the click of the camera as well as for the click between the child and their environment. KLIK is a participatory action research project, which aims to improve the health and resilience of children living in a disadvantaged neighborhood. Ideas and plans are developed to promote the health of children through partnerships and the participation of children and other stakeholders within the neighborhood. Children's experiences form the basis of bottom-up health promotion, and photography is the common thread throughout the process. Bottom-up health promotion begins by exploring issues of concern to particular groups or individuals and regards some improvement in their overall power or capacity as the important health outcome.

Study conducted by co-author Tineke Abma, with colleagues Janine Schrijver and Femke Boelsma, VU University, Amsterdam.

The presumption that research, which prizes the perspectives and priorities of the "researched," will find practical application cannot be guaranteed (O'Higgins et al. 2010). Nevertheless, PHR has developed in such a way that, regardless of what the research achieves, the very act of participating in the research is likely to have been positive for the participants (ICPHR 2013). This is not to suggest that PHR is synonymous with, or guarantees a positive experience but rather, it optimizes the likelihood of meaningful engagement. This may involve an opportunity to work through difficult issues, respecting children's right to express and develop an understanding of their life experiences. In other studies, research methods that engender fun create a genuine desire to remain engaged for all those involved, so that PHR does not conclude with a sigh but with a roar of glee and a positive memory of the process.

Diverse methods can be used to enable children to generate research ideas and collect data (see Table 7.1). They include visual methods, such as mind maps, photos, and drawings; oral methods, including storytelling and interviewing; mobile methods, including tour guides; and arts-based methods, including role playing and puppetry. The options are almost endless – they simply require the use of a technique, like a game, that will help to stimulate and share ideas and then to identify potential solutions. Children are often easy to engage in play and creative methods because these forms of expression are important parts of their daily activities. Irish children highlighted that fun was an important part of what "makes and keeps them well" (Sixsmith et al. 2007). The detail presented in Table 7.1 is not exhaustive, nor are the suggested foci, techniques, or descriptions mutually exclusive – the table simply serves as a "platter" to whet the research appetite.

What Are Some of the Challenges?

The first challenge of PHR with children is to provide a space for children's real participation, while securing their other rights, especially protection. As advocates of children's agency, participatory adult researchers must enable all stakeholders (including community members) to understand and respond to children's voices and ideas (Black et al. 2015). However, the interdependency of children's rights, when operationalized, highlights the challenge of fulfilling them all without prioritizing one over others, lest they be compromised (Woodhead 2010; Lansdown 2010; Black and Busch 2016; Chakraborty et al. 2012). For instance, some authors have found that ethics committees will typically be wary of research involving children and err on the side of caution (Chakraborty et al. 2012); yet this might overlook children's right to participate. In case study 1, the adult researchers had to negotiate with the university ethics committee to override the standard ethics protocol to deidentify children's contributions and instead allow the children's work to be attributed to them in the art gallery (Black and Busch 2016). Thus, engagement with, and agreement from, research gatekeepers to involve children in research is paramount to allow children to be given a voice and be heard. This can be difficult if legal guardians assume child protection is synonymous with confidentiality and/or anonymity.

Table 7.1 Some useful techniques for PHR with children

Focus	Description	Techniques	Reference
Children's exploration of their space and environment	Children lead the exploration and representation of the spaces and environments relevant for them. The identification of important issues for children is carried out either by direct interaction with these spaces or by focusing on children's perspectives, ideas, and feelings about them	Mind maps, guided tours, mobile methods, mapping exercises	Block et al. (2017, 2014), Clark and Moss (2001), and Pascal and Bertram (2009)
Children's audio-visual and corporal expression	Children identify, explore, and express their own views, feelings, and ideas through the creation of or response to images, music, dance, among others. This can involve the exploration of their own bodies and sensibility	Art, collage, model making, child-led photography, music, dance, videoing	Barker and Weller (2003), Pascal and Bertram (2009), Burke (2005), Hart (1997), Lancaster and Broadbent (2010), Sinclair (2000), Greenfield (2004), and Schalkers et al. (2015)
Children's creation of spaces for citizenship	Children participate in spaces for citizenship that are like those currently used by adults in local, national, or international politics. Issues are presented and debated, and proposals for changes are made	Youth citizens' panels, management committees, advisory groups, youth forums	Franklin and Sloper (2006), Sinclair (2000), and Smith et al. (2002)
Children's development of narratives	Children use their creativity to identify narratives/stories through verbal or written language and/or recreating them using their own bodies and expression	Storytelling, drama work, puppetry, chronicled lifeline drawing, diaries, story writing	Malone and Hartung (2010), Sinclair (2000), Barker and Weller (2003), Clandinin and Connelly (2004), Lancaster and Broadbent (2010), and Ulvik and Gulbrandsen (2015)
Children's involvement in collective dialogue and meaning-making techniques	Children, as creators of meaning, explore their own perspectives, and those of others via reciprocal dialogue where concepts, beliefs, behaviors, assumptions, and identities, among others, are questioned. This process helps to build the relationships necessary for relational research, where children inquiry into their own lives, and how they can make a for difference for themselves, each other, and their community	Conversational groups, "symmetrical" and "reflexive" dialogues, ongoing group work, role plays, spider diagrams	Barker and Weller (2003), Clark and Moss (2001), Pascal and Bertram (2009), Sinclair (2000), Punch (2002b), and Cartmel and Casley (2014)
Children's involvement in traditional research techniques	Children, as part of a team of co-researchers, use tools and techniques from different fields and disciplines in (social) science to gather research data	Focus groups, questionnaires, interviews, peer-led research	Mutch and Gawith (2014) and Sinclair (2000)
Children's involvement in media and communication	Children experiment and express their views using mass media to reach out and validate their opinions to the wider community	Websites, print journalism, electronic publishing, radio production	Hart (1997), Sinclair (2000), Lancaster and Broadbent (2010), and Weller (2006)

It becomes further complicated when legal guardians are not present, which might require support from an independent third party. Kirrily Pells (2010) highlighted the difficulties for Rwandan orphans who have adult roles as the heads of their household and/or as carers of younger siblings, yet are still excluded from community decision-making (Pells 2010).

Role redefinition and power sharing in PHR require adult and child researchers to interpret and react to each other's behavior in a different way. This is part of an interactive meaning-making process, which unfolds over time in different spaces and between those occupying different social and generational positions (Gladstone 2015). In a participatory digital storytelling project with young Canadians, co-author Brenda Gladstone noted:

> In previous studies, I have been ambivalent about 'my role' and tried to avoid naming it; but the children in the group 'called me out' using humour, naming me, 'Seen but not Heard', which I think speaks to children's agency using means other than direct talk to challenge adults. (Berman and MacNevin 2017)

When invited to partake in PHR, children can choose to engage for a range of reasons. They might have a belief in the research aim, an aversion to schoolwork, and/or a preference for fun and enjoyment. Yet, despite an adult researcher's best intentions, children might perceive PHR as yet another adult-initiated, boring process (Greene and Hogan 2005) or assume they will not be listened to anyway and thus decide not to engage. These assumptions might be addressed through meaningful dialogue with children, inviting them to recognize the principles of PHR.

However, PHR is not for the fainthearted; giving children the power to make their own decisions can challenge the adult researcher. Influenced by conventional notions of the adult-child relationship, the adult researcher might assume child subversion of the participatory process, if children decline to participate (Gallacher and Gallagher 2008), change the focus of the discussion (Ozer et al. 2010), or question and challenge adult authority (Woodhead 2010). For instance, in a participatory study with children with diabetes conducted by co-author Christine Dedding and colleagues (2015), one child demonstrated their capacity to challenge adult assumptions about their health experiences:

It's my life;
my life doesn't look like that.

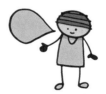

Similarly, in a study con-
ducted by co-author Siobhan O'Higgins and colleagues, children's proposals to improve their health at a primary school in Ireland demonstrated that they do not always agree with adults' ideas and plans for a study or even among themselves (Nic Gabhainn et al. 2010, see Fig. 7.3). All participants' comments were included in the schema created by the children to fully represent the ideas that had been

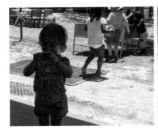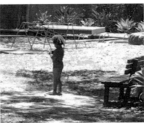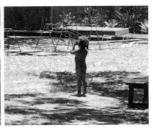

Fig. 7.3 These images show the involvement and enjoyment of very young children in taking photos to collect data. The children, aged between 15 months and 4 years, became adept at using the camera as part of a participatory research study of spaces in a child care center in Queensland, Australia. "I find it hard to describe the intensity of the children's participation; for me, the visual images give a stronger sense of the engagement" (Personal communication from researcher Jennifer Cartmel). In a related study, children in School Age Care were asked to take 15 photographs of play experiences that they felt were important (Bell 2013). From the outset, the exuberant use of the cameras by the children highlighted their intent for implicitly renegotiating the original parameters of the study (they took 675 photos including 53 of "out of bounds" and forbidden areas). The children in the study were enthusiastic participants who were unashamedly and openly willing to stretch the boundaries

debated and presented in previous workshops. Some ideas were explicitly labeled as "stupid" by the final group of children, probably against the adult researcher's wishes! These comments, though labeled as stupid by one group, were kept in all stages of the research and reported on; they too were treated respectfully by the researchers (Fig. 7.4).

Children's real participation means acknowledging their right to participate in the way they choose. Adult researchers often shy away from participatory research for fear of losing methodological control – yet, this willingness to let go and value child researchers' contributions from where they are at helps to ensure the process is truly participatory, and the data generated will be rich and meaningful for those involved.

Despite children's observable sense of agency, children in Western societies are generally under constant surveillance as parents and professionals work toward understanding children's needs and abilities (Mayall 2002). It appears that the meta-narratives about adult-child relationships hinder processes that enable children's participation. Therefore, it is important to examine how adult views of adulthood and childhood shape their ability to listen to children's perspectives and to conceptualize what needs to be disrupted in these dominant views. For example, in the Talking Circle project conducted by co-authors Jennifer Cartmel and Marilyn Casley (2014), an authentic dialogical process helped the adults to build relationships with children and lessen the power imbalance (Cartmel and Casley 2014):

> [University] students were continually telling me how amazed they were at how quickly they were able to build relationships with the children. Many of the students expressed difficulty they had in letting go of the power, as most felt they needed to take control of the group rather than letting things happen as the sessions unfolded. (University academic field-notes)

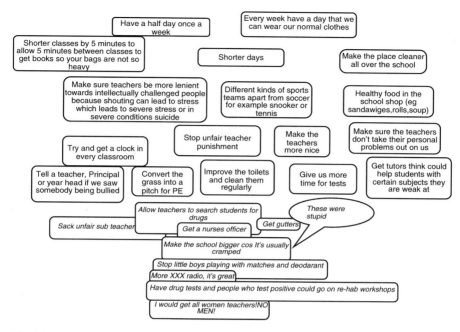

Fig. 7.4 Schema elaborated by sixth graders in Ireland about their peers' ideas for a healthier school

This allowed the adults to engage in deep learning about and with the children. The children eventually took ownership of the Talking Circle process, recognizing others' ideas and opinions. Furthermore, both the children and adults reported increased confidence and communication skills. Power can therefore be an instrument of both oppression and liberation. As noted by Michael Gallagher (2008), "Participatory techniques may provide interesting ways to intervene in games of power, but they do not provide a way to transcend such games" (p. 147). Adults involved in PHR with children must, therefore, reflect on their own expectations. If the aim is to enable children to shift from passive compliance to active citizenship, are the adults prepared to accommodate an additional shift for children to (further) develop as social agents, where they might critique the current systems (Westheimer and Kahne 2004)?

As an approach that focuses on the redefinition of roles and power asymmetries, PHR with children is intrinsically a relational process. This highlights the need for adult facilitators to develop skills for managing group dynamics. For instance, Samantha Punch (2002a) suggested that five is an ideal number of participants that provides enough flexibility and space for negotiation between adult and child researchers.

There also needs to be scope within and support from participating organizations, like schools, to accommodate potentially negative feedback from child researchers and/or respond to their suggestions for change (Ray 2010). The adult researcher, as a facilitator, has a responsibility to ensure there is support for PHR and its potential outcomes before it begins and to provide feedback and alternatives when children's proposals cannot be fulfilled to prevent frustration and disillusionment (Shier 2001). In some cases, it may be advisable to shift the PHR from restrictive environments that include disciplinary and instructive programs to more creative and responsive spaces. Mary Kellett (2010b) offered an example of a research study undertaken by an 11-year-old girl whose father had a disability. The girl recorded and reported on their experiences negotiating different forms of transport as they traveled around their city together in their daily lives. One of the adults supporting the child researcher arranged for her to present her findings to the UK Government's transport department, which responded by introducing a range of measures to increase the accessibility of buses in the public transport system. Similarly, in a study conducted by Kids in Action member Harry Shier (2015) and a team of child researchers in Yukul, Nicaragua, the children chose to conduct research on alcohol and associated violence in their community. They presented their work to their village, local government, and the national government's Family Life and Security Commission, which prioritized the issue for local action. Local police, national television networks, and local government supported the initiative, which resulted in reduced liquor licenses, shut down of unlicensed cantinas, and illegal liquor being confiscated. "Local government and party officials admitted they had been aware of the problem for years, but it wasn't until the children came forward with their research that they felt forced to act on it" (p212).

Given that PHR is shaped by its context, the models and standards for good practice when working with children must be flexible. They must have the elasticity to accommodate varied social (including familial) and cultural situations (Shier 2015; Porter et al. 2010; Maglajlic 2010), as well as the disparate organizational structures and climates of different institutions, such as schools (Kohfeldt et al. 2011; Ozer et al. 2010). These and other contextual elements might promote and/or diminish children's capacities to be active and creative throughout the whole process, and/or at particular stages. Children's roles within their families may generate practical challenges, such as conflicting values, limited time, and excessive burden. The threat of disrupting conventional power hierarchies might also threaten adults. However, even in bounded contexts where there are significant power constraints, children can still experience considerable empowerment and influence their environments (Ozer et al. 2013).

PHR with children operates within local protocols, including (but not limited to) legislation and the relevant human research ethics guidelines regarding consent and confidentiality. Recognizing the latter as guidelines, rather than directives, it can be helpful to understand how legislation might be operationalized within the context of a study. Consider, for instance, PHR to improve the well-being of young people with substance use issues. Initial challenges might include how these individuals might be invited to participate in such a study and whether the consent of parents or guardians is required. In New South Wales, Australia, legislation allows those over 14 years to legally consent to their own general medical or dental treatment (Redfern Legal Centre 2014) – this recognizes the personal agency and decision-making capacity of young people. Correspondingly, the National Statement on Ethical Conduct in Human Research states:

An ethical review body may approve research to which only the young person consents if it is satisfied that he or she is mature enough to understand and consent, and not vulnerable through immaturity in ways that would warrant additional consent from a parent or guardian. (NHMRC, ARC & AVCC 2014)

Yet, what of the young person with substance use issues who is yet to inform others of their substance use for fear of discipline or harm? Although the National Statement encourages consent to be obtained from both the child when appropriate and their parent or legal guardian, it also prizes "the child or young person's safety, emotional and psychological security, and well-being." This suggests a need to situate the ethics of PHR within a context that is complicated by personal, social, and institutional factors.

Knowledge about guidelines should thus be complemented with a situated ethics approach that acknowledges the complexity of real-life contexts and responds to emerging issues (Piper and Simons 2005). For example, in the Stepping Out study in Australia, conducted by co-author Lisa Gibbs and colleagues, child researchers helped to develop the data collection methods for a study of child independent mobility (Nansen et al. 2015). They suggested the adult researchers follow them to study how they travel to and from school. This method highlighted many aspects to children's transition to independence, which had not been identified in focus group discussions with the children and their parents. However, there were times when the adult researchers had to shift from passive observers to protective adults to stop children from stepping out onto busy roads when the children seemed to relax their safety practices because an adult was present.

In recognition of PHR principles, adult researchers must also revisit ethical issues and standards that are common to all research involving children. Principles such as obtaining informed consent are put under scrutiny because, in the context of PHR, who should provide consent? Can children and parents be fully informed before a project commences if it is to evolve, as is the case in PHR? In the previously mentioned digital storytelling project with young Canadians, the adult researchers used a two-stage consent process. The first involved consenting to make the story; the second involved sharing it, to what extent, in what formats, and with whom (Gladstone and Stasiulis in press). Progressive consent is a useful ethical technique in PHR with children by regularly providing opportunities for child researchers to reflect on their well-being, needs, and preferences within the research process. This includes exploring questions with children like: Do I want to continue my participation in this project? How do I want to participate in, or contribute to, this project? What are the advantages and disadvantages associated with this decision – for me and/or others – both now and in the long term?

The authorship, ownership, and dissemination of the research must also be questioned: Can the project be separated from the research? Can the research truly be deidentified? What if children want to claim their own work? What knowledge should be shared only within the research setting versus the wider audience (Clark 2010)? PHR encourages a shift from institutional "ownership" of research (Kirshner and O'Donoghue 2001) to the inclusion of participants in decision-making and the interpretation and application of findings (Mayall 1994). In the aforesaid storytelling project, young people told stories about their parents' mental health difficulties.

However, because their parents would not have the opportunity to vet or comment on the stories, the team worked with the young researchers to use pseudonyms to deidentify the data. This demonstrates how decisions on the representation of findings can influence the afterlife of the research and its impact on those it represents, as well as those who can effect change (Matthews and Sunderland 2013; Mazzei and Jackson 2012). The adult and child researchers can co-develop a knowledge translation and dissemination plan to ensure research findings are represented ethically, information about the research and its findings is tailored for different audiences (Gladstone and Stasiulis in press), and there is due recognition of all contributors, notably children, on all outputs, including academic publications.

Finally, there is the issue of the sustainability, because as children increase in age and maturity, they might cease to be considered as children during the project. This can affect the continuity of long-term projects (Lansdown 2010; Ozer et al. 2010) and how children perceive and look back on the process and results. For example, a child researcher once proud to be in a video might later be ashamed of what they might now perceive as childish behavior. Although time-limited consent can help to address this possibility, it can be difficult to honor if project outputs are shared through social media.

What Is Required of the Adult Facilitator?

PHR with children does not abdicate adults of their responsibilities (Woodhead 2010). As advocates for child agency, adult researchers enter PHR with the task of relinquishing (at least part of) their adult-centric views and power (Sinclair 2000). However, this does not imply a passive role, or that child researchers are expected to make decisions that should be under the charge of professionals. Adults must promote the spaces, culture, and climate that enable, if not encourage, children to participate, build their capacities, and make informed contributions that can evolve over time (Lundy and McEvoy 2012b).

Alison Clark and Peter Moss (2001) suggested that listening to children is not limited to the spoken word but includes the many ways that children express themselves. Adult researchers must therefore take the time to build rapport with child researchers to truly understand what is happening to children and how they attribute meaning to this situation (Sarti et al. in press). They must learn to listen to what children say, rather than assume what is best for them (Petrie 2011). This approach recognizes adult researcher limitations to understand another's life.

Apart from listening to children and witnessing their actions, adults promote child agency by facilitating, encouraging, and providing scaffolding support. The adult role thus provides a temporary supportive framework that becomes less necessary as children become more familiar and confident with the research process (Woodhead 2010; Clark 2010; Lambert and Clyde 2000). Power is shared by acknowledging and respecting differences between all researchers (Malone and Hartung 2010; Sinclair 2000). This includes recognizing both children's and adults' skills, expertise, and contributions to the process of co-learning (Rinaldi 2005;

Rogoff et al. 2002). In this way, children can teach adults (Malone and Hartung 2010), and adults can provide children with the support needed to further their skills. This democratization of knowledge places both adults and children as active meaning makers who work in collaboration (Freire 1972).

PHR demands a constant reflective practice, where adults continually reflect on their actions, relationships, values, intentions, and ethical foundations. Despite adults' efforts to listen to children, the structural view of children, based on age and maturity, can constrain children's participation and silence their voices (James and James 2012; Mason and Hood 2011). Age is still regarded as the key definitional marker of children's status, ignoring the agency they bring to their social context and their lives (James and James 2012; Mason and Hood 2011). Reflexivity can enable an adult researcher to connect local protocols, or procedural ethics, with their research in practice, or micro-ethics (Guillemin and Gillam 2004; Komesaroff 1995). Reflexivity assumes an ongoing self-awareness and self-analysis in relation to methodological practice and thus encourages the adult researcher to constantly adapt to a changing context (Ebrahim 2010; Finlay 2002).

To help navigate and manage some of the challenges associated with PHR with children, some guidance is available. For instance, co-author Christine Dedding et al. (2013) developed principles to guide adult facilitators involved in participatory research with children and young people, to support and sustain reflexivity and optimize quality (see Table 7.2). Similarly, Harry Shier (forthcoming) co-devised an analytical tool to aid decision-making about when, how, and who to engage in research relating to children's lives.

Table 7.2 Guidelines for responsible participatory research with children and young people, developed by the Dutch-Belgian (Flemish) platform researching children (Dedding et al. 2013)

1. The opinions of children and young people will be listened to in research, and opportunities will be created for genuine dialogue between children, young people, and adult researchers
2. Participatory research is more than expressing opinions; it also involves action and change
3. Children and young people should have equal opportunities to participate in research. Particular attention should be paid to children who are living in vulnerable situations and to children with special needs
4. The perspective and experiences of children and young people are the focus of the research. The research concerns issues which are important to children and young people
5. Before starting participatory research, the necessary conditions (time, means) to ensure meaningful participation are guaranteed
6. Children and young people are voluntarily participants in the research and will be openly and adequately informed about the research, before and throughout the research process
7. Adult researchers who are responsible for the implementation of participatory research have the capacities from either education or experience to perform this kind of research
8. Adult researchers guarantee the integrity and safety of children and young people participating in the research
9. The research methods are adapted to the specific interests, competences, and needs of children and young people. There is time and space for children and young people to explore and test their ideas during the process
10. Adult researchers value the experiences of children and young people and desire to improve their circumstances based on the findings of the research

Conclusion

Involving children in PHR can provide opportunities to understand their perspectives, reveal their competencies and needs, and empower them to make a meaningful contribution to issues affecting their lives. It is underpinned by a rights-based approach, where children's evolving capacities and expertise are valued. In PHR, children are not just research participants – they are co-researchers. This raises a range of potential challenges and ethical issues, including the nature of child engagement; the role of adults; methods to promote child agency, while ensuring children's safety is not compromised; and ensuring due recognition of their contributions in project outputs for different audiences. The flexibility of PHR accommodates culture and context and the different interests, needs, and capacities of the children involved. Children's right to alter or deny the participatory process and to critique current systems is a way to potentially achieve impacts and outcomes that are more relevant and useful for the children and the challenges they face.

References

Alderson, P. (2001). Research by children. *International Journal of Social Research Methodology, 4*(2), 139–153.

Arnstein, S. R. (1969). A ladder of citizen participation. *Journal of the American Institute of Planners, 35*(4), 216–224.

Barker, J., & Weller, S. (2003). "Is it fun?" developing children centred research methods. *International Journal of Sociology and Social Policy, 23*(1/2), 33–58.

Bell, K. (2013). *What is the experience of play for children in one school age care service?* Brisbane: Griffith University.

Berman, R., & MacNevin, M. (2017). Adults researching with children. In X. Chen, R. Raby, & P. Albanese (Eds.), *The sociology of child and youth studies in Canada: Categories, inequalities, engagement*. Toronto, ON.:: Canadian Scholars Press.

Black, A., & Busch, G. (2016). Understanding and influencing research with children. In B. Harreveld, M. Danaher, B. Knight, C. Lawson, & G. Busch (Eds.), *Constructing methodology for qualitative research: Researching education and social practices, Palgrave studies in education research methods* (pp. 219–235). London: Palgrave MacMillan.

Black, A., Busch, G., & Hayes, M. (2015). Reducing the marginalization of children: Relational knowledge production and the power of collaboration. In K. Trimmer, A. Black, & S. Riddle (Eds.), *Mainstreams, margins and the spaces in-between: New possibilities for education research, Research in Education Series*. UK: Routledge.

Block, K., Gibbs, L., Snowdon, E., & MacDougall, C. (2014). *Participant-guided mobile methods: Investigating personal experiences of communities following a disaster, SAGE research methods. Cases*. London: SAGE 2014.

Block, K., Gibbs, L., & MacDougall, C. (2017). Participant-guided mobile methods. In P. Liamputtong (Ed.), *Research methods in health social sciences*. Springer.

Boddy, J. (2011). The supportive relationship in 'Public care': The relevance of social pedagogy. In C. Cameron & P. Moss (Eds.), *Social pedagogy and working with children and young people* (pp. 105–124). London: Jessica Kingsley Publishers.

Burke, C. (2005). "Play in focus": Children researching their own spaces and places for play. *Children, Youth and Environments, 15*(1), 27–53.

Cameron, C. (2013). Cross-national understandings of the purpose of professional child relationships: Towards a social pedagogical approach. *International Journal of Social Pedagogy, 2*(1), 3–16.

Cargo, M., Grams, G. D., Ottoson, J. M., Ward, P., & Green, L. W. (2004). Empowerment as fostering positive youth development and citizenship: An evaluator's reflections. *American Journal of Health Behavior, 27*(Suppl 1), S66–S79.

Cartmel, J., & Casley, M. (2014). Talking circles: Building relationships with children. *Communities, Children and Families Australia, 8*(1), 67.

Chakraborty, K., Nansen, B., Gibbs, L., & MacDougall, C. (2012). Ethical negotiations: Committees, methods and research with children. *International Journal of Children's Rights, 20*(4), 541–553.

Charles, C., & DeMaio, S. (1993). Lay participation in health care decision making: A conceptual framework. *Journal of Health Politics, Policy and Law, 18*(4), 881–904.

Clandinin, D. J., & Connelly, F. M. (2004). *Narrative inquiry: Experience and story in qualitative research*. Hoboken: Wiley.

Clark, A. (2010). Young children as protagonists and the role of participatory, visual methods in engaging multiple perspectives. *American Journal of Community Psychology, 46*(1–2), 115–123.

Clark, A., & Moss, P. (2001). *Listening to young children: The mosaic approach* (2nd ed.). London: NCB.

Darbyshire, P., MacDougall, C., & Schiller, W. (2005). Multiple methods in qualitative research with children: More insight or just more? *Qualitative Research, 5*(4), 417–436.

Dedding, C., Jurrius, K., Moonen, X., & Rutjes, L. (Eds.). (2013). *Kinderen en jongeren actief in wetenschappelijk onderzoek. Ethiek, methoden en resultaten van onderzoek met en door jeugd [Children and young people active in scientific research: Ethics, methods and results of research with and by youth]*. Houten: Lannoo Campus.

Dedding, C., Reis, R., Wolf, B., & Hardon, A. (2015). Children's agency in the clinical encounter. *Health Expectations: An International Journal of Public Participation in Health Care and Health Policy*. https://doi.org/10.1111/hex.12180.

Ebrahim, E. B. (2010). Situated ethics: Possibilities for young children as research participants in the South African context. *Early Child Development and Care, 180*(3), 289–298.

Feingold, P. C. (1976). *Toward a paradigm of effective communication: An empirical study of perceived communicative effectiveness*. Doctorate, Purdue University, West Lafayette, IN.

Finlay, L. (2002). "Outing" the researcher: The provenance, process, and practice of reflexivity. *Qualitative Health Research, 12*(4), 531–545.

Foster-Fishman, P., Deacon, Z., Nievar, M. A., & McCann, P. (2005). Using methods that matter: The impact of reflection, dialogue and voice. *American Journal of Community Psychology, 36*(3/4), 275–291.

Franklin, A., & Sloper, P. (2006). Promoting participation for children and young people: Some key questions for health and social welfare organisations. *British Journal of Social Work, 36*, 723–741.

Freire, P. (1972). *Pedagogy of the oppressed*. Harmondsworth: Penguin Books.

Gallacher, L. A., & Gallagher, M. (2008). Methodological immaturity in childhood research? Thinking through 'participatory methods'. *Childhood, 15*(4), 499–516.

Gallagher, M. (2008). 'Power is not an evil': Rethinking power in participatory methods. *Children's Geographies, 6*(2), 137–150.

Gladstone, B. M. (2015). Thinking about children of parents with mental illnesses as a form of intergenerational practice. In D. M. A. Reupert, J. Nicholson, M. Seeman, & M. Göpfert (Eds.), *Parental psychiatric disorder: Distressed parents and their families* (3rd ed., pp. 85–95). Cambridge University Press, UK.

Gladstone, B. M., & Stasiulis, E. (in press). Digital story-telling method. In P. Liamputtong (Ed.), *Handbook of research methods in health social sciences* (Vol. 1). Singapore: Springer.

Greene, S., & Hogan, D. (Eds.). (2005). *Researching children's experience: Approaches and methods*. London: Sage Publications.

Greenfield, C. (2004). Transcript: "Can run, play on bikes, jump on the zoom slide, and play on the swings": Exploring the value of outdoor play. *Australian Journal of Early Childhood, 29*(2), 1–5.

Guillemin, M., & Gillam, L. (2004). Ethics, reflexivity, and "ethically important moments" in research. *Qualitative Inquiry, 10*(2), 261–280.

Hart, R. A. (1997). *Children's participation: The theory and practice of involving young citizens in community development and environment care.* London: Earthscan.

Hart, J., Newman, J., & Ackermann, L. (2004). *Children changing their world: Understanding and evaluating children's participation in development.* London: Plan.

Hart, R. A., Jensen, B. B., Nikel, J., & Simovska, V. (2008). Stepping back from 'the ladder': Reflections on a model of participatory work with children. In A. Reid (Ed.), *Participation and learning: Perspectives on education and the environment, health and sustainability* (pp. 19–31). Netherlands: Springer.

International Collaboration for Participatory Health Research (ICPHR). (2013). *What is participatory health research?* Berlin: International Collaboration for Participatory Health Research (ICPHR).

Israel, B. A., Parker, E. A., Rowe, Z., Salvatore, A., Minkler, M., López, J., et al. (2005). Community-based participatory research: Lessons learned from the Centers for Children's Environmental Health and Disease Prevention Research. *Environmental Health Perspectives, 113*, 1463–1471.

James, A., & James, A. (2012). *Key concepts in childhood studies, Sage key concepts series* (2nd ed.). London: Sage Publications.

Kellett, M. (2010a). Rethinking children and research: Attitudes in contemporary society. In *New childhoods.* London: Continuum International.

Kellett, M. (2010b). Small shoes, big steps! Empowering children as active researchers. *American Journal of Community Psychology, 46*, 195–203. https://doi.org/10.1007/s10464-010-9324-y.

Kirshner, B. R., & O'Donoghue, J. L. (2001). *Youth-adult research collaborations: Bringing youth voice and development to the research process.* Paper presented at the Annual Meeting of the American Educational Research Association, Seattle, WA, 10–14 Apr 2001.

Kohfeldt, D., Chhun, L., Grace, S., & Langhout, R. D. (2011). Youth empowerment in context: Exploring tensions in school-based yPAR. *American Journal of Community Psychology, 47*(1–2), 28–45.

Komesaroff, P. (1995). From bioethics to microethics: Ethical debate and clinical medicine. In P. Komesaroff (Ed.), *Troubled bodies: Critical perspectives on postmodernism, medical ethics and the body* (pp. 62–86). Melbourne: Melbourne University Press.

Lambert, E. B., & Clyde, M. (2000). *Re-thinking early childhood: Theory and practice.* Southbank: Thomson Learning Australia.

Lancaster, Y. P., & Broadbent, V. (2010). *Listening to young children* (2nd ed.). Berkshire: Open University Press.

Lansdown, G. (2010). The realisation of children's participation rights: Critical reflections. In B. Percy-Smith & N. Thomas (Eds.), *A handbook of children and young people's participation: Perspectives from theory and practice* (pp. 11–23). Milton Park: Routledge.

Lester, S., & Russell, W. (2008). *Play for a change.* London: National Children's Bureau.

Liegghio, M., Nelson, G., & Evans, S. D. (2010). Partnering with children diagnosed with mental health issues: Contributions of a sociology of childhood perspective to participatory action research. *American Journal of Community Psychology, 46*(1–2), 84–99.

Lundy, L., & McEvoy, L. (2012a). Childhood, the United Nations convention on the rights of the child and research: What constitutes a 'rights-based' approach? In M. Freeman (Ed.), *Law and childhood studies* (Vol. 14, pp. 75–91). Oxford: Oxford University Press.

Lundy, L., & McEvoy, L. (2012b). Children's rights and research processes: Assisting children to (in)formed views. *Childhood, 19*(1), 129–144.

Maglajlic, R. A. (2010). Participation of children through PAR. *American Journal of Community Psychology, 46*, 204–214. https://doi.org/10.1007/s10464-010-9322-0.

Malone, K., & Hartung, C. (2010). Challenges of participatory practice with children. In B. Percy-Smith & N. Thomas (Eds.), *A handbook of children and young people's participation: Perspectives from theory and practice*. Abingdon: Routledge.

Mason, J., & Hood, S. (2011). Exploring issues of children as actors in social research. *Children and Youth Services Review, 33*(4), 490–495.

Matthews, N., & Sunderland, N. (2013). Digital life-story narratives as data for policy makers and practitioners: Thinking through methodologies for large-scale multimedia qualitative datasets. *Journal of Broadcasting and Electronic Media, 57*(1), 97–114.

Mayall, B. (1994). *Children's childhoods: Observed and experienced*. London: Falmer Press.

Mayall, B. (2002). *Towards a sociology for childhood: Thinking from children's lives*. Maidenhead: Open University Press.

Mazzei, L. A., & Jackson, A. Y. (2012). Complicating voice in a refusal to "let participants speak for themselves". *Qualitative Inquiry, 18*(9), 745–751.

Moss, P., & Petrie, P. (2002). *From children's services to children's spaces*. Abingdon: RoutledgeFalmer.

Mutch, C., & Gawith, E. (2014). The New Zealand earthquakes and the role of schools in engaging children in emotional processing of disaster experiences. *Pastoral Care in Education, 32*(1), 54–67. https://doi.org/10.1080/02643944.2013.857363.

Nansen, B., Gibbs, L., MacDougall, C., Vetere, F., Ross, N. J., & McKendrick, J. (2015). Children's interdependent mobility: Compositions, collaborations and compromises. *Children's Geographies, 13*(4), 467–481.

NHMRC (National Health and Medical Research Council), ARC (Australian Research Council), & AVCC (Australian Vice-Chancellors' Committee). (2014). *National statement on ethical conduct in human research*. Canberra: Commonwealth of Australia.

Nic Gabhainn, S., O'Higgins, S., & Barry, M. (2010). The implementation of social, personal and health education (SPHE) in Irish schools. *Health Education, 110*, 452–470.

O'Higgins, S., & Nic Gabhainn, S. (2010). Youth participation in setting the agenda: Learning outcomes for sex education in Ireland. *Sex Education: Sexuality Society and Learning, 10*(4), 387–403.

O'Higgins, S., Nic Gabhainn, S., & Sixsmith, J. (2010). Adolescents' perceptions of the words 'health' and 'happy'. *Health Education, 110*(5), 367–381.

Ozer, E. J., Ritterman, M. L., & Wanis, M. G. (2010). Participatory action research (PAR) in middle school: Opportunities, constraints, and key processes. *American Journal of Community Psychology, 46*(1–2), 152–166.

Ozer, E. J., Newlan, S., Douglas, L., & Hubbard, E. (2013). "Bounded" empowerment: Analyzing tensions in the practice of youth-led participatory research in urban public schools. *American Journal of Community Psychology, 52*, 13–26. https://doi.org/10.1007/s10464-013-9573-7.

Pascal, C., & Bertram, T. (2009). Listening to young citizens: The struggle to make real a participatory paradigm in research with young children. *European Early Childhood Research Journal, 17*(2), 249–262.

Pells, K. (2010). No one ever listens to us': Challenging obstacles to the participation of children and young people in Rwanda. In B. Percy-Smith & N. Thomas (Eds.), *A handbook of children and young people's participation: Perspectives from theory and practice*. Abingdon: Routledge.

Petrie, P. (2011). *Communication skills for working with children and young people: Introducing social pedagogy*. London: Jessica Kingsley Publishers.

Piper, H., & Simons, H. (2005). Ethical responsibility in social research. In B. Somekh & C. Lewin (Eds.), *Research methods in the social sciences* (pp. 56–63). London: Sage Publications.

Porter, G., Hampshire, K., Bourdillon, M., Robson, E., Munthali, A., Abane, A., et al. (2010). Children as research collaborators: Issues and reflections from a mobility study in Sub-Saharan Africa. *American Journal of Community Psychology, 46*(1–2), 215–227.

Punch, S. (2002a). Interviewing strategies with young people: The "secret box", stimulus material and task-based activities. *Children & Society, 16*(1), 45–56.

Punch, S. (2002b). Research with children: The same or different from research with adults? *Childhood, 9*(3), 321–341.

Ramsden, V., Martin, R., McMillan, J., Granger-Brown, A., & Tole, B. (2015). Participatory health research within a prison setting: A qualitative analysis of 'paragraphs of passion'. *Global Health Promotion, 22*(4), 48–55. https://doi.org/10.1177/1757975914547922.

Ray, P. (2010). The participation of children living in the poorest and most difficult situations. In B. Percy-Smith & N. Thomas (Eds.), *A handbook of children and young people's participation: Perspectives from theory and practice.* Abingdon: Routledge.

Redfern Legal Centre. (2014). *The law handbook: Your practical guide to the law in New South Wales* (13th ed.). Pyrmont: Redfern Legal Centre.

Rinaldi, C. (2005). Documentation and assessment: What is the relationship? In A. Clark, A. Kjørholt, & P. Moss (Eds.), *Beyond listening: Children's perspectives on early childhood services* (pp. 17–28). Bristol: Policy Press.

Rogoff, B., Bartlett, L., & Goodman Turkanis, C. (2002). *Learning together: Children and adults in a school community.* Oxford: Oxford University Press.

Salmon, A., Browne, A. J., & Pederson, A. (2010). 'Now we call it research': Participatory health research involving marginalized women who use drugs. *Nursing Inquiry, 17*(4), 336–345. https://doi.org/10.1111/j.1440-1800.2010.00507.x.

Sarti, A., Schalkers, I., Bunder, J. F. G., & Dedding, C. (2017). Around the table with policymakers: Giving voice to children in contexts of poverty and deprivation. *Action Research Journal.* 1476750317695412, http://doi.org/10.1177/1476750317695412.

Schalkers, I., Dedding, C., & Bunders, J. (2015). "[I would like] a place to be alone, other than the toilet" – Children's perspectives on paediatric hospital care in the Netherlands. *Health Expectations: An International Journal of Public Participation in Health Care and Health Policy, 18*, 2066–2078. https://doi.org/10.1111/hex.12174.

Shier, H. (2001). Pathways to participation: Openings, opportunities and obligations. *Children and Society, 15*(2), 107–117.

Shier, H. (2015). Children as researchers in Nicaragua: Children's consultancy to transformative research. *Global Studies of Childhood, 5*(2), 206–219. https://doi.org/10.1177/2043610615587798.

Shier, H. (forthcoming). An analytical tool to help researchers develop partnerships with children and adolescents. In I. R. Berson, M. J. Berson, & C. Gray (Eds.), *Participatory methodologies to elevate children's voice and agency (Research in Global Child Advocacy).* Charlotte: IAP.

Sinclair, R. (2000). Young people's participation. In *Research in practice, making research count.* London: Department of Health.

Sinclair, R. (2004). Participation in practice: Making it meaningful, effective and sustainable. *Children and Society, 18*, 106–118.

Sixsmith, J., Nic Gabhainn, S., Fleming, C., & O'Higgins, S. (2007). Childrens', parents' and teachers' perceptions of child wellbeing. *Health Education, 107*(6), 511–523.

Smith, L. T., Smith, G. H., Boler, M., Kempton, M., Ormond, A., Chueh, H. C., et al. (2002). "Do you guys hate Aucklanders too?" youth: Voicing difference from the rural heartland. *Journal of Rural Studies, 18*(2), 169–178.

van Staa, A. L., Jedeloo, S., Latour, J. M., & Trappenburg, M. J. (2010). Exciting but exhausting: Experiences with participatory research with chronically ill adolescents. *Health Expectations, 13*(1), 95–107.

Tizard, B., & Hughes, M. (2002). *Young children learning, Understanding children's worlds* (2nd ed.). Malden: Blackwell Publishing.

Treseder, P. (1997). *Empowering children and young people: Training manual.* London: Save the Children and Children's Rights Office.

Ulvik, O. S., & Gulbrandsen, L. M. (2015). Exploring children's everyday life: An examination of professional practices. *Nordic Psychology, 67*(3), 210–224.

UNCRC. (1989). United Nations convention on the rights of the child. G.A. res. 44/25, annex, 44 U.N. GAOR Supp. (No. 49) at 167, U.N. Doc. A/44/49 (1989), entered into force September 2 1990. /C/93/Add.5 of 16 July 2003.

Veale, A. (2005). Creative methodologies in participatory research with children. In S. Greene & D. Hogan (Eds.), *Researching children's experience: Approaches and methods* (pp. 253–272). London: Sage Publications.

Wallerstein, N., Sanchez-Merki, V., & Dow, L. (2002). Freirian praxis in health education and community organizing. In M. Minkler (Ed.), *Community organizing and community building for health* (pp. 195–211). New Brunswick: Rutgers University Press.

Weller, S. (2006). Tuning-in to teenagers! Using radio phone-in discussions in research with young people. *International Journal of Social Research Methodology, 9*(4), 303–315.

Westheimer, J., & Kahne, J. (2004). What kind of citizen? The politics of educating for democracy. *American Educational Research Journal, 41*(2), 237–269.

Wong, N., Zimmerman, M. A., & Parker, E. A. (2010). A typology of youth participation and empowerment for child and adolescent health promotion. *American Journal of Community Psychology, 46*(1–2), 100–114.

Woodhead, M. (2010). Foreword. B. Percy-Smith, N. Thomas, A handbook of children and young people's participation: Perspectives from theory and practice (xix–xxii). Milton Park: Routledge.

Part II
Regional Perspectives

Chapter 8
PartKommPlus: German Research Consortium for Healthy Communities—New Developments and Challenges for Participatory Health Research in Germany

Michael T. Wright, Reinhard Burtscher, and Petra Wihofszky

Participatory Research in Germany

Participatory forms of research in Germany were initially based on the *action research* of Kurt Lewin.[1] The German-Jewish scientist emigrated from Germany to the United States after being banned from civil service at the start of the Nazi period in 1933. Lewin wanted to harness social science research for the purpose of emancipation and the promotion of democracy. The distinction he made between "action research" and "basic social research," on the one hand, and "pure science," on the other (Lewin 1946), foretells the divide that has characterized the German debate on participatory research since the beginning. His claim that action research need not be "less scientific" stands in contrast to the German social science tradition which has focused on high-level theory building and social structure; applied forms of research have not had an equal status, receiving relatively little funding and often seen as not being research in the true sense (Altrichter and Posch 2010).

The German reception of Lewin's action research approach followed some two decades after its introduction in the United States. Toward the end of the 1960s, a broad and critical discussion of theory and method took place in Germany; it followed a heated dispute over positivism within sociology and occurred alongside the student movement's ongoing critique of mainstream society and science. It was in this context that action research became popular in the early 1970s—particularly in

---

[1] The historical development of participatory research in Germany is based on the work of von Unger et al. (2007).

Members of the PartKommPlus Research Consortium

M. T. Wright (✉) · R. Burtscher
Catholic University of Applied Sciences, Institute for Social Health, Berlin, Germany
e-mail: michael.wright@khsb-berlin.de

P. Wihofszky
Faculty of Social Work, Health Care and Nursing Sciences, Esslingen University of Applied Sciences, Esslingen am Neckar, Germany

© Springer International Publishing AG, part of Springer Nature 2018   117
M. T. Wright, K. Kongats (eds.), *Participatory Health Research*,
https://doi.org/10.1007/978-3-319-92177-8_8

the fields of education, sociology, social work, critical psychology, and political science. Action research seemed to be the ideal way to implement—in a new practice-based, empirical approach—theoretically formulated critiques of the scientific and research establishment. Other important sources for German action research in the 1970s included the Critical Theory of the Frankfurt School, Niklas Luhmann's social systems theory, the approach of the Brazilian educator and theorist Paulo Freire, and the work of the French psychoanalyst and anthropologist George Devereux (Haag et al. 1972; Horn 1979).

The first German action researchers had reformist ambitions, some of them Marxist in nature. The new research strategy was embedded in a fundamental critique of the "widespread societal contradictions in the political economic system of late capitalism" (Haag et al. 1972, p. 23), often with the hope of contributing to processes of radical change in society. Proponents of action research feared, however, that "under society's existing contradictions, which include private control over both the means of production and their political regulation, the methods of action research—despite all intentions to the contrary—could be exploited for other purposes" and "absorbed by the hegemony" (Haag et al. 1972, p. 41). Thus, the political context of research and science also became a topic of discussion, and researchers were asked continually to engage in a reflective process on their own work and methods. These calls for self-reflection also had another source, namely, the much broader discussion at that time on methodology, which challenged the traditional subject-object relationship of the researcher and the researched. Moreover, the self-reflection of researchers was viewed as a methodological imperative necessitated by the influence of the researcher's subjectivity as well as the inevitable influence of the research participants (Devereux 1976; Gstettner 1979; Horn 1979).

There were differences between the various manifestations of action research in Germany. For example, not all action researchers drew from historical materialism or articulated their approach as part of a Marxist critique of capitalism. The ambition to produce insights and theory within the context of action research also was a point of difference. Some concepts of action research as a "problem-oriented and problem-solving research strategy" saw no explicit need to construct theory beyond analysis of the concrete problem at hand (Pieper 1972; Kramer et al. 1979). Still others explicitly claimed the need and right to pursue theoretical questions, as well.

Action research generated lively debates in Germany and drew a good deal of criticism, both from within and outside of action research circles. A study of first-generation action researchers in Germany concluded that action research had fallen into a state of "demise" after a "brief period of interest" (Altrichter and Gstettner 1993). From 1972 to 1982 approximately 400 German-language publications on action research appeared; in the early 1990s, the place of action research was negligible. Altrichter and Gstettner explain the demise having been caused by the following weaknesses:

1. Action research was based on amorphous concepts and ill-defined goals, premises, and methods.
2. In spite of action research's basic goal of social critique, very little social theory was actually formulated.
3. The transformative potential of research to bring about reform was overestimated.
4. The relationship between the "researchers and the researched" was "too simplistic and optimistic," resulting in power differences not being taken into account.
5. Despite all of the criticism of "science as usual" by action researchers, they retained a good degree of faith in the usual research practice, establishing hierarchies and permitting learning processes in one direction only.
6. There was much infighting and competition among action researchers, preventing the establishment of a scientific and practice community.
7. The changing sociopolitical environment also took its toll as the student movement began to disintegrate and the era of reform gave way to a politically conservative period.
8. Action researchers in Germany cultivated few international contacts and were thus unaffected by newer developments and discussions in other countries.

Now, more than two decades after Altrichter and Gstettner's study, participatory forms of research are again on the rise, largely influenced by European action research traditions and *community-based participatory research* as practiced in North America. This development has gone hand-in-hand with an increasing investment in applied research in the social sciences; a growing emphasis on cooperative relationships between academic institutions, practitioners, and civil society in problem-centered research; and a shift toward a service user focus in research on structures in the healthcare and social welfare systems. Participatory research is gaining prominence particularly in the fields of health (Wright et al. 2013), disability studies (Buchner et al. 2011), community psychology (Hermann et al. 2004), education (Schemme and Novak 2017), and technical fields (Bürger schaffen wissen. Die Citzen Science Plattform 2017, Bergmann and Schramm 2008). The new generation of action researchers are well-networked nationally and internationally in cooperative structures, including the German Network for Participatory Health Research (PartNet), the Participation Research Network (*Netzwerk Teilhabeforschung*), and the Citizen Science Platform (*BürgerSchaffenWissen*). PartNet is the regional partner of the International Collaboration for Participatory Health Research (ICPHR) for the German-speaking countries. There remains a critical stance regarding the degree to which participatory forms of research have the ability to transform society and to involve marginalized communities, given the deeper social-structural issues and the power dynamics inherent in the reproduction of social inequality (e.g., Frielinghaus 2016).

The Research Consortium PartKommPlus: Background

PartKommPlus—German Research Consortium for Healthy Communities—is the largest participatory research project to date in Germany. It is one of seven consortia on health promotion and prevention being funded by the Federal Ministry for Education and Research in the Prevention Research Program.[2] The consortium is a project of the German Network for Participatory Health Research (PartNet). It was founded in order to investigate the factors determining the successful implementation and maintenance of integrated municipal strategies (IMS) for health promotion and how to engage a wide range of stakeholders, particularly vulnerable communities, in such strategies. IMS, more commonly known in Germany as "prevention chains" (*Präventionsketten*) are intended to provide a coordinated approach to health promotion during the entire life span, with a particular focus on vulnerable communities. The need to establish IMS as an integral part of population-based health promotion was identified more than 20 years ago. The concept was first taken up by the Healthy Cities movement which was formed in Europe to implement the WHO Ottawa Charta on Health Promotion. IMS are currently a cornerstone of health policy on health promotion in Germany. They aim to involve all sectors of the social welfare, educational and healthcare systems, civil society, and the general public in designing long-term strategies to improve and maintain the health of the population. Local stakeholders, including NGOs and local authorities, are supported by coordinators located at the regional Associations for Health Promotion (AHP) or a similar body found in each of the 16 states in Germany. Based on our experience and a literature search prior to our initial proposal, we identified issues of governance and engagement (participation) as being areas where there is a particular need for improvement.

An important development over the last 2 years at the policy level is the national Law on Prevention (*Präventionsgesetz*) which took effect in 2016. The law requires all states to develop health promotion and prevention strategies and provides new funding mechanisms for these strategies, predominantly through the statutory health insurance companies. This includes supporting the Associations for Health Promotion and similar structures as they assist municipalities in setting up and maintaining IMS. The governance structures require strong forms of cooperation among a wide group of stakeholders, making the work of the PartKommPlus consortium even more relevant and affirming the focus of our work.

The Structure of PartKommPlus

The consortium consisted originally of five subprojects conducting locally-based participatory research studies in eight different municipalities located in 6 of the 16 states in Germany: Baden-Württemberg, Berlin, Brandenburg, Hamburg, Hesse, and Lower Saxony. The selection of the subprojects was a result of both convenience (building on existing networks and partnerships) and the intention to

---

[2] Grant numbers 01EL1423A to 01EL1423H. Funding period: 2015–2018

Table 1 The projects in PartKommPlus

Project title (with abbreviation)	Focus
Parents asking parents: from model project to municipal roll-out (ElfE²)	Parent peer research to promote the participation of vulnerable families in pre-schools
Participatory evaluation of the prevention chain in Braunschweig (PEBS)	A participatory evaluation of the Braunschweig network to prevent poverty among families with children
Development of municipal health promotion strategies (KEG)	Developing municipal strategies for health promotion through a dialogue between research and practice
Health promoting neighborhoods (Age4Health)	Engaging vulnerable older people in developing local health promotion strategies
People with intellectual disabilities and health promotion programs (Health!)	Inclusion of people with intellectual disabilities in health promotion strategies
Municipalities and health insurance funds—cooperating for healthy local environments (K³)	Governance in municipal health promotion strategies with the focus on the cooperation between health insurers and public authorities
Participatory epidemiology: from data to recommendations (P&E)	Participatory approaches to epidemiology and health monitoring
Integration & synthesis (I&S)	Synthesis and dissemination of the work of the consortium

maximize variation in terms of the types of municipalities (large and small, rural and urban), regional distribution, the communities served, and the participatory methods being employed. Over time, two additional subprojects have developed. The focus of the work of these two partners is participatory epidemiology and participatory health reporting as a basis for local municipal health strategies (P&E) and questions of governance in municipal strategies of health promotion (K³). Each of the subprojects is a participatory research process in its own right, focusing on different topics and employing different methods in widely differing settings and constellations of stakeholders (see Table 1).[3]

The knowledge gained from these projects is being brought together in the subproject called Integration and Synthesis. The synthesized knowledge is being transferred throughout the country by way of the Cooperation Network "Equity In Health" (EIH) through its Internet platform *inforo* and other channels.

We began with a relatively conventional structure with a coordinating body in charge of integrating and synthesizing the data from the original five projects taking place at the local level. The data collection was intended to take place at the colloquia scheduled twice a year, each lasting 3 days and focusing on a topic related to the overarching research questions and being attended by representatives from each of the five local projects. In addition, interviews were to be conducted with people taking part in the five projects, and other local data was to be gathered so as to address questions of governance and monitoring. The idea was to draw together systematically data from each of the five subprojects and to discuss these data at the colloquia, so as to answer the overarching research questions of the consortium.

---

[3] Detailed information on the subprojects can be found at www.partkommplus.de.

This plan did not work, for two primary reasons: firstly, the five projects felt that they were being made the objects of researchers from outside of the local context. They felt that they were being called to deliver data but that they did not have sufficient control over what data was collected or how it would be analyzed. Several attempts were made to be more transparent about the central data collecting process and to include the five projects in that process, until we concluded that the problem was a structural one. Secondly, participatory research is at its heart a local process. In PartKommPlus the research processes at the municipal level are focused on maximizing the participation of the various stakeholders, thereby enabling a broad ownership of the local projects. Building trust and ownership at the local level stands in contrast to a central and, for many partners, abstract and geographically remote process of data synthesis.

Over the last year, we have decentralized our data collection and analysis strategy at the consortium level, thus departing from our initial structure. This bottom-up, inductive approach has led to identifying topics in which different constellations of lead institutions and stakeholders from the various projects bring together what they have learned about a topic of common interest. And each of these subgroups is deciding how they will work together and what they will produce as a result. For example, a group of peer researchers may come together to produce a list of criteria for participating in research. Whereas, a group of academic researchers may write a journal article on how participatory health research differs methodologically from other forms of health promotion research. Or a group of practitioners and academic researchers may design a tool for helping municipalities in setting up local strategies. Thus, not all subprojects are involved in all topics, and the option is also available for a subproject to work on a specific topic which only applies to its focus area. The result will not be a neat data synthesis from which answers to all research questions can be formulated but rather a diverse assortment of various types of knowledge, products, and forms of reflection and analysis regarding municipal strategies of health promotion and participation. This will provide findings and forms of reporting which are most relevant for the stakeholders without excluding the opportunity for more conventional academic treatments of the data.

We have continued meeting twice a year at the colloquia, but the focus has shifted to capacity building through mutual support, skill building, and the exchange of ideas, for example, by sharing lessons learned at the local level. Peer supervision and input provided by national and international experts have been particularly useful. The subprojects have also taken on a larger role in determining the focus and structure of the colloquia, including an increasing involvement of their local partners. We are currently examining the question of whether a true community of inquiry can be established at the consortium level, given the challenges described here. More likely we can characterize our colloquia as temporary communities of inquiry in which new knowledge is generated with an immediate transfer value for the practice and research processes of those present. In any case, the colloquia are serving their intended function of promoting the quality of the research processes taking place at the local level.

The Goals of PartKommPlus

As stated earlier, PartKommPlus was founded to investigate the factors determining the successful implementation and maintenance of integrated municipal strategies for health promotion (IMS) and how to engage a wide range of stakeholders, particularly vulnerable communities, in such strategies. Our work is guided by the principles of participatory health research (PHR). This focus has been adjusted and refined over time in response to the experiences of the local projects.

The term IMS, anchored in urban planning and in health policy, reflects a general trend toward integrated planning and service delivery in the governmental sector. Accordingly, the stakeholders interested in IMS tend to be from local and regional authorities. However, as noted above, the term IMS is not commonly used but rather "prevention chains." For the majority of stakeholders not working in a planning capacity, the terms IMS and prevention chain are abstract and of no immediate interest. These same stakeholders are, however, interested in health promotion at the municipal level, including issues related to cooperation and participation. Our use of the term IMS to describe our work was thus a barrier to engaging local people in the research process. This is, in itself, an important finding from our research: The use of IMS as an overarching term is not effective in mobilizing professionals or other engaged citizens for the cause of health promotion. As a consequence, we have modified our focus to be on municipal health promotion strategies, more generally, while maintaining the governmental planning perspective as an important element in developing effective and sustainable health promotion.

We have encountered a similar problem with PHR. It has been difficult to engage local stakeholders in projects with the word "research" in the title. This is due to the fact that participatory forms of research are relatively unknown in Germany and that research is seen as something that is done exclusively by academics. The German scientific tradition is also characterized by a sharper distinction between research vs. everyday life and professional practice than is found, for example, in English-speaking countries. It also has been difficult for the academic researchers in our consortium to accommodate a broader definition of research, given their own socialization, which has presented an additional challenge. This experience represents an important finding regarding the barriers to establishing PHR in a German context which are related to the history of participatory approaches to research in Germany, as described above: There is a great need for capacity building within the practice and scientific communities in Germany. Much of our work in the first funding phase has been focused on building that capacity.

To address these issues, we have refocused our research on the topic *participation in municipal health promotion strategies*. In line with the international discussion, we define participation as not just taking part but rather as having influence on central aspects of one's living and work environments. We are focusing specifically on the following issues which are raised in the context of attempting to make participation a reality at the municipal level:

- *Cooperation and coordination (governance)*: Local authorities are challenged to provide a form of oversight which is based on cooperation and consensus and which coordinates, both vertically between levels (administrative level, intermediate level, district level, project level) and horizontally between the various functional departments and disciplines. This presumably requires specific forms of governance which we want to actively promote and to describe, based on systematic reflection with the various stakeholders.

- *The forms of participation among the various stakeholders*: The various stakeholders—local authorities, civil society, social service and health providers, and local citizens—can influence municipal strategies in different ways. We are looking at the various forms which this influence can take.
- *The impact of participation on municipal strategies of health promotion*: The various forms of participation on the part of the stakeholders can presumably have different effects on the municipal strategies, for example, in terms of the focus of the strategy, the measures taken at the local level, and their outcomes. We seek to describe these impacts.
- *The contribution of participatory health research to municipal strategies*: The consortium is applying various forms of participatory research to support the development and maintenance of municipal strategies. We are looking at how this form of research can contribute to the work at the local level and reflecting on this contribution with the various stakeholders.
- *Participatory epidemiology and health reporting (surveillance and monitoring)*: Data on the health of the population is a basis for all public health activities. Here we are looking at how participatory forms of data collection and analysis can support municipal and regional strategies in their work.
- *Cooperation within a research consortium* applying participatory research principles: Participatory research projects are commonly local in scope. Within PartKommPlus we seek to bring together the knowledge gained from local studies to contribute to a national strategy. To do this, we are developing ways of working together in a participatory fashion and are reflecting specifically on our own participatory process.

These goals have a direct connection to concrete issues related to municipal health promotion strategies and thus are of interest to a wide group of stakeholders. This provides a stronger basis for participatory research projects at the local level, as compared to our original goals and questions. In addition, the new goals focus our work on the topic of participation in research and practice at the municipal level. This topic is tangible and also relevant from both a practical and theoretical perspective. And it highlights the strength of our work which is about participatory methods and processes. Our original research questions and goals were disjointed, not offering a clear connection between research and practice for many outsiders. And our objective to identify general indicators and contributing factors for successful IMS was too broad. Our research will offer new knowledge on methods and processes of participation and cooperation which are important components of successful IMS, but not on other factors such as funding or broader policy issues.

In the next funding phase (2018–2021), we will continue with our focus on participation in municipal health promotion, as specified by the above goals. The emphasis will, however, shift from capacity building for PHR within the municipal context to issues of transfer and sustainability.

Ongoing Challenges

Participatory research takes place within *communities of inquiry* which, when based in *communities of practice*, can lead to change. Building communities of inquiry at both the local and consortium levels has been a challenge. At the local level, the focus has been on engaging a wide range of stakeholders, including many disadvantaged communities and over-extended professionals. The projects have explicitly sought to reach communities who profit less from the usual health promotion measures and are therefore often called "hard-to-reach." Within these communities are people whose participation in society is generally less, due to multiple factors related to social status, education, and immigration. The local projects were therefore not only confronted with the aforementioned challenges related to the topic of the research (IMS) and the unknown approach of PHR but also with the task of engaging groups of people (practitioners and local citizens) in resource-poor settings who are faced with multiple stressors. In spite of these challenges, all local projects were able to establish communities of inquiry in cooperation with various groups of stakeholders. And they were able to set up projects following the goals as outlined in their proposals for the first funding phase. Changes in design were, however, necessary in all cases and timelines needed to be adjusted to accommodate the participatory process.

At the consortium level, we are confronted with the task of building a community of inquiry comprised of people from the local projects and others from the broader community of practitioners involved in municipal health promotion. Typically, participatory research takes place at the local or regional levels, so we have no model internationally on which to base community building at the national level. Because of the innovative nature of this task, this has been the topic of most interest in the presentations we have made at international conferences. We have been in a process of experimentation to find forms of working together which not only maximize the participation of each lead institution in decision-making at the consortium level but which also bring the voices of local people into the work of the consortium as a whole. The latter has proven to be the larger of the two challenges but also the most rewarding in terms of the mutual learning process.

Conclusion

PartKommPlus provides an important opportunity to investigate the implementation of a core concept of health promotion—integrated municipal strategies—on a large scale. In addition, it is an attempt to scale up PHR, an approach most commonly associated with local communities, so as to address the issue of health promotion at the population level. Finally, PartKommPlus will support the establishment of PHR in Germany as a means for researching health promotion. In this way, PartKommPlus will contribute to both the national and international discussions on participation as both a local strategy and a research process in the interest of health promotion.

References

Altrichter, H., & Gstettner, P. (1993). Aktionsforschung – ein abgeschlossenes Kapitel in der Geschichte der deutschen Sozialwissenschaft? *Sozialwissenschaftliche Literatur Rundschau, 26*, 67–83.

Altrichter, H., & Posch, P. (2010). Reflective development and developmental research: Is there a future for action research as a research strategy in German-speaking countries? *Educational Action Research, 18*(1), 57–71.

Bergmann, M., & Schramm, E. (2008). *Transdisziplinäre Forschung. Integrative Forschungsprozesse verstehen und bewerten*. Frankfurt: Campus.

Buchner, T., Koenig, O., & Schuppener, S. (2011). Gemeinsames Forschen mit Menschen mit intellektueller Behinderung. Geschichte, Status quo und Möglichkeiten im Kontext der UN-Behindertenrechtskonvention. *Teilhabe, 1*, 4–11.

Bürger schaffen wissen. Die Citzen Science Plattform. (2017). Grünbuch Citizen Science Strategie 2020 für Deutschland. www.buergerschaffenwissen.de

Devereux, G. (1976). *Angst und Methode in den Verhaltenswissenschaften*. Munich: Hanser.

Frielinghaus, F. (2016). *Stadtteilkämpfe: und die (Un)Möglichkeiten ihrer Erforschung*. Norderstedt: Books on Demand.

Gstettner, P. (1979). Distanz und Verweigerung. Über einige Schwierigkeiten, zu einer erkenntnisrelevanten Aktionsforschungspraxis zu kommen. In K. Horn (Ed.), *Aktionsforschung: Balanceakt ohne Netz? Methodische Kommentare* (pp. 163–205). Frankfurt: Syndikat.

Haag, F., Krüger, H., Schwärzel, W., & Wildt, J. (Eds.). (1972). *Aktionsforschung: Forschungsstrategien, Forschungsfelder und Forschungspläne*. Munich: Juventa.

Hermann, A., Partenfelder, F., Raabe, S., Riedel, B., & Ruszetzki, R. (2004). "Miteinander statt übereinander" – Ergebnisse einer Begleitstudie zum Weddinger Psychoseseminar und Erfahrungen mit Forschungspartizipation psychoseerfahrener Teilnehmer/innen an dieser Studie. *Journal für Psychologie, 12*(4), 295–325.

Horn, K. (Ed.). (1979). *Aktionsforschung: Balanceakt ohne Netz? Methodische Kommentare*. Frankfurt: Syndikat.

Kramer, D., Kramer, H., & Lehmann, S. (1979). Aktionsforschung: Sozialforschung und gesellschaftliche Wirklichkeit. In K. Horn (Ed.), *Aktionsforschung: Balanceakt ohne Netz? Methodische Kommentare* (pp. 21–40). Frankfurt: Syndikat.

Lewin, K. (1946). Action research and minority problems. In *Resolving social conflicts: Selected papers on group dynamics* (pp. 201–216). New York: Harper & Brothers.

Pieper, R. (1972). Aktionsforschung und Systemwissenschaften. In F. Haag, H. Krüger, W. Schwärzel, & J. Wildt (Eds.), *Aktionsforschung: Forschungsstrategien, Forschungsfelder und Forschungspläne* (pp. 100–116). Munich: Juventa.

Schemme, D., & Novak, H. (2017). *Gestaltungsorientierte Forschung. Erprobte Ansätze im Zusammenwirken von Wissenschaft und Praxis*. Berlin: BIBB Bundesinstitut für Berufsbildung.

von Unger, H., Block, M., & Wright, M. T. (2007). *Aktionsforschung im deutschsprachigen Raum. Zur Geschichte und Aktualität eines kontroversen Ansatzes aus Public Health Sicht*. In der Reihe "Discussion Papers". Berlin: Wissenschaftszentrum Berlin für Sozialforschung.

Wright, M. T., Nöcker, G., Pawils, S., & Walter, U. (2013). Partizipative Gesundheitsforschung – ein neuer Ansatz für die Präventionsforschung. *Prävention und Gesundheitsförderung, 8*(3), 119–121.

Chapter 9
Participatory Health Research: An Indian Perspective

Wafa Singh

Introduction

The world today is living in contesting times. While we continue to make significant progress in terms of economic development, our human development parameters do not have a very happy story to narrate. This has been particularly true for India. As per the gross domestic product (GDP) rankings released by the World Bank in 2015, India secured the 7th position, among a total of 199 countries (World Bank 2015), while it ranked at 131 out of the 188 countries, as per the UNDP's (United Nations Development Program) Human Development Report 2016 (UNDP 2016). This clearly points toward the fact that we have faltered in our development agendas, which has focused narrowly on economic growth rather than on the well-being of people.

While a focus on economic development is undoubtedly important for any nation, this should not make us forget the most important resource for a country, namely, its citizenry. It is the human resources which actually build a nation and contribute to its development. In this context, a discussion on the health of the people is most pertinent. However, in the Indian context, this aspect loses traction, as is evident by some of the health statistics of the country. The World Health Report of 2016 recently released by the World Health Organization (WHO) shows that despite being placed roughly in the middle of the South-East Asian Region (SEAR)—one of the worst performing regions in health after Africa—in terms of gross national income per capita, India figures in the bottom slots for most health-related parameters within the group (WHO 2016).

So, *how do we improve the health scenario in the country? What practices can we adopt that can help the health sector cater to the needs of the citizens?*

W. Singh (✉)
Society for Participatory Research in Asia (PRIA), New Delhi, India
e-mail: wafa.singh@pria.org

© Springer International Publishing AG, part of Springer Nature 2018
M. T. Wright, K. Kongats (eds.), *Participatory Health Research*,
https://doi.org/10.1007/978-3-319-92177-8_9

Such multilevel health complexities and crosscutting challenges demand the production of *new knowledge in the field of health*, one which is linked to the Sustainable Development Goals (SDGs). Thus, there is a need for *creation of new knowledge through research in the health sector*. However, the magnitude of the problem at hand demands much more than what traditional health research approaches have been offering. It calls for viewing the *processes* of health research, beyond traditional notions of being top-down and driven by scientific agencies and health institutions. Although they are important stakeholders in the process, we need to realize that an initiative like health research cannot exclude the very people for whom it is meant. The involvement of people in research which is meant to achieve better health outcomes for them is as essential as the participation of experts. This lays the foundation for *participatory health research (PHR)*, which signifies an innovative approach to health research, in being *participatory, bottom-up, and sustainable and ensuring the generation of new knowledge on a variety of health parameters.*

Contextual Framework

Health research is the generation of new knowledge using scientific methods for improving and maintaining the health of the population and specific communities, including identifying important health issues and how to address them effectively and efficiently. The wide-scale implications and potential of health research on communities make the knowledge generated in the process a public good. Viewing health research from this perspective, it should ideally involve all people and organizations having a stake in health and social development in different stages of the research process. This includes research institutions, universities, governments, professional organizations, civil society, healthcare institutions, health workers, and—most importantly—the people who are directly faced with the health issues being researched. This is the essence of PHR (ICPHR 2013).

Here, the primary underlying assumption is that participation on the part of those whose lives or work is the subject of the study fundamentally affects all aspects of the research. The engagement of these people in the study is an end in itself and is the hallmark of PHR, recognizing the value of each person's contribution to the co-creation of knowledge in a process that is not only practical but also collaborative and empowering (ICPHR 2013; Onwuegbuzie et al. 2009). PHR is based on the premise that creating healthier communities and overcoming complex societal problems require collaborative solutions that bring communities and institutions together as equal partners and build upon the assets, strengths, and capacities of each. Therefore, it focuses on social, structural, and physical environmental inequities through active involvement of community members, organizational representatives, and academic researchers in all aspects of the research process. Partners contribute their expertise to enhance understanding of a given phenomenon and integrate the knowledge gained with action to benefit the community involved (ICPHR 2013).

Doing so, PHR aims at the "creation of new knowledge" which is local, collective, co-created, dialogical, and diverse. As in other forms of participatory research, the people whose life or work is being studied have the opportunity to articulate their local (indigenous) knowledge and to question and expand on that knowledge through the participatory research process (ICPHR 2013). So, the collective research process is conducted in such a way that knowledge is produced in an ongoing dialogue among the participants on all aspects of the research process. The various perspectives of the participants need to be incorporated into this dialogue.

Andrea Cornwall documents that the conceptual research framework introduced by health workers regarding the impact of contraceptives on women's bodies did not fit into the knowledge local women had about their bodies (Koning and Martin 1996). This resulted in both the stakeholders feeling inadequate in the research process. However, when the local women drew individual drawings of their bodies and functions, this exercise helped both groups to visualize, discuss, and understand the different frameworks. It also led to the adoption of a mutually agreeable and acceptable research framework (Koning and Martin 1996). Further, by collecting, analyzing, and interpreting evidence, PHR provides new knowledge to inform pathways and policies for improving the function of health systems. PHR is also motivated by contradiction, such as that between how things are currently understood and how they are in reality (Loewenson et al. 2014). For instance, an excessive focus on physical and biological determinants of ill-health makes us miss the fact that people's chances of staying healthy are also shaped by social structures and systems (Loewenson et al. 2014).

There are several reasons behind PHR as a methodology gaining traction across the globe: first, there is an increasing recognition of the gap between the concepts and models professionals use to understand and interpret reality and the concepts and perspectives of different groups in the community (Koning and Martin 1996). The biomedical interpretation and understanding of diseases, supported by studies carried out in laboratories, is in many cases different from the understanding embedded in a local culture or history. Second, many factors—cultural, historical, socioeconomic, and political—which are difficult to measure have a crucial influence on the outcomes of interventions and efforts to improve the health of the people (Koning and Martin 1996).

This chapter focuses on PHR in India and how this field of action has been contributing to the health scenario of the country. In particular, a comparison is made between how two sets of institutions, i.e., governmental organizations and nongovernmental organizations (NGOs), have been responding and how the latter have been spearheading this area of intervention in public health. Supporting evidence is provided in the form of a detailed analysis of PHR initiatives undertaken by two NGOs (PRIA and SARTHI). Finally, the chapter closes with a discussion and conclusions.

PHR in India

In India, PHR is still an uncommon practice, when viewed at a larger country-level scale. There are many examples of the use of participatory methods and techniques for agricultural research or community-based rural development programs.

However, the use of participatory research methods in the field of health is still limited, and the majority of health research continues to be top-down and driven by technical institutions. Participation by community stakeholders in health research is an aspect still not recognized by public institutions. This is evident from a detailed analysis of the missions and policies of the government of India, where though health research emerges as an important parameter, PHR is conspicuous by its absence in all such policies and programs. Another aspect worth noting is that although participation as a concept emerges in "healthcare" in general, its application in "research" is missing.

However, an interesting emerging trend is that while PHR is not yet considered an important area of intervention by the government and the policy sector, the NGOs in the country have been actively pursuing it for furthering the objectives of sound community health. Many NGOs have used PHR as a paradigm for improving the health of communities. This has been done in the context of project-based work or targeted interventions in a particular area of community health. The following sections reflect on how the government and the NGOs have been responding to health research in general and PHR in particular. This reflection is supported by evidence from governmental policy documents and the interventions made by NGOs, respectively.

Role of Government

According to the Indian Economic Survey 2016–2017, *the country's public spending on health is just over 1% of the country's gross domestic product (GDP), which is much below the world average of 5.99%* (GoI 2017). This has been a major reason behind the abysmal state of public health systems in the country. The governmental policies have also not been able to lift the health sector out of its poor operational state. In the context of research in particular, the policies have focused on exclusive, top-down approaches; the government has been viewing the area of health research as an exclusive field of work, one which is a prerogative of only specialized public research institutions.

This is evident from the recent policy statements issued by the Ministry of Health and Family Welfare (MoHFW) and the Department of Health. For instance, the National Health Policy of 2017 accords importance to health research as it calls for increased investment in the same, considering the important role health plays in the development of a nation. It also endorses strengthening research institutes under the Department of Health Research for this purpose (MoHFW 2017). The policy supports strengthening health research in India on the following fronts: *health systems and services research, medical product innovation (including point of care diagnostics and related technologies and internet of things), and fundamental research in all areas relevant to health such as physiology, biochemistry, pharmacology, microbiology, pathology, molecular sciences, and cell sciences.* While research has been viewed as top-down and exclusive, the word "participation" does, however, make an appearance in policy but only in the area of community health planning, monitoring, and evaluation. Further, although the policy documents talk about inclusive partnerships with communities and not-for-profit agencies, their role in health research has been missing.

Similarly, the framework of implementation of the National Health Mission (NHM) 2012–2017 also ascribes the responsibility of health research solely to public health education and research institutions (MoHFW 2014). This framework also views participation as only limited to healthcare in general. It says that, "States shall work with NGOs to build capacities of Village Health Sanitation and Nutrition Committees (VHSNC) members for making village health plans and increasing community participation. Particular emphasis will be on strengthening the capacity of members in understanding their roles in relation to development, implementation and monitoring of convergent action plans" (MoHFW 2014). Thus, participation only extends to community healthcare and community participation in VHSNC for health planning, monitoring, and evaluation. Further in the policy document, health research figures in the 25th position out of a total of 28 agenda items. Health research also does not figure under the goals set by the National Health Mission 2017. The implementation framework for the National Health Mission does mention a grant-in-aid to NGOs (amounting to 5% of the NHM budget) for providing "implementation support, undertake service delivery in remote areas, community monitoring, capacity building, for innovations in community processes, implementation research, impact assessments and research." However, there is not much evidence of this translating into actual implementation, with PHR again being conspicuous by its absence in all such directives.

The 3-year action agenda published in 2017 by the National Institution for Transforming India (NITI Aayog), a governmental think tank, also follows the same agenda and ideology. It talks about setting up of research consortia for diseases of high priority, bringing together all major national and international stakeholders for developing new tools (drug, diagnostics, and vaccines). It says that, "Indian Council of Medical Research (ICMR) academy and regional center for excellence should expand the number of postgraduate degrees that are offered. At least 20 academic or research institutions should be identified at the regional level to act as hubs capable of training a minimum of 500 doctors every year" (NITI Aayog 2017). While the policy talks about the operationalization of research and diagnostic labs, there is again no mention of participation in health research processes.

Key Takeaways

- *The policy documents view research as the sole prerogative of research institutions, such as the Indian Council of Medical Research (ICMR), National Institute of Health and Family Welfare (NIHFW), Indian Institute of Health Management Research (IIHMR), etc. It has, therefore, projected health research as a top-down process with no participation involved.*
- *The absence of health research as a whole from the NHM goals and its appearance at the bottom of NHM 2012–2017 bears testimony to the fact that policy prescriptions for health have gone wrong in their priority setting.*

- *The complete absence of PHR in all policy documents and directives gives evidence that this area of research is still not viewed as a valid, reliable, or acceptable area in the field of health research, especially by the governmental sector.*
- *Participation is still only taken as a superficial aspect. Although there is a mention of collaboration with NGOs or the private sector, it appears as a mere token. This is also evident from the meager budget accorded to these aspects or the areas of healthcare to be catered by such collaboration.*

Role of NGOs

The NGO sector in India has grown rapidly in the last couple of decades and has had an increasing impact in the developmental processes in the country. One targeted area of their intervention has been public health. NGOs have worked with communities and have designed their initiatives in a collaborative manner to achieve the objectives of sound public health in the interest of moving toward an efficient, reliable, and responsive healthcare system in the country. Faced by monetary constraints, often such interventions have been at a small scale. Further, the lack of appropriate skills and training has also constrained the efforts, but the NGOs have remained committed toward this end. With limited resources and capacity but abundance of will and a clear-cut vision, NGOs in India have been playing a crucial role in initiating and implementing PHR in the country. Cornwall and Jewkes (1995) report about PHR processes undertaken by Indian NGOs, where rural women and traditional birth attendants address reproductive health concerns. Here, we present case studies of two NGOs in India who have demonstrated much potential in the field of PHR, striving to engage and involve communities in finding solutions to their health issues.

The Work of PRIA and SARTHI

Society for Participatory Research in Asia (PRIA)

PRIA, since its inception in 1983, has pioneered the concept of participatory research (PR) in bringing about social change among the marginalized in India. It has also used the concept of PR in furthering the objectives of community health. PRIA has engaged extensively in the field of occupational health and safety (OHS) studies for over two decades, starting from the early 1980s and continuing up till the early 2000s.

In the early 1980s, when PRIA started its intervention on OHS, there was very little awareness regarding occupation-related diseases. Workers, while being aware of the kind of problems and adverse circumstances at the workplace, were not able to articulate and consolidate their knowledge to put it to any collective or relevant use (PRIA 2004). While they were aware of suffering from health problems and hostile working environs, they were unaware of the causal factors and causative agents. It was within such a context that the efforts begun toward creating a form of industrial development with a difference, namely, where the health of workers rightly assumes importance (PRIA 2004). Most importantly, the intention was to recognize the relevance of worker's experiential knowledge.

Therefore, in the year 1983, PRIA began to address the issue of OHS using PHR with the focus of involving all concerned parties in developing a consensual method of working for the mutual benefit of all. For instance, in Odisha (a state in East India), participatory researchers at PRIA engaged in an OHS study of a cement plant which was operating under hazardous conditions. Hundreds of workers and community members living around the factories suffered from respiratory disorders (Jaitli and Kanhere 2005). A major complication was that their disorders had been misdiagnosed as tuberculosis, an ailment which is not caused by occupational health hazards. This resulted in a twofold challenge for the participatory health researchers at PRIA: one, to challenge and explode the myth about tuberculosis, and, two, to demonstrate the real cause of the worker's ailments and arrive at solutions to safeguard their health.

As a first step, a 2-day workshop was organized with the representatives of the local trade union, workers, and other community members, for the mutual sharing of information. The local people and the workers provided information about the working conditions in the area and also a detailed description of their ailment. The researchers present at the workshop shared information about occupational health hazards, legislation to safeguard the workers' rights, and prevention techniques. At the end of the discussion, a detailed and open-ended questionnaire was prepared which covered aspects such as occupational history, symptoms, legal provisions, and the availabilities of appropriate facilities at the workplace. The responsibility of data collection was entrusted to a group who was selected from those present at the workshop. The time allocated for data collection was 15 days during which the data collectors were expected to collect as much information as possible (Jaitli and Kanhere 2005). At the end of this exercise, a study report was prepared jointly by the researchers and the data collectors.

The outcome of this experience was that workers became more aware of their suffering and the causes of their ailments. A high degree of sensitization took place, not only among the workers, but also among the community members. The PHR process also brought to light the fact that the workers were actually suffering from *silicosis*, a lung disease caused due to silica dust. The emerging lesson here is that PHR enables the stakeholders involved to reach a deeper understanding of occupational health hazards, bringing hidden problems out in the open. In the process, the workers involved also became capable of articulating their knowledge in front of experts. PHR, therefore, is not just about conducting research to ensure safety and occupational health but also affects the way the participatory researchers view themselves, the workers, and the role of researchers in improving the latter's lives. This example bears testimony to the fact that if we as participatory researchers are interested in uplifting people and communities, the opportunities in the field of PHR are immense.

Social Action for Rural and Tribal In-habitants of India (SARTHI)

SARTHI is a voluntary organization which started its operations in 1980 in Gujarat (a state in Western India). In the late 1980s, the trajectory of SARTHI's work gradually began to focus on the status of women in the area, which was quite discouraging. The latter were subjected to exploitation in terms of work overload, desertion, domestic violence, etc. Further, the declining sex ratio in the area, coupled with rampant poverty, malnutrition, and illiteracy, made their case even worse. This resulted in SARTHI developing its first women's health program in the year 1988. The women's health program in the pilot phase had three distinct parts, chronologically implemented: maternal and child health components, participatory research on traditional medicines, and training in gynecology through a self-help approach.

The component on PHR for improving women's health was implemented in several phases. The problems were first identified by the local women, and SARTHI responded by enabling the participation of women as well as obtaining extensive external support. This resulted in creating an alternative model of woman-centered, holistic healthcare at the primary level. An essential part of the introductory work had to do with creating spaces for the local women to start sharing their stories (Khanna 1996). Through workshop sessions, women were encouraged to speak up on their health concerns, ranging from menstruation to childbirth.

Through workshops with traditional healers, village meetings with elders, participatory field exercises with schoolchildren, and field visits with local women in the forests, identification of flora traditionally used to treat common health problems (especially women's gynecological problems) was carried out (Khanna 1996). This process resulted in building a sense of empowerment among local women, as they began to realize the wealth of traditional medicinal knowledge they had. Validation of this was done by a Shodhini (a feminist network in India, doing action research on alternative healing practices based on traditional remedies) botanist, who revealed that almost 80% of the remedies documented by the local women had a strong phytochemical/botanical basis (Khanna 1996). This resulted in further reinforcement. As a result of this PHR approach, the village people began making conscious efforts to propagate medicinal plants and revitalize the knowledge systems of traditional medicines for their primary healthcare needs.

Furthermore, the self-help workshops for training in social and gender-sensitive gynecology were also based on a PHR approach. A team of 11 people (including 8 arogya sakhis,[1] 2 program planners, and 1 facilitator) met regularly each month for 3 days over the course of more than a year, demonstrating a classic example of PHR. In this group, there was no distinction between the researcher and the

---

[1] Arogya means being healthy and sakhi means a friend. Therefore, the term arogya sakhis is used for women selected from the villages who play the role of "health friends" for rural women and girls. They play a crucial role in facilitating conversations with the rural women and girls on their health problems, access to information, health services, practices, and more.

researched. The group of 11 women, 8 of whom were locals, came together as equal members of self-help groups. The research question, i.e., how to treat common health problems of women, was defined jointly. The data were generated by each providing information on her own body and life experiences. The analysis and planning for follow-up action were also done collectively (Khanna 1996). This exercise had a transforming effect on the entire group, where all became more conscious and aware of their health and their rights, ultimately changing the way they responded to critical situations.

SARTHI's women's health program and the application of PHR to achieve health outcomes for rural women emerge as a best practice example. SARTHI's ability to understand the local realities as well as the importance of the bottom-up approach for better healthcare and service resulted in transformed outcomes for the local women's community with respect to their health. Simple approaches of PHR when applied judiciously can have paramount impacts on the people involved, as in this example. This in itself is a major lesson for the policy drivers of the country, who still see health research as an exclusive and top-down area of work.

Key Takeaways

- *The PHR practices by Indian NGOs present a model of how to use this paradigm for furthering development objectives. Through employing simple tools of participatory research in the field of health, the cases of NGOs point toward the need of demystifying the area of health research. This can be done by ensuring people's participation in ways that benefit them as well as the implementing agency.*
- *The variety of settings in which PHR can be applied—such as occupational health, implementation of national programs, community health and sanitation projects, etc.—opens up a plethora of opportunities wherein this paradigm can be used for ensuring sound health outcomes of communities.*
- *The kinds of PHR being undertaken by NGOs indicate that it is time they be viewed not as superficial partners in healthcare management but rather as equal partners in a full-fledged health research process.*
- *The PHR model applied by NGOs can also be scaled up, given that they receive adequate support from governmental agencies and funding bodies. It can then serve as a basis for important inputs to future policy health documents and therefore play a key role in popularizing and validating the practice of PHR in the country.*

Discussion

The aforementioned account helps us in appreciating the fact that PHR can redefine health as an essential component of people's development. It contributes to the vast knowledge systems of indigenous practices of healthcare and helps mainstream this knowledge, thereby contributing to its validity and appropriateness in the era of modern medicine and medical technologies. It also bridges the gap between knowledge and practice by embedding problem-solving and action in research methods (Loewenson et al. 2014). This clearly emerged from the SARTHI case study, where women's traditional knowledge on remedies for ailments led to a sense of mutual empowerment. The PRIA case study demonstrated that PHR also contributes to the demystification of medical terminologies and methods for treatment. For practitioners and promoters of PHR, there is a need for demystifying modern knowledge, technology, and medicine which make people dependent patients, as opposed to being active agents in pursuit of their own health (Tandon 1996). However, the process does not come easy. Among the three main challenges that emerge are:

- *Dynamics of power relations*

PHR requires equal participation of the local community and the external researchers. However, years of subjugation and dominance by the "more powerful" result in mental barriers in the local community who begin to believe that they are incapable of any knowledge generation and see themselves only as passive recipients of handed-down knowledge. Overcoming this challenge requires efforts to build relations of mutual trust, based on respect for the other's values and belief systems. For instance, in the PRIA case study, it took time for the workers to become comfortable with external researchers, and much mutual relationship building effort was necessary before the participants started sharing their experiences.

- *Unlearning and relearning on the part of researchers*

As much difficult as it is for people to *learn* how to contribute to knowledge creation; equally challenging for researchers is to *unlearn* the belief that they have all the answers. As researchers are often used to imposing their own knowledge and beliefs; giving up of this position is not an easy proposition. This requires unlearning of what they have learnt about research as a process and "relearning" values and principles of research as a method of co-generation of knowledge where all stakeholders are considered as equals. The PRIA case study is a model example in this regard, where the disease that was diagnosed by medical experts (that of tuberculosis) based on their academic expertise was actually wrong. It was only after a joint consultation with the workers that the correct diagnosis of silicosis was made.

- *Devising suitable methods of data collection*

Data collection needs to be cleverly intertwined with a series of dialogue and discussions aimed at eliciting people's opinions and voices. It should be a technique to facilitate mutual exchange, rather than just a one-way process of extracting information for research purposes. For instance, in the SARTHI case study, posing questions to women on indigenous medicines in a conventional way did not bear fruit, as the medicines were considered sacred and thus could not be directly named. A better way was to accompany the women to the forests and to document the indigenous medicinal plants when they pointed them out.

Conclusion

The importance of people's health in a country's development agenda is paramount. Sound health brings with it a number of benefits which are directly or indirectly related to a country's well-being, such as increased productivity, educational achievement, increased life expectancy, etc. On the other hand, poor health results in a vicious cycle of malnutrition, decreased productivity, decreased life expectancy, and increased inequities. Therefore, it is essential for a country to focus on health research for addressing the health issues identified by the people by placing the latter at the center of the research process. This would however require strategic actions and a clear vision and mission. Some recommendations in this regard are as follows:

- Firstly, there is a need to move beyond "traditional" notions of research toward more open and inclusive research, one which incorporates multiple dimensions of health and involves all relevant stakeholders.
- Secondly, the policymakers need to push for policy reforms to encourage PHR for finding sustainable solutions to health issues faced by communities. National health research policies could provide a framework for the institutional strengthening of PHR.
- Thirdly, as any PHR initiative involves several partners and the process is subdivided into various stages, adequate funding is crucial for its successful conduct. Governmental and other research funding bodies (foundations, research institutions) should find ways of supporting PHR from a monetary perspective.
- Lastly, capacity building in PHR needs to be done through proper training of stakeholders, built on pedagogical principles like orientation toward research ethics and values, a deep understanding of power and partnerships, incorporation of multiple modes of inquiry, development of the researcher as a facilitator, and a balance between classroom activities and field practice (Tandon and Singh 2016).

To sum up, it can be easily said that with the kind of benefits it carries and the opportunities currently present, PHR in India has the potential to snowball into a potent development tool. There is a need to encourage this field of research by having a facilitative environment and by scaling up the positive efforts at a broader level. This can further lead to far-reaching impacts on individuals, communities, institutions, and governments alike, playing a crucial role in ensuring *Health for All*.

References

Cornwall, A., & Jewkes, R. (1995). What is participatory research. *Social Science & Medicine, 41*(12), 1667–1676.

Government of India (GoI) (2017). Economic Survey 2016–17. Available via INDIA BUDGET. http://indiabudget.nic.in/es2016-17/echapter.pdf. Accessed 6 Jan 2018.

International Collaboration for Participatory Health Research (ICPHR) (2013). What is Participatory Health Research (Position paper no. 1). Available via ICPHR. http://www.icphr. org/uploads/2/0/3/9/20399575/ichpr_position_paper_1_defintion_-_version_may_2013.pdf. Accessed 6 Jan 2018.

Jaitli, H., & Kanhere, V. P. (2005). Occupational health and participatory research. In R. Tandon (Ed.), *Participatory research: Revisiting the roots* (pp. 67–73). New Delhi: Mosaic Books.

Khanna, R. (1996). Participatory action research (PAR) in Women's health: SARTHI, India. In K. K. Koning & M. Martin (Eds.), *Participatory research in health: Issues and experiences* (pp. 62–69). South Africa: National Progressive Primary Health Care Network (NPPHCN) & Zed Books.

Koning, K. D., & Martin, M. (1996). Participatory research in health: Setting the context. In K. K. Koning & M. Martin (Eds.), *Participatory research in health: Issues and experiences* (pp. 1–18). South Africa: National Progressive Primary Health Care Network (NPPHCN) & Zed Books.

Loewenson, R. et al. (2014). Participatory Action Research in Health Systems: A Methods Reader. Available via EQUINETAFRICA. http://www.equinetafrica.org/sites/default/files/uploads/ documents/PAR%20Methods%20Reader2014%20for%20web.pdf. Accessed 6 Jan 2018.

Ministry of Health & Family Welfare Government of India (2014). Framework for Implementation: National Health Mission 2012–2017. http://nhm.gov.in/images/pdf/NHM/NHM_Framework_ for_Implementation__08-01-2014_.pdf. Accessed 6 Jan 2018.

Ministry of Health & Family Welfare Government of India (2017). National Health Policy (NHP) 2017. https://www.nhp.gov.in/NHPfiles/national_health_policy_2017.pdf. Accessed 6 Jan 2018.

NITI Aayog Government of India (2017). India; Three Year Action Agenda (2017–18 to 2019–20). Available via NITI Aayog. http://niti.gov.in/writereaddata/files/coop/IndiaActionPlan.pdf. Accessed 6 Jan 2018.

Onwuegbuzie, A. J., Burke, J. R., & Collins, K. M. T. (2009). Call for mixed analysis: A philosophical framework for combining qualitative and quantitative approaches. *International Journal of Multiple Research Approaches, 3*(2), 114–139.

PRIA. (2004). *Occupational health in India.* New Delhi: PRIA.

Tandon, R. (1996). The historical roots and contemporary tendencies in participatory research: Implications for health care. In K. Koning & M. Martin (Eds.), Participatory Research in Health: Issues and Experiences (pp. 19–26). New Jersey: Zed Books.

Tandon, R., & Singh, W. (2016). Comparative analysis of case studies. In R. Tandon, B. Hall, W. Lepore, & W. Singh (Eds.), *Knowledge and engagement: Building capacity for the next generation of community based researchers* (pp. 253–287). New Delhi: PRIA/University of Victoria.

United Nations Development Program (UNDP) (2016). Human Development Report 2016. Available via UNDP. http://hdr.undp.org/sites/default/files/2016_human_development_report. pdf. Accessed 6 Jan 2018.

World Bank (2015). Gross Domestic Product (2015). Available via WORLD BANK. http://data-bank.worldbank.org/data/download/GDP.pdf. Accessed 6 Jan 2018.

World Health Organization (2016). World Health Report; Statistics 2016. Available via WHO. http://www.who.int/gho/publications/world_health_statistics/2016/en/. Accessed 6 Jan 2018.

Chapter 10
Participatory Health Research in Latin America: Scientific Production on Chronic Diseases

Francisco J. Mercado-Martínez, Leticia Robles-Silva, and Bernardo Jiménez-Domínguez

> *The reliability of a science lies not so much in the positive rigor of its thinking, but in the contribution made by its practice in the collective search for knowledge that will make human beings … more fair, free, critical, creative, participatory, co-responsible, and expressing solidarity*
>
> —Carlos Brandão (2005:45)

Participatory research generated in the Global South, particularly in Latin America, has been part of the international research scene for decades. The best known contributions are those made by Paulo Freire and Orlando Fals-Borda, whose ideas gave rise to the participatory action research tradition (PAR) in the 1970s and 1980s (Hall 1992; Kemmis and McTaggart 2005). Participatory research has been applied in most Latin American countries across different fields, mainly in education and social development (Fals-Borda 1987; Flores-Kastanis et al. 2009), but since the early 1980s, it has been commonly used in the health field (Fals-Borda 1992).

Epidemiological conditions in Latin America at the time were characterized by infectious and nutritional diseases, and so participatory health research (PHR) focused on these problems (Organización Panamericana de la Salud 1998); however, chronic noncommunicable diseases have drawn the attention of PHR scholars in Latin America in recent years due to a shift in the epidemiological landscape. Such conditions have high rates of morbidity and mortality and detrimental effects on the lives of individuals and society (Organización Panamericana de la Salud 2016). And although it is known that there has been PHR on chronic diseases, there is little knowledge about the approaches, directions, and specific types of research in this particular area.

F. J. Mercado-Martínez (✉)
Depto Salud Publica, Universidad de Guadalajara, Guadalajara, Jalisco, Mexico

L. Robles-Silva · B. Jiménez-Domínguez
Universidad de Guadalajara, Guadalajara, Jalisco, Mexico

© Springer International Publishing AG, part of Springer Nature 2018   139
M. T. Wright, K. Kongats (eds.), *Participatory Health Research*,
https://doi.org/10.1007/978-3-319-92177-8_10

The objective of this chapter is thus to examine the PHR carried out on chronic noncommunicable diseases in Latin America. This review focuses on the characteristics of participatory interventions through an examination of the diversity of practices labelled as "participatory" as these practices have been applied in projects focused on chronic noncommunicable diseases. Our analyses focused on the approaches used, for what purpose, who was involved, and which variants of participation were applied in practice.

The chapter is divided into three sections. The first section describes the origins and emergence of participatory research and its variants in Latin America during the second half of the twentieth century. The second section gives an account of existing literature reviews on PHR in the region. The third section describes PHR specifically on chronic noncommunicable diseases in the Latin American countries.

Origins of Participatory Research in Latin America

The intellectual roots of participatory research usually date back to the work of Lewin (1946); however, this author had a marginal influence on its development in Latin America. Participatory research emerged in this region in the 1960s amid a political and intellectual context rich in ideas and proposals for social action, creating a liberation movement. This included popular education, liberation theology, popular social movements, and participatory research. The common feature was the emancipatory advocacy for the oppressed. The liberation movement was driven by authors such as Paulo Freire, Gustavo Gutiérrez, Leonardo Boff, Orlando Fals-Borda, and Joao Bosco Pinto (Brandão 1984). Its development should also be understood as part of the region's resistance in a Cold War era of social tensions and coups, in which the people opposed and resisted through a multitude of social, political, and cultural movements and in which academia was also involved. In this context of turmoil and social unrest, regardless of variations in terminology and specific practices, Latin American participatory research is recognized as part of a Marxist tradition going beyond Kurt Lewin's action research (Brandão 2005), but later going also beyond dogmatic Marxism.

A variety of approaches[1] to participatory research were developed in Latin America during the period from the 1960s to the 1980s. In Brazil and Chile, *thematic research* took shape based on work by Paulo Freire (Osorio 2015) as did *militant research*, which also developed on a common Freirean base of supporting agricultural workers (Freire 1998). Very close to this was *militant observation* which primarily serves the oppressed, and can only be developed together with them, for its purpose and goal is to stimulate the autonomous organization and creativity of this group (Oliveira and Oliveira 1975). Additional roots of this work are

---

[1] Fals-Borda (2001) notes that there are various schools, trends, or streams of participatory research. Other authors refer to approaches, types, or tendencies. In this text we use the term "approaches."

found in the Southern tradition of *participatory research* (Fals-Borda 1991) and *action research*. In Mexico and Central America, in turn, a methodology called *systematization of experiences* was developed in popular education projects (Jara 2012). Paulo Freire and Orlando Fals-Borda were among the most important figures; however, other researchers gave these areas great impetus in particular countries, such as Roscisca Darcy de Oliveira and Miguel Darcy de Oliveira in *militant observation*, Carlos Rodriguez Brandão and Pedro Demo in *participatory research*, and Jean-Marie Michel Thiollent in *action research* in Brazil. Francisco Vio Grossi in Chile and Anton de Shutter and Carlos Nuñez in Mexico also contributed to the development of *participatory research*.

Of the various approaches, the one most used at that time was participatory action research. Its origins date back to the creation of an independent research center by Orlando Fals-Borda, together with two Colombian intellectuals, Gonzalo Castillo and Augusto Libreros, during a meeting in Geneva, Switzerland on July 6, 1970. This center promoted a participatory research method that was called the *social action and research circle*, known as *La Rosca* (Colombian neologism meaning *the circle*). It was based on concepts such as critical reclaiming of local experiences and the systematic return of knowledge (Jiménez 2002). According to Fals-Borda and Rahman (1992), at that time, PAR was distinguished by its anti-corporate activism. This was the reason that a number of academics left their jobs to carry out militant research, using imbedded observation as a radical version of participatory observation, inspired by what Fals-Borda ironically termed a "Talmudic" Marxism.

PAR brought together academics located in what are now identified as epistemologies of the Global South. Paulo Freire, who had been welcomed in Switzerland as an exile of Brazil's military dictatorship, was central, just as his iconic book *Pedagogy of the Oppressed* was about to be published. Another was Rodolfo Stavenhagen who worked in Geneva and, before returning to Mexico, wrote a text on how to decolonize the applied social sciences. However, other intellectual roots can be found in a diverse set of authors, among them Piotr Kropotkin, Georg Lukacs, Antonio Gramsci, Edmund Husserl, José Ortega y Gasset, Agnes Heller, Henri Lefebvre, and Paul Feyerabend.

The theoretical foundations of PAR are brought together in a book that came out of the "World Congress for Participatory Convergence" held in Cartagena, Colombia in 1977 (Fals-Borda 1998). Among its key concepts are experience, common sense, and the integration of academic knowledge and popular knowledge through horizontal participatory experience in a dialogic relationship. Participation is conceptualized as the voluntary and experiential breaking of the asymmetrical relationship of submission and dependence. To achieve this, a type of science based on equal participation and symmetrical reciprocity is proposed, in which the subject of the research becomes a committed actor (Fals Borda et al. 1987). This way of doing science combines an evaluation structure that is critical of knowledge and of the social and cultural context to be transformed and an extensive epistemology that assimilates fairness into liberation (Fals-Borda 1998).

Since the early 1980s, another perspective has been incorporated into participatory research, namely, the *Italian Labor Model*. This model was integrated into an alternative proposal for research in the workplace that called for the active and necessary participation of workers in the development of health evaluations (Laurell et al. 1992). This proposal became widespread throughout Latin America, especially among academics with a Marxist or critical theoretical background, and in union and partisan movements (Loewenson et al. 2014).

These are the intellectual and political roots of participatory research in Latin America, which has given it an important influence in various aspects of society, all of them linked to various protest movements that advocate for oppressed communities, the poor and subordinate groups, except for the *Italian Labor Model*, which is closer to the labor movement.

Participatory Health Research in Latin America: The State of the Art

There have been few reviews of the scientific production of participatory health research in Latin America in spite of its undeniable presence in the region. One pioneering review is the anthology by Vejarano (1983), which includes experiences in the field of health. The author presents the work of 53 researchers from 8 countries in the region who participated in the Second Latin American Seminar on Participatory Research (Patzcuaro, Mexico, 1982). This author argued that the theoretical foundation and richest experiences in Latin America were developed under the contributions of Paulo Freire, Orlando Fals-Borda, Roscisca Darcy de Oliveira, Ramiro Beltrán, and Frank Gerace and the areas of expertise were adult education and rural development. Only the work of Rodríguez (1983) was in the field of health. According to this author, health was not an auspicious field for the practice of participatory research because it was dominated by people with medical training and because health care institutions had a formalized hierarchical structure. Nevertheless, she promoted a participatory approach in an environmental health program to reduce gastrointestinal diseases in rural and poor urban areas (Rodríguez 1983).

Pasteur and Blauert (2000) of the Institute of Development Studies, University of Sussex, published a review titled "Participatory Monitoring and Evaluation in Latin America." Among their findings they highlight that most projects were carried out together with indigenous and rural populations, particularly in rural and social development programs in Colombia, Peru, and Bolivia. A variety of methodologies were found, *participatory rural appraisal* being highlighted. Researchers from developed countries participated in these projects, and funding also came from these countries through development agencies. In addition, there was involvement by non-governmental and governmental organizations in the countries where the projects were carried out. This participatory research focused on environmental, agricultural, water, and housing issues and, to a lesser extent, on health. Most projects related to health concerned infectious and nutritional deficiency diseases.

Another review focused on emerging evaluations in the health field in Latin American and Iberian countries carried out in the 1990s and 2000s (Mercado-Martinez et al. 2008). This review described work with participatory, qualitative, critical, hermeneutical, bottom-up, collaborative, and cross-disciplinary methodologies used for program evaluation. Of the 70 papers reviewed, the most common type of evaluation was participatory, most referring to studies carried out in Brazil, Mexico, and Colombia. As with the other reviews, their primary interest was in programs and services for people with infectious and deficiency diseases.

The review by Grittem et al. (2008), in contrast, only considered the Brazilian publications using the action research approach in the nursing field. According to their findings, the studies were related to public health, obstetrics, and psychiatry topics and were carried out in hospitals and in nursing education. More recently, Thiollent and Toledo (2012) published a paper which reflected on the feasibility and implementation of participatory methodologies and action research in the area of health also in Brazil. Nevertheless, these authors emphasized the participatory action research approach. The authors show how such research has been used to promote health, health care system organization, and training of human resources, as well as to promote research and community-based programs in the universities.

In sum, the above mentioned reviews show that participatory research has been used in the health field in Latin America since the 1980s, although not in all countries of the region. The initiatives have focused on infectious and nutritional deficiency diseases, but do not include applications of participatory research to other diseases, such as chronic noncommunicable diseases or mental disorders. Finally, no particular approach stands out in these reviews.

Participatory Health Research on Chronic Noncommunicable Diseases in Latin America

Twenty-six articles on participatory research on chronic noncommunicable diseases in Latin America were found in this review,[2] and four approaches were identified[3]: participatory action research, action research, community-based participatory

[2] This literature review focuses on articles on empirical studies carried out in the Latin American countries. The electronic bibliography databases searched were Index Medicus, SciELO and Redalyc, and the Google Scholar's database. The following keywords were used: participatory research, participatory visual method, community-based participatory research, participatory health research, participatory action research, and participatory action. These keywords were combined with Boolean commands and the keyword Latin America and the name of each country in the region. We also used a berrypicking/evolving search mode employing two strategies, citation searching and backward chaining through the reference list Bates 1989.

[3] Each article was assigned to a participatory approach according to what its authors themselves

research, and participatory research. Table 10.1 shows a summary of the characteristics of the studies according to their approach.

The Participatory Action Research Approach

Two studies in Chile and one in Colombia were associated with this approach. Their theoretical referents were the Northern tradition citing Kurt Lewin and the Southern tradition citing Orlando Fals-Borda (Krause 2003; Ortiz et al. 2008) as well as other authors as Ernest Stringer and Gloria Pérez Serrano from action research (Krause 2003). It is worth noting that Prieto and Amaya (2014) did not explicitly cite any particular author. Being the most cited author, Fals-Borda's main claim is that participatory action research is a process aimed at initiating and promoting a radical change based on an awareness-building process that includes scientific research, adult education, and political action (Fals-Borda 1987). The aim of these studies goes according with such premise; so the aim of Krause (2003) was to empower a patient self-help group to change their relationship with health workers. The goal of Ortiz et al. (2008) was to sensitize medical students about the experience of being a person with a chronic disease to change their attitudes when interacting with them. Meanwhile, Prieto and Amaya (2014) intended to modify the patient's knowledge on hypertension and its risk factors.

The academic partners were professors at public universities, medical and psychology researchers in the case of the Chilean study (Krause 2003), research assistants (Ortiz et al. 2008), and nursing students in Colombia (Prieto and Amaya 2014). The non-academic partners were adult and elderly patients at a teaching hospital (Krause 2003), university workers with risk factors for cardiovascular disease (Prieto and Amaya 2014), and medical students (Ortiz et al. 2008). The academic partners initiated the whole process and defined all research stages and strategies.

Non-academic partners participated in a variety of ways: university workers participated in dialogical workshops according to the principles of Freire and were asked to suggest the topics for the workshops (Prieto and Amaya 2014); the self-help group participated in workshops designed on the basis of a psycho–social assessment using qualitative and quantitative techniques and strategies based on community psychology, the theory of social support for community interventions, and sessions where legal advice was given to individuals and the group (Krause 2003). Medical students were involved by accompanying patients, who acted as educators, to convey their experiences in a series of meetings. The participatory interaction was between the student and the person with the disease, but not with the

---

declared in the methodology section. The PHR characteristics analyzed were the approach or tradition behind the research, which authors' framework were used, the purpose of the study, the participants involved, and the level of participation.

Table 10.1 Characteristics of participatory health research on chronic diseases in Latin America according to their approaches

Reference	Tradition and author(s) referred	Country/disease	Purpose of participation	Academic (Ac) and non-academic (NAc) partners/ level of participation	Intervention features
Participatory action research (PAR) approach					
Krause (2003)	*Participatory action research* Orlando Fals-Borda Kurt Lewin Action research Gloria Perez Serrano Ernest Stringer	Chile Crohn's disease	To empower a self-help group	Ac: a psychology researcher Participation: in all research phases NAc: sick people participating in a self-help group in a teaching hospital Participation: in the workshops	*Workshops* a. Thematic expositions b. Community dynamics c. Legal advise
Ortiz et al. (2008)	*Participatory action research* Orlando Fals- Borda Kurt Lewin	Chile Chronic diseases	To modify their perceptions on the illness experience	Ac: medicine professors and research assistants Participation: in all research phases NAc: students of medicine Participation: in the intervention	Accompaniment of chronically ill individuals
Prieto and Amaya (2014)	No author nor approach	Colombia Cardiovascular disease	To modify knowledge about the disease	Ac: nursing professors and nursing students Participation: students are in charge of the workshop NAc: university workers with risk factors Participation: in the workshop	*Dialogic workshop* a. Thematic expositions b. Presentation of experiences c. Dialogic sessions

(continued)

Table 10.1 (continued)

Reference	Tradition and author(s) referred	Country/disease	Purpose of participation	Academic (Ac) and non-academic (NAc) partners/ level of participation	Intervention features
Action research (AR) approach					
Andrade and Rodrigues (2002)	*Action research* Michel Thiollent	Brazil	To improve the quality of nursing care increasing the knowledge about family's experience	Ac: nursing professors Participation: in all research phases NAc: families of sick people who attend a public hospital Participation: in the sessions	Sessions a. Interchange of experiences
		Stroke			
Ataíde and Damasceno (2006)	*Action research* Michel Thiollent	Brazil	a. To improve self-care changing knowledge and behavior b. To empower sick people	Ac: nursing professors Participation: in all research phases NAc: sick people who attend primary health care Participation: only in the educational sessions	*Educational sessions* a. Participatory dialog
		Diabetes			
Ávila-Schwerter et al. (2016)	No author	Chile	To improve health care elaborating a therapy guide	Ac: public and sexual health researchers Participation: in all research phases NAc: health professionals of a tertiary hospital and health workers Participation: in all phases after the guide design	*Workshops* a. Delphi method b. Sessions to modify and take co-joint decisions
		Thyroid cancer			

Carvalho et al. (2004)	*Action research* Michel Thiollent	Brazil Osteoporosis	a. To improve self-care increasing people's health knowledge b. To become a promoter of health knowledge in the community	Ac: medicine and nutrition researchers Participation: in all research phases NAc: healthy old people who attend a third age university Participation: in the educational sessions	*Educational sessions* a. Exposition b. Group dynamics
Cesarino and Casagrande (1998)	*Action research* Michel Thiollent *Emancipatory education* Paulo Freire	Brazil Chronic kidney disease	To improve self-care changing people's health knowledge and behavior	Ac: nursing professors Participation: in all research phases NAc: sick people who attend a teaching hospital Participation: in the educational sessions	*Awareness education* a. Discussion circles b. Problematizing situations
Lima et al. (2016)	*Qualitative method* Augusto Triviños	Brazil Chronic kidney disease	To improve nursing care through health promotion	Ac: nursing professors and research assistants Participation: in all research phases NAc: sick people who attend a public hospital and health workers of such hospital Participation: in the sessions	*Sessions* a. Interchange of experiences

(continued)

Table 10.1 (continued)

Reference	Tradition and author(s) referred	Country/disease	Purpose of participation	Academic (Ac) and non-academic (NAc) partners/ level of participation	Intervention features
Luce et al. (1990)	*Action research* Michel Thiollent	Brazil Diabetes	To improve self-care through the acquisition of health knowledge	*Ac:* nursing professors and research assistants Participation: in all research phases *NAc:* sick people and their families who attend a teaching hospital Participation: in the educational sessions *NAc:* head nurse Participation: interactive participation in all phases	*Educational sessions* a. Expositions b. Delivery of educational material
Moura et al. (2014)	*Qualitative method* Maria Cecilia Minayo	Brazil Chronic kidney disease	To cope better with the hospitalization process through capacity building	*Ac:* psychology, medicine, and nursing professors Participation: in all research phases *NAc:* sick children and adolescents in a public teaching hospital Participation: in the workshop	*Workshop* a. Registration of experiences in a book b. Interchange of experiences
Rêgo et al. (2006)	*Action research* Michel Thiollent *Emancipatory education* Paulo Freire	Brazil Diabetes	a. To improve self-care through enhancing capacity b. To become a promoter of health knowledge in the community	*Ac:* nursing professors Participation: in all research phases *NAc:* sick people who attend primary health centers Participation: in the educational sessions	Health education a. Dialogical and participatory sessions

Sabóia and Valente (2010)	*Action research* René Barbier	Brazil Diabetes	To improve self-care increasing sick people health's knowledge	*Ac:* nursing professors Participation: in all the research phases *NAc:* individuals with diabetes attending a primary health center and nursing students Participation: in the educational sessions	*Health education* a. Exposition of topics b. Discussion of topics among health professionals, students, and sick people
Souza et al. (2015)	*Qualitative method* Marli André	Brazil Cervical cancer	To increase sick people's knowledge regarding risk factors	*Ac:* nursing professors Participation: in all research phases *NAc:* sick people attending a primary health center Participation: in the educational sessions	*Popular education* a. Dialogic sessions b. Group dynamics
Community-based participatory research (CBPR) approach					
Abuelo et al. (2014)	CBPR Meredith Minkler Nina Wallerstein	Peru Cancer	To decrease barriers in the screen/treat and vaccination program	*Ac:* medical researchers from the USA, Mexico, and Peru Participation: in all phases of the design and prevention strategy *NAc:* community health leaders Participation: in the modification of the strategy	*Training program* a. Thematic exposition b. Session to talk about the strategy implementation

(continued)

Table 10.1 (continued)

Reference	Tradition and author(s) referred	Country/disease	Purpose of participation	Academic (Ac) and non-academic (NAc) partners/level of participation	Intervention features
Berger-González et al. (2016)	CBPR Barbara Israel et al. Meredith Minkler Nina Wallerstein	Guatemala Cancer	a. To promote a co-learning process between indigenous specialists, western doctors, and scientists regarding cancer treatment b. To empower indigenous Mayan medical specialists	Ac: medical researchers from Switzerland and the scientific advisory board NAc: Mayan elders of the traditional medical system Participation: Ac and NAc partners participate in all phases of the elaboration and implementation process	*Workshops* a. Interactive process to interchange knowledge based on a transdisciplinarity approach b. Conjoint design of methods, instruments, and strategies of the research
Levinson et al. (2013)	CBPR Meredith Minkler Nina Wallerstein	Peru Cancer	To decrease barriers in the screen/treat and vaccination program	Ac: medical researchers from the USA, Mexico, and Peru Participation: in all research phases NAc: population of a rural community, community-health leaders, midwife, health technician, and nurse Participation: in the modification of the strategy	*Training program* a. Thematic exposition b. Interchange of ideas to implement the strategy

Martín et al. (2010)	CBPR Meredith Minkler Nina Wallerstein	Puerto Rico Asthma	To design a culturally tailored management intervention	*Ac:* researchers from Puerto Rico and the USA Participation: in all research phases *NAc:* familial caregivers of low-income urban people Participation: in the educational sessions *NAc:* medical practitioners and stakeholders of the Public Health Department Participation: in the workshops	*Educational sessions* a. Thematic exposition b. Session with experts *Workshops* a. Meetings

Participatory research (PR) approach

Ferretti et al. (2014)	*Action research* Michel Thiollent	Brazil Cardiovascular disease	a. To increase health knowledge b. To become a promoter of health knowledge in their community	*Ac:* public health and nutrition professors and physiotherapy students Participation: in all research phases *NAc:* healthy old people attending a primary health center Participation: in the educational sessions	*Health education* a. Educational intervention
Noronha (1986)	*Participatory action research* Orlando Fals-Borda *Emancipatory education* Paulo Freire	Brazil Cancer	To improve self-care increasing sick people's knowledge	*Ac:* nursing professor Participation: in all research phases *NAc:* sick people attending a school hospital Participation: in the educational sessions	*Liberating education* a. Presenting experiential situations b. Provision of information

(continued)

Table 10.1 (continued)

Reference	Tradition and author(s) referred	Country/disease	Purpose of participation	Academic (Ac) and non-academic (NAc) partners/ level of participation	Intervention features
Santos and Lima (2008)	None	Brazil Hypertension	a. To modify risk factors adopting healthy lifestyles b. To become a promoter of health knowledge in the community	*Ac:* nursing professors and postgraduate students Participation: in all research phases *NAc:* workers of a public university Participation: in the educational sessions	*Educational workshops* a. Group dynamics b. Training c. Use of educational health technologies
Santos et al. (2011)	*Qualitative method* Pedro Demo	Brazil Hypertension	To modify risk factors adopting healthy behaviors	*Ac:* nursing and physical education professors Participation: in all research phases *NAc:* parents of healthy kindergarten children Participation: in the educational workshops	*Educational workshops* a. Educational technology in health b. Thematic exposition and discussion
Silva et al. (2015)	*Action research* Michel Thiollent	Brazil Diabetes	To elaborate an instrument to evaluate competences for the clinical practice	*Ac:* medicine professors Participation: in all research phases and the instrument design *NAc:* students of medicine and medical specialists Participation: in discussing and modifying the instrument	*Workshop in a virtual environment* a. Dialogic relationships b. Knowledge confrontation c. Knowledge reflection

Spinato et al. (2010)	None	Brazil Hypertension	a. To modify risk factors acquiring healthy behaviors b. To become a promoter of health knowledge in the community	*Ac*: nursing and physiotherapy professors and Ph.D. students Participation: in all research phases *NAc*: sick people attending a hospital Participation: in the educational workshops	*Educational workshops* a. Socialization of experiences b. Exposition c. Healthy behaviors practice
Torres et al. (2010)	*Action research* Michel Thiollent *Emancipatory education* Paulo Freire	Brazil Diabetes	To learn health education to use in the clinical practice	*Ac*: nursing and public health professors Participation: in all research phases *NAc*: health professionals in primary health centers Participation: in the workshops	*Training workshops* a. Dialogic sessions b. Socialization of experiences c. Ludic dynamics d. Expert panel
Torres et al. (2012)	None	Brazil Diabetes	To improve self-care increasing sick people's knowledge and capacity building	*Ac*: nursing professors and students Participation: in all research phases *NAc*: sick people attending health services Participation: in the educational sessions	*Educational sessions* a. Ludic dynamics b. Texts and poems reading c. Experiences telling d. Exchange of recipes

academic partners, who only recorded changes before and after the meetings (Ortiz et al. 2008).

The three studies were centered on capacity building through a process of co-learning where non-academics shared their knowledge and experiences in order to create a new understanding. Although the intervention was controlled by the academic partners, the non-academics developed an interactive participation.

The Action Research Approach

Ten studies carried out in Brazil and one in Chile are associated with the Southern tradition of action research. According with Thiollent and Toledo (2012), action research is focused on research with the explicit action of an actor or a set of actors and the use of participatory methods. It has two main objectives: (a) problem-solving and (b) knowledge-building. In theory, action research is guided by a change in democratic values, such as in issues of citizenship, struggle against discrimination, humanization of care, and emancipation. Six Brazilian studies cite as a methodological and theoretical reference the work of the Franco-Brazilian researcher Michel Thiollent, while another cites the French researcher René Barbier. Three studies refer to general works on qualitative methodology, authored by Brazilian scholars such as Augusto Triviños, Maria Cecilia Minayo, and Marli André, who classify action research as a qualitative method following Carlos Brandão and René Barbier. The Chilean study does not cite any author in reference to the action research approach (Ávila-Schwerter et al. 2016).

The purpose of these studies was to promote the health of the patients or individuals with risk factors – diabetes, chronic renal failure, and cancer – living in urban areas. Their intention was to convey information about the characteristics of the disease, its risk factors, and the treatment so that people could better direct their actions and take responsibility for their self-care; another goal was that the participants would become health knowledge multipliers in their communities (Ataíde and Damasceno 2006; Carvalho et al. 2004; Cesarino and Casagrande 1998; Luce et al. 1990; Moura et al. 2014; Rêgo et al. 2006; Sabóia and Valente 2010; Souza et al. 2015). Other studies were interested in improving the quality of services, so their target groups were primary health care and teaching hospital workers. Their purpose was to modify the knowledge of these professionals about the condition of the patients, to improve health care (Andrade and Rodrigues 2002; Lima et al. 2016) or to develop a management model for comprehensive care of cancer patients (Ávila-Schwerter et al. 2016). The goals of these studies are related to making changes in health knowledge and behavior; they are not interested in increasing or constructing community capacities.

The authors, as academic partners, were professors at public universities, some only of nursing (Andrade and Rodrigues 2002; Ataíde and Damasceno 2006;

Cesarino and Casagrande 1998; Lima et al. 2016; Luce et al. 1990; Rêgo et al. 2006; Souza et al. 2015), while others were nursing professors together with students (Sabóia and Valente 2010) or of multidisciplinary teams – medicine, psychology, public health, and nutrition (Ávila-Schwerter et al. 2016; Carvalho et al. 2004; Moura et al. 2014). Non-academic partners, in turn, were the patients and their families who participated in two of the studies (Andrade and Rodrigues 2002; Luce et al. 1990). But nurses (Luce et al. 1990; Rêgo et al. 2006; Souza et al. 2015; Lima et al. 2016) and medical specialists at the hospital also participated as non-academic partners.

In most studies, the non-academic partners only participated in the educational intervention phase in order to change or acquire new knowledge. The academic partners planned and carried out all stages of the investigation, as well as evaluated the educational needs of the non-academic partners, using qualitative techniques such as participant observation (Cesarino and Casagrande 1998; Moura et al. 2014; Souza et al. 2015), focus groups (Ataíde and Damasceno 2006), or questionnaires (Carvalho et al. 2004). From the information gathered by these means, the academic partners designed the educational sessions, supported by contents of health education, health promotion, or popular education. In most studies, the patients interacted with the academic partners in the sessions, based on a participatory dialog and group dynamics of community psychology. Another form of participation was when the patients, in addition to attending educational sessions, were consulted on issues to be included in the educational interventions based on Freire's principles of liberating education (Rêgo et al. 2006; Sabóia and Valente 2010). The participation of health workers was of two types. One was an interactive participation where the academic partners modified, analyzed, and evaluated the intervention and the development of the research (Luce et al. 1990; Ávila-Schwerter et al. 2016). The other consisted in the provision of information and the exchange of experiences with the academic partners, so that they could plan and implement the intervention (Andrade and Rodrigues 2002; Lima et al. 2016). This form of participation could be named participation by consultation (Cornwall 2008), since the professionals, or academic partners, defined the problems, gathered the information, and controlled the decision-making process.

The Community-Based Participatory Research (CBPR) Approach

Four studies were aligned with the Northern tradition of CBPR, being inspired by the work of Minkler and Wallerstein (2008) and Israel et al. (2005). This tradition takes the perspectives that participation involves research, action, and education in a collaborative democratic process, with the aim to improve the community members' lives. The researchers and the community members negotiate information and capacities in both directions to pursue mutual knowledge: researchers transfer tools for community members to analyze their conditions and take informed decisions on actions; meanwhile community members transfer their expert content and meanings to researchers (Wallerstein and Duran 2003).

The abovementioned studies include poor and powerless people as target groups and the studies' purpose was to improve the health of specific populations and the quality of the services by addressing organizational issues. The aim of the study with indigenous Mayan medical specialists in Guatemala was to promote a co-learning process between the indigenous specialists, Western medical doctors, and scientists regarding the treatment of cancer in indigenous people, and to empower indigenous Mayan medical specialists (Berger-González et al. 2016). Two studies with community health workers in poor rural communities in Peru had the goal of improving the quality of services by addressing barriers in a mother/child screen/ treat-and-vaccinate program for cervical cancer prevention (Abuelo et al. 2014; Levinson et al. 2013). The fourth study sought to improve the health of asthmatic children in low-income families in Puerto Rico through a culturally tailored asthma management intervention (Martín et al. 2010).

The academic partners were medical and psychology researchers from both within and outside Latin America, USA–Mexico–Peru, USA–Puerto Rico, and Switzerland. Only the study by Berger-González et al. (2016) involved another type of academic partner, a scientific advisory board composed of European, American, and Guatemalan researchers. None of the studies included individuals with chronic diseases as non-academic partners, but some included people who interfaced directly with people with such conditions, these being members of the community, as in the case of the elders in the indigenous Mayan medical system (Berger-González et al. 2016) or community health workers (Abuelo et al. 2014; Levinson et al. 2013). The other non-academic partners were medical practitioners and family caregivers (Martín et al. 2010).

There was only one study in which both academic and non-academic partners participated in all stages of the research process. This was the study by Berger-González et al. (2016) in which all parties worked together during several workshops to define, negotiate, and reach a consensus on the design and methods of each phase of the investigation. In the other studies, the academic partners decided a priori the intervention while the non-academic partners only were involved in one phase of the study, but such involvement was an interactive participation with the academic partners. The community health workers in Peru modified and adapted the strategies for the advertisement, recording, delivery of samples, reporting results, and vaccination of the women during the training program (Abuelo et al. 2014; Levinson et al. 2013). The same was true of the medical practitioners who participated in developing the intervention (Martín et al. 2010). Family caregivers were the only partners who did not participate interactively, being passive recipients of a multidisciplinary panel meeting (Martín et al. 2010).

These studies, driven by interactive participation, developed a strategy of either sharing ownership of the intervention, joint problem-solving, or involvement in making decisions. As a result, academics and non-academics shared almost equal participation during the project development.

The Participatory Research Approach

There were eight studies carried out in Brazil in which the authors claim they used a participatory approach. These studies are based more on the principles of several PHR approaches than on one particular approach. For example, some authors cite Thiollent in reference to action research (Ferretti et al. 2014; Silva et al. 2015; Torres et al. 2010, 2012), but others cite Fals-Borda in reference to PAR (Noronha 1986), and others refer to general qualitative methodological works that allude to participatory research (Santos and Lima 2008), and two even do not reference any author on participatory research (Santos et al. 2011; Spinato et al. 2010). In this respect, the authors only claim an adhesion to the participation principles, but not to a particular approach of participatory research.

The purpose of some studies was that individuals with diabetes and arterial hypertension or with risk factors would recognize their self-management or their lifestyles as a problem in order to and modify them. To achieve this, they sought to change their knowledge and behavior to adopt healthy behaviors. To encourage self-care, the researchers focused on the transmission of knowledge about the disease, its risk factors, and treatment (Ferretti et al. 2014; Noronha 1986; Torres et al. 2012). In contrast, other studies that were interested in the adoption of healthy behaviors or lifestyles used health promotion models for bringing about changes in nutrition and physical activity (Santos and Lima 2008; Santos et al. 2011; Spinato et al. 2010). Two more studies focused on health professionals. One designed a tool to assess medical students' level of knowledge about diabetes (Silva et al. 2015); and the other, linked to health education, intended to improve the clinical management of diabetes (Torres et al. 2010).

The academic partners in these studies were professors at public universities; some participated in multidisciplinary groups (nursing, public health, nutrition, physiotherapy, physical education, and medicine); others were professors of nursing or medicine and master's or doctoral students (Spinato et al. 2010; Torres et al. 2012). The non-academic partners were of three types. One type were adult patients of public health services (Noronha 1986; Spinato et al. 2010) or private health services (Torres et al. 2012); the second type were elderly and healthy people such as university workers (Santos and Lima 2008), parents of preschool children (Santos et al. 2011), and elderly people receiving primary care (Ferretti et al. 2014); and the last type were members of health care center teams (Torres et al. 2010), medical students, and medical specialists (Silva et al. 2015).

In the studies that used this approach, none of the issues were chosen by the non-academic partners, since they only participated in a single stage of the research. The academic partners initiated the study, defined the problem, and identified the needs of the non-academic partners. The latter was done through questionnaires or semi-structured interviews (Noronha 1986; Santos et al. 2011; Spinato et al. 2010), the information gathered from previous studies (Santos and Lima 2008), or the curriculum requirements of their education program in the case of students and medical professionals (Torres et al. 2010). Non-academic partners were only consulted in two studies, when were asked to suggest topics for the educational intervention (Ferretti et al. 2014; Torres et al. 2012). Based on this information, the academic partners devised solutions supporting their proposals for popular education (Ferretti et al. 2014), health promotion (Santos and Lima 2008; Santos et al. 2011), or Freire's consciousness-raising education (Noronha 1986; Spinato et al. 2010; Torres et al. 2010, 2012).

Participation by non-academic partners was limited to the educational intervention phase where they interacted with their academic partners. The interventions were workshops, exhibitions, group or recreational sessions, or educational technology. They were based on life-experience situations and personal stories and then continued with dialog, reflection, and critical thinking as part of the workshop. If the intention was to change behaviors, participant training, such as doing a particular physical activity, was included. The only study that included interactive participation between academic and non-academic partners was one in which they cooperated in the design of an instrument to assess their clinical skills for diabetes diagnosis and treatment. Digital technologies were used to facilitate joint participation by students, medical specialists, and academic partners through a dialogical interaction in which they structured, evaluated, corrected, and improved the assessment tool (Silva et al. 2015).

To sum up, the studies included in this approach are characterized by a combination of passive and functional participation, in which the participation can be seen as simply a pretense. Non-academic participants were involved in a process of consultation, but without any shared decision-making. At the end, they were the passive targets of academic projects.

Final Considerations

Our PHR findings on chronic noncommunicable diseases in Latin America demonstrate the continuity of the Southern tradition into the twenty-first century. Several findings from this review regarding the practices of this tradition in the region stand out. The studies are located in only a few countries – Brazil, Colombia, Chile, Peru, and Guatemala – which are the countries that have a prior tradition of participatory research. The absence of PHR projects in the rest of Latin America is surprising, particularly Mexico, given its prominence in this subject area for several decades (Castillo-Burgete et al. 2008; Rodríguez and

Hernández 1994).[4] This indicates the need to extend the review to books, doctoral theses, and gray literature to provide a broader picture of the research on chronic noncommunicable diseases.

The origins of participatory health research in Latin America are recognized in these studies, showing the continuity of such research into the field of chronic noncommunicable diseases. The researchers not only use the approaches that gave rise to the Southern tradition in Latin America but also continue to reference authors such as Paulo Freire, Michell Thiollent, and Carlos Brandão. Nevertheless, a shift was found in regard to the participatory approaches; action research has become the most commonly used, displacing participatory action research and Fals-Borda as the classical references in Latin America. Furthermore, the presence of CBPR, due to the influence of foreign academics, gives evidence of the incursion of the Northern tradition into Latin America. Future work should review research in other medical fields, such as health promotion education, to confirm the transition observed here.

Transformations were also observed in the practice of participation in these projects. Those people who form part of the "community" are no longer the poor or the powerless, as was the case when participatory research began in Latin America; now there are a variety of actors, and it is not always the sick individuals who make up the target groups. Health care workers, professionals, and students have become subjects of interest in many of these projects. The academic partners, in turn, are also scholars from Latin America as well as from the Northern countries, and they are no longer independent of institutions, as in the past.

Another important change relates to different types of participation according to the actors' involvement. If the term "participatory" is applied to a study, it should mean that all participants are actively involved in all aspects of the research process (ICPHR 2013), but this is not always the case, as non-academic partners are generally involved in only one phase of the study, particularly when such partners are chronically sick people. Some studies implemented top-down forms of participation that involved academic partners exploring the needs of non-academic partners and developing independent strategic plans to address them. In such cases, there was no opportunity for non-academic partners to become involved in decision-making and action-taking, and their participation was limited to that of being passive recipients of a service. Collaborative forms of participation only occurred when the non-academic partners were medical practitioners, including practitioners of traditional medicine. Given these differences, it is necessary to conduct a deeper examination into the social contexts that explain such situations, as well as to explore ways of strengthening the participation of stakeholders.

---

[4] Libertad Hernández Landa was raped and murdered in August 1998 after being threatened as a result of her participatory research work on pederasty and child exploitation. This case is one of the Latin American experiences that illustrates the risks faced by committed researchers that go beyond value neutrality in their research practice.

References

Abuelo, C. E., Levinson, K. L., Salmeron, J., Vallejos, C., Vallejos, M. C., & Belinson, J. (2014). The Peru cervical cancer screening study (PERCAPS): The design and implementation of a mother/daughter screen, treat, and vaccinate program in the Peruvian jungle. *Journal of Community Health, 39*(3), 409–415.

Andrade, O., & Rodrigues, R. (2002). Abordagem holística do sistema de cuidado familiar do idoso com acidente vascular cerebral. *Revista Ciência, Cuidado e Saúde, 1*(1), 185–191.

Ataíde, M., & Damasceno, M. (2006). Fatores que interferem na adesão ao autocuidado em diabetes. *Revista Enfermagem UERJ, 14*(4), 518–523.

Ávila-Schwerter, C., Torres-Andrade, M. C., Méndez, C., & Márquez-Manzano, M. (2016). Modelamiento del proceso clínico para manejo de usuarios con cáncer tiroideo diferenciado en el Hospital Base Valdivia, Chile. *Revista Calidad Asistencial, 31*(4), 190–195.

Bates, M. J. (1989). The design of browsing and berrypicking techniques for the online search interface. *Online Review, 13*(5), 407–424.

Berger-González, M., Stauffacher, M., Zinsstag, J., Edwards, P., & Krütli, P. (2016). Transdisciplinary research on cancer-healing systems between biomedicine and the Maya of Guatemala: A tool for reciprocal reflexivity in a multi-epistemological setting. *Qualitative Health Research, 26*(1), 77–91.

Brandão, C. (1984). *Repensando a pesquisa participante*. Sao Paulo: Editora Brasiliense.

Brandão, C. (Ed.). (2005). Participatory research and participation in research: A look between times and spaces from Latin America. *International Journal of Action Research, 1*(1), 43–68.

Carvalho, C., Fonseca, C. C., & Pedrosa, J. (2004). Educação para a saúde em osteoporose com idosos de um programa universitário: Repercussões. *Cadernos de Saúde Pública, 20*(3), 719–726.

Castillo-Burgete, M. T., Viga, M. D., & Dickinson, F. (2008). Changing the culture of dependency to allow for successful outcomes in participatory research: Fourteen years of experience in Yucatan, Mexico. In P. Reason & H. Bradbury (Eds.), *The SAGE handbook of action research. Participative inquiry and practice* (2nd ed., pp. 522–533). Los Angeles: SAGE Publications.

Cesarino, C., & Casagrande, L. D. (1998). Paciente com insuficiência renal crônica em tratamento hemodialítico: Atividade educativa do enfermeiro. *Revista Latino-Americana de Enfermagem, 6*(4), 31–40.

Cornwall, A. (2008). Unpacking 'participation': Models, meanings and practices. *Community Development Journal, 43*(3), 269–283.

Fals Borda, O., Brandão, C., & Cetrulo, R. (1987). *Investigación participativa*. Montevideo: Instituto del Hombre.

Fals-Borda, O. (1987). The application of participatory action-research in Latin America. *International Sociology, 2*(4), 329–347.

Fals-Borda, O. (1991). Some basic ingredients. In O. Fals-Borda & M. A. Rahman (Eds.), *Action and knowledge. Breaking the monopoly with participatory action-research* (pp. 3–12). New York: The Apex Press.

Fals-Borda, O. (1992). Evolution and convergence in participatory action-research. In J. S. Frideres (Ed.), *A world of communities: Participatory research perspectives* (pp. 14–19). North York: Captus University Publications.

Fals-Borda, O. (1998). *Participación popular: Retos del futuro*. Bogotá: Universidad Nacional de Colombia.

Fals-Borda, O. (2001). Participatory (action) research in social theory: Origins and challenges. In P. Reason & H. Bradbury (Eds.), *Handbook of action research: Participative inquiry and practice* (pp. 27–37). London: Sage Publications.

Fals-Borda, O., & Rahman, M. A. (1992). La situación actual y las perspectivas de la investigación-acción participativa en el mundo. In M. C. Salazar (Ed.), *La investigación-acción participativa. Inicios y desarrollos* (pp. 205–223). Bogotá: Editorial Magisterio.

Ferretti, F., Gris, A., Mattiello, D., Rosane, C., Teo, P., & Sá, C. (2014). Impacto de programa de educação em saúde no conhecimento de idosos sobre doenças cardiovasculares. *Revista de Salud Pública, 16*(6), 807–820.

Flores-Kastanis, E., Montoya-Vargas, J., & Suárez, D. H. (2009). Investigación-acción participativa en la educación latinoamericana. Un mapa de otra parte del mundo. *Revista Mexicana de Investigación Educativa, 14*(40), 289–308.

Freire, P. (1998). *Pedagogy of freedom: Ethics, democracy, and civic courage*. Oxford: Rowman & Littlefield.

Grittem, L., Meier, M. J., & Zagonel, I. P. (2008). Pesquisa-ação: uma alternativa metodológica para pesquisa em enfermagem. *Texto & Contexto Enfermagem, 17*(4), 765–770.

Hall, B. L. (1992). From margins to center? The development and purpose of participatory research. *The American Sociologist, 23*(4), 15–28.

International Collaboration for Participatory Health Research (ICPHR). (2013). *Position paper 1: What is participatory health research? Version: Mai 2013*. Berlin: International Collaboration for Participatory Health Research.

Israel, B. A., Parker, E. A., Rowe, Z., Salvatore, A., Minkler, M., López, J., et al. (2005). Community-based participatory research: Lessons learned from the centers for children's environmental health and disease prevention research. *Environmental Health Perspectives, 113*(10), 1463–1471.

Jara, O. (2012). *La sistematización de experiencias: Práctica y teoría para otros mundos posibles*. San José: Centro de Estudios y Publicaciones Alforja, Consejo de Educación de Adultos de América Latina e Intermon-Oxfam.

Jiménez, B. (2002). Investigación-acción participante: una dimensión desconocida. In M. Montero (Ed.), *Psicología social comunitaria. Teoría, método y experiencia* (pp. 103–137). Guadalajara: Universidad de Guadalajara.

Kemmis, S., & McTaggart, R. (2005). Participatory action research. Communicative action and the public sphere. In N. K. Denzin & Y. Lincoln (Eds.), *The SAGE handbook of qualitative research* (3th ed., pp. 559–604). Thousand Oaks: Sage.

Krause, M. (2003). The transformation of social representations of chronic disease in a self-help group. *Journal of Health Psychology, 8*(5), 599–615.

Laurell, A. C., Noriega, M., Martínez, S., & Villegas, J. (1992). Participatory research on workers' health. *Social Science & Medicine, 34*(6), 603–613.

Levinson, K., Abuelo, C., Chyung, E., Salmeron, J., Belinson, S. E., Vallejos, C., et al. (2013). The Peru cervical cancer prevention study (PERCAPS): Community-based participatory research in Manchay, Peru. *International Journal of Gynecological Cancer, 23*(1), 141–147.

Lewin, K. (1946). Action research and minority problems. *Journal of Social Issues, 2*(4), 34–46.

Lima, M., Galiza, F. T., Xavier, F. R., Medeiros, J. R., Moura, F. E., & Araújo, L. L. (2016). Cultura de aprendizagem em nefrologia. *Revista de Enfermagem da Universidade Federal do Piauí, 5*(1), 73–78.

Loewenson, R., Laurell, A. C., Hogstedt, C., D'Ambruoso, L., & Shroff, Z. (2014). *Investigación acción participativa en sistemas de salud: Una guía de métodos*. Ottawa: TARSC, AHPSR, WHO, IDRC-Canada, EQUINET Harare.

Luce, M., Padilha, M., Almeida, R. L., & Silva, M. (1990). O preparo o autocuidado do cliente diabético e família. *Revista Brasileira de Enfermagem, 43*(1, 2, 3/4), 36–43.

Martín, C., Andrade, A., Vila, D., Acosta-Pérez, E., & Canino, G. (2010). The development of a community-based family asthma management intervention for Puerto Rican children. *Progress in Community Health Partnerships: Research, Education, and Action, 4*(4), 315–324.

Mercado-Martinez, F. J., Tejada-Tayabas, L. M., & Springett, J. (2008). Methodological issues in emergent evaluations of health programs: Lessons from Iberoamerica. *Qualitative Health Research, 18*(9), 1277–1288.

Minkler, M., & Wallerstein, N. (Eds.). (2008). *Community-based participatory research for health: From process to outcomes* (2nd ed.). San Francisco: Wiley.

Moura, F., Júnior, A. L., Dantas, M., Araújo, G., & Collet, N. (2014). Playful intervention with chronically-ill children: Promoting coping. *Revista Gaúcha de Enfermagem, 35*(2), 86–92.

Noronha, R. (1986). Experiência participativa mobilizadora de enfermagem: Condições previas para o autocuidado. *Revista Brasileira de Enfermagem, 39*(1), 34–43.

Oliveira, R., & Oliveira, M. (1975). *The militant observer: A sociological alternative, IDAC Document 9.* Geneva: The Institute.

Organización Panamericana de la Salud. (1998). *La salud en las Américas. Publicación Científica 569.* Washington, DC: Organización Panamericana de la Salud.

Organización Panamericana de la Salud. (2016). *Aplicación de modelos para mejorar las decisiones en materia de política sanitaria y económica en las Américas: El caso de las enfermedades no transmisibles.* Washington, DC: OPS.

Ortiz, A., Beca, J. P., Salas, S. P., Browne, F., & Salas, C. (2008). Acompañamiento del enfermo: Una experiencia de aprendizaje sobre el significado de la enfermedad. *Revista Médica de Chile, 136*(3), 304–309.

Osorio, J. (2015). De la investigación participativa fundacional a la investigación-acción participativa pro-común: Ensayo memorial desde la historia de la educación popular latinoamericana y las redes del CEAAL. *La Piragua. Revista Latinoamericana y Caribeña de Educación y Política, 41*(noviembre), 29–34.

Pasteur, K., & Blauert, J. (2000). *Participatory monitoring and evaluation in Latin America: Overview of the literature with annotated bibliography* (Vol. 18). Sussex: Institute of Development Studies.

Prieto, B. N., & Amaya, M. C. (2014). Estrategia educativa en salud cardiovascular para trabajadores de una institución educativa. *Revista Científica Salud Uninorte, 30*(1), 44–51.

Rêgo, M. A., Nakatai, A. Y., & Bachion, M. M. (2006). Educação para a saúde como estratégia de intervenção de enfermagem às pessoas portadoras de diabetes. *Revista Gaúcha de Enfermagem, 27*(1), 60–70.

Rodríguez, A. (1983). Investigación participativa en el campo de la salud pública. In G. Vejarano (Ed.), *La investigación participativa en América Latina. Antología* (pp. 221–228). Patzcuaro: CREFAL.

Rodríguez, L., & Hernández, L. (1994). *Investigación participativa.* Madrid: Centro de Investigaciones Sociológicas.

Sabóia, V. M., & Valente, G. S. (2010). A prática educativa em saúde nas consultas de enfermagem e nos encontros com grupos. *Revista de Enfermagem Referência, 3*(2), 17–26.

Santos, Z. M., & Lima, H. (2008). Tecnologia educativa em saúde na prevenção da hipertensão arterial em trabalhadores: Análise das mudanças no estilo de vida. *Texto & Contexto Enfermagem, 17*(1), 90–97.

Santos, Z. M., Caetano, J., & Moreira, F. G. (2011). Atuação dos pais na prevenção da hipertensão arterial: Uma tecnologia educativa em saúde. *Ciência & Saúde Coletiva, 16*(2), 4385–4394.

Silva, E., Taleb, A., & Costa, N. M. (2015). Ambiente virtual de avaliação de competências no manejo do diabetes mellitus. *Revista Brasileira de Educação Médica, 39*(3), 470–478.

Souza, K., Paixão, G. P., Almeida, E., Sousa, A., Lirio, J., & Campos, L. (2015). Educação popular como instrumento participativo para a prevenção do câncer ginecológico: Percepção de mulheres. *Revista CUIDARTE, 6*(1), 892–899.

Spinato, I., Monteiro, L., & Santos, Z. M. (2010). Adesão da pessoa hipertensa ao exercício físico: Uma proposta educativa em saúde. *Texto & Contexto Enfermagem, 19*(2), 256–264.

Thiollent, M., & Toledo, R. F. D. (2012). Participatory methodology and action research in the area of health. *International Journal of Action Research, 8*(2), 142–158.

Torres, H., Amaral, M., Amorim, M. M., Cyrino, A., & Bodstein, R. (2010). Capacitação de profissionais da atenção primária à saúde para educação em diabetes mellitus. *Acta Paulista de Enfermagem, 23*(6), 751–756.

Torres, H., Barroso, R. A., Peixoto, S., Baciliere, J., & Morgan, B. (2012). Promoção da saúde e portadores de diabetes mellitus de uma operadora de plano de saúde. *Revista Enfermagem UERJ, 20*(2), 752–757.

Vejarano, G. (Ed.). (1983). *La investigación participativa en América Latina. Antología.* Patzcuaro: CREFAL.

Wallerstein, N., & Duran, B. (2003). The conceptual, historical, and practice roots of community based participatory research and related participatory traditions. In M. Minkler & N. Wallerstein (Eds.), *Community-based participatory research for health* (pp. 27–52). San Francisco: Jossey-Bass.

Chapter 11
Participatory Health Research with Older People in the Netherlands: Navigating Power Imbalances Towards Mutually Transforming Power

Barbara C. Groot and Tineke A. Abma

Foreword

Mrs. Caring (pseudonym) is a Dutch older woman in her 90s living in a nursing home. When we met her for the first time, she said that—despite her limited mobility and hearing problems—everything was fine. At a later visit, Mrs. Caring took part in a lively conversation with a group of women her age during which they were emotionally voicing their concern about the bad meals. Mr. Daring (pseudonym) is an articulate Dutch man aged 73, living at home in a suburb of Amsterdam. He and a group of other active older baby boomers are involved in an age-friendly project to improve their neighbourhood. When they find out that the professionals involved are taking the credit for what the older people have done, Mr. Daring is eager to assert control.

As a participatory researcher, how do you create room for a greater say in service delivery by older people admitted to a nursing home? How do you support older people who are commonly seen as passive and silent, and who often do not dare to 'complain', like Mrs. Caring, fearing repercussions? And what do you do as a researcher when you enter into a situation in which the research project ownership on the part of the older people concerned—a key principle in participatory health research (PHR)—is threatened by unintended actions on the part of professionals, as in the case of Mr. Daring? In both situations prevailing power imbalances run counter to the democratic ideal of mutually sharing and transforming power in PHR.

In this chapter we present the approach we took in two studies with older people from different generations. We will share the challenges we encountered and the lessons learned about the use of PHR in sharing power, facilitating dialogue and

B. C. Groot (✉) · T. A. Abma
Department Medical Humanities, VU University Medical Centre, Amsterdam Public Health Institute, Amsterdam, The Netherlands
e-mail: b.groot@vumc.nl; t.abma@vumc.nl

© Springer International Publishing AG, part of Springer Nature 2018
M. T. Wright, K. Kongats (eds.), *Participatory Health Research*,
https://doi.org/10.1007/978-3-319-92177-8_11

mutual learning between stakeholders. We will show how we navigated tacit tensions between stakeholders and how we tried to ensure that all voices are heard and genuine dialogue and action take place in a context in which the voices of older people tend to be marginalized.

But first, we will describe briefly the Dutch regional context in the Netherlands. Then we will provide an impression of the intellectual history of PHR in the Netherlands and provide key insights and approaches that have inspired us and are informing our Dutch practice.

Regional Context: The Netherlands and the So-Called Participation Society

In many European countries, healthcare reforms are taking place to deal with the aging population and economic crisis (European Commission 2014, 2016). The Netherlands is intending to transform itself from a welfare state to a 'participation society', a concept introduced by a neo-liberal government.

The transformation to this so-called participation society consists of reforms in different interrelated areas: a normative reorientation, a shift from residential to non-residential care, decentralization of responsibilities and expenditure cuts (Maarse and Jeurissen 2016). Firstly, the normative reorientation is more or less identical to what is happening in many European welfare states that are cutting back their responsibilities in care and emphasizing 'self-sufficiency' for care needs (Grootegoed 2013). Secondly, the government is supporting a shift from residential to non-residential care. This transition is in line with the trend of *aging in place* (Wiles et al. 2012), a popular concept in current aging policy. Finally, in 2015 a transition in the organizational and financial structure of healthcare took place in the Netherlands. The transition was accompanied by a budget cut of 25% for support and home care. The budget cuts put the aim of aging in place and participation under great pressure.

Given this context, we are critical of the notion of participation that is being proposed. Participation seems more like a form of co-optation and a unilateral form of power. Under these circumstances, we think PHR is urgently needed to redress power imbalances and work towards the mutual sharing of power to transform socially unjust situations.

PHR in the Netherlands

Intellectual History

The tradition of PHR in the Netherlands goes back to the 1960s when the student revolts and democratic ideals stimulated the inquiry into *action research* (AR). In the 1970s and 1980s, a whole array of AR approaches was developed under various names such as decision-making or utilization-focused research (*beslissingsgericht onderzoek* in Dutch) and practice-based research (*praktijkonderzoek* in Dutch). What all those approaches had in common was the aim to improve the practical impact and use of scientific research. An articulate group of scholars criticized some of these approaches for being positivist and managerialist in orientation, coining the term *handelingsonderzoek* after the German term of Heinz Moser *handlungsforschung* (Boog 2007). Dutch *handelingsonderzoek* scholars are, for example, Bos (2016), Donk and Van Lanen (2012), Jacobs (2001), Lieshout (2013), Snoeren (2015) and Weerman (2016).

In recent years there has been a movement to increase the participation of people whose lives are affected by health issues by consulting them over the course of developing and implementing health research studies. People affected by the issue being studied are, for example, consulted in advance regarding research topics and priorities (Abma and Broerse 2010; Caron-Flinterman 2005; Dedding 2009; Elberse 2012; Nierse and Abma, 2011; Schipper 2012; Teunissen 2014; de Wit 2014). This has led to an increasing repertoire of more innovative data collection methods to engage study participants in a more active way in research, for instance, as co-researchers (Bindels et al. 2014; de Wit et al. 2013). More widely, however, it continues to be more likely in health research that those without lived experience and other external players lack the commitment to addressing epistemic injustice (Fricker 2013) and social inequalities in health provision. Epistemic injustice captures the kind of discrimination arising when unfair biases cause people to underestimate the credibility of knowledge of members of often socially disadvantaged groups. PHR takes a more radical view and includes moving beyond understanding of the individual in order to address societal and structural injustices through a mutual sharing of power.

Our Approach to PHR

Our work is inspired by a hermeneutic-dialogical tradition from responsive evaluation (Abma 2005a, b; Abma and Widdershoven 2005, 2006; Guba and Lincoln 1987; Stake 1975, 2004; Widdershoven 2001). Central elements to this tradition are a variety of different perspectives, narratives, storytelling, relationality, interactivity, ongoing dialogues and mutual understanding. Recently, art has become an element in our approach, inspired by performative social science (Gergen and Gergen 2016) with the purpose of performing social transformation. The goals of our PHR approach are the mutual sharing of power, social change and learning and encouraging all stakeholders to extend their horizon by appropriating new perspectives (Abma and Stake 2001; Widdershoven 2001). We see a need for a relational empowerment (Vander Plaat 1999) based on the acknowledgement that people exist in relation to each other and are empowered in that context.

Our dialogical approach to PHR has three different phases. It starts by collecting experiences of those whose life (or work) is the subject of the study. We collect the experiences together with people whose life (or work) is at stake or these people collect the experiences themselves. These experiences, captured in stories, photography and/or other forms of art, present the complexity of human life and work and are the starting point for mutual learning processes (Baur 2012). All data collection methods focus on individuals or homogeneous groups of stakeholders with shared interests, as a way to deal with power imbalances (Abma 2005a, b). In this phase of collaboration, creative methods of analyses are used, for example, the collaborative creative hermeneutical analysis method (CCHA) (Lieshout and Cardiff 2011) or participatory visual analysis methods. The aim of this phase is to deepen a mutual understanding of the issues faced by the different groups of stakeholders in a safe and mutually encouraging environment (Abma and Widdershoven 2005).

The second phase of the dialogical approach is the start of the ongoing dialogue between different stakeholders about the issues that matter to them. By means of dialogue sessions (Abma et al. 2001), storytelling workshops (Abma 1998, 2003; Abma and Widdershoven 2005) and working conferences (Oguz et al. 2015), stakeholders are encouraged to extend their horizon by appropriating new perspectives. Photographs, music or other performances bring the lifeworld of the people who are the focus of the research literally into the room. In this phase, we are also inspired by Appreciative Inquiry (Cooperrider and Srivastva 1987; Cooperrider et al. 2008). This 'strength-based' approach encourages hope and optimism and focuses on similarities, including shared interests. It gives room for the resilience and potential of stakeholders that might otherwise be overshadowed by frustration and difference (Baur et al. 2010). The final and ongoing phase is about collaborative action and monitoring of the outcomes of the collaborative process in the previous phases.

Stories from the Field

Here we illustrate our approach in two research projects with older people of different age groups and generations. Needs and aspirations for being involved in research differ between generations, as we sensed in projects involving different generations. Every generation is united by memories, historical periods, language, habits, beliefs and life lessons (Howe and Strauss 2007). Different major societal events during the formative years have a lasting influence on the world views of the members of each generation (Diepstraten et al. 1999). The lens of generations helps to understand the dynamics and needs for the facilitation of older people in PHR projects.

When we look at research with older people in the Netherlands, we speak about the Pre-War Generation (born 1901–1930), the Silent Generation (born 1930–1940) and the Protest Generation (born 1940–1955), also called Baby Boom Generation (Becker 1992). In this chapter we tell a story of one project working with the Pre-War and the Silent Generations and one working predominantly with the Protest Generation. The baby boomers are legendary for their political resistance to the 'capitalist system' and for embracing norms and values that accentuate freedom, democratization, equality and political involvement. The other two generations share traditional norms and values that stress a solid work ethic, temperance, thrift and a desire for law and order (Diepstraten et al. 1999).

A Case of Mutual Inquiry for Healthy, Tasty Meals

Fostering Dialogue in a Residential Setting: Participatory and Local

We turn to Mrs. Caring, a woman from the Silent Generation, who we met a few years ago in a PHR study with the aim to involve older people in decision-making processes concerning their life and well-being in a nursing home (Baur & Abma, 2012). The features of this study that distinguish PHR from other research paradigms are that the study was 'participatory' (conducted together with those who are the subject of the study) and 'locally situated' (grounded in the reality of daily life in a specific place and time) (ICPHR 2013a). It namely concerned a small home with 129 apartments for older people who could still live independently but who are in need of some kind of support due to frailty. We brought together a group of residents, all from the Silent or Pre-War Generations, to set their agenda. The study was therefore 'collectively owned', also a distinguishing feature of PHR (ICPHR 2013a). After a series of conversations, a core action group of seven women aged 82–92 decided to work on improving meals. All had some degree of physical limitation and suffered from illness and/or poor vision, hearing problems and decreased mobility.

Eight meetings were held with this action group over a 7-month period. We encouraged the group to explore the problems they had identified. In later gatherings, the group was encouraged to look for solutions by inviting them to make a collage and a series of photographs to show their dreams and wishes. It was at this stage that the participants came up with a name for themselves: the Taste Buddies. A meeting was set up for the entire resident community in order to establish whether the other residents shared the same concerns and solutions. We also organized homogeneous meetings with kitchen staff and with the restaurant staff who served the meals.

In the next stage, dialogue meetings with heterogeneous groups were held. First, the action group met with the team leader and local manager to discuss their experiences with the meals and to explore where there might be room for improvement. Later, the Taste Buddies met with team leaders, kitchen staff, restaurant staff, the local manager and a resident council member to discuss their ideas for improvement. A collage helped the Taste Buddies to present the plans for improvement.

Transformation Through Human Agency Amongst the Older Women

Initially the Taste Buddies discussed a broad set of subjects for improvement, including not feeling at home, not being able to go out, feeling dependent and experiences of loss and grief. One theme stood out as particularly meaningful for them:

the dissatisfaction over the meals. This issue was not high on the local manager's list of priorities; he was more concerned with care-related topics.

Originally, the interaction in the group consisted of a careful exploration of shared experiences about meals, downplaying anything negative. After a while, the group began to feel more comfortable with each other and felt empowered by discovering that their discontent about meals was mutual. However, sharing negative experiences resulted in stagnation. The colourful collage the group made together put an end to this negativism and the associated downward spiral since they had to envision the ideal situation in which anything was possible. There was a renewed sense of joy and hope. The Taste Buddies began to express an activist attitude and was more future-oriented. The group had jointly learned in a very natural way, with help of the academic researcher as facilitator, how to transform their discontent into constructive advice for improvements in their quality of life. In terms of PHR, we call this feature 'transformation through human agency' (ICPHR 2013a).

Collage and Photographs on Dreams and Wishes

Over time, the women developed into a cohesive group in which they supported each other to keep going. Whenever one of them expressed doubt about the feasibility of their dreams, the others gently motivated her to stay positive. Trust was an important aspect of their process, as they had found a place in this group where they could speak freely about their concerns and dissatisfaction. This is reflected in the quote from Mrs. Caring when assuring her fellow participants that criticism was acceptable in an atmosphere of mutual encouragement: '*After all, we're here by ourselves, we can talk freely about this*'. This relates to two ethical principles of PHR 'mutual respect' and 'personal integrity' (ICPHR 2013b).

Engaging Others, Finding Common Ground and Action

For the kitchen and restaurant staff, the project was an opportunity to share their ideas about the meals. Early in their meetings, participants were critical and negative about developments in the organization and their own lack of influence. For example, some restaurant staff pointed out that the kitchen staff did not appreciate their ideas for improving dinner time. An appreciative approach was used by us for these meetings: the participants were asked to think about what could be done to make improvements and about what they could do to contribute towards the wellbeing of the residents. Furthermore, we introduced the participants in these groups to the issues and ideas of the Taste Buddies. They soon realized that they shared the same concerns and dreams. This process could be typified as 'active learning': learning from each other, an ethical principle of PHR (ICPHR 2013b). At the final meeting, the Taste Buddies, kitchen staff, team leader, local manager, resident council members, volunteers and restaurant staff all got together to share their views. They first discussed the perspectives and values of the Taste Buddies as reflected in the photos they had taken. The other participants recognized these issues very well. For example, one of the kitchen staff said: *'Yes, that's something we often talk about, that the combination* [of different parts of the menu] *is not always good'*. The professionals came up with their own examples of these issues and discussed their dissatisfaction about the meals. There was openness, and the result was a feeling of mutual understanding and recognition, and this led to all participants' arriving at agreements about practice improvements. The result is 'collective action' to 'make a difference', two ethical principles of PHR (ICPHR 2013b).

Collaborative Action and Monitoring Changes

The next step was to create plans for actions. This was done in collaboration between management, staff and older residents. The local kitchen in the care facility was reopened, a cook was hired, meals became more fresh and adjusted to the seasons, and the ambiance was improved.

The Taste Buddies decided to continue as a group. They monitored the changes and were not only successful in terms of the concrete actions they implemented but also in bringing about a change in their own perceptions of self and how they were seen and named by their environment. While these women were initially a bit shy and insecure, through a process of relational empowerment, they became more self-confident and proud. The story of the Taste Buddies has become part of the corporate story in the larger organization (this residential care home is part of a holding of five residential care homes), is told over and over and functions as a success story for others (staff, management) willing to change their relation with older people. Other facilities adopted a similar strategy to engage older people and implemented local changes as well (Baur et al. 2013). The project has increased our understanding of direct democracy.

A Case in the Age-Friendly City Amsterdam: Who Owns the Project?

Facilitating Participation in the Neighbourhood

Back to Mr. Daring, a baby boomer living independently with his wife in a suburb of Amsterdam. We met him in an Age-Friendly City PHR project in Amsterdam in 2016, aiming to research and improve the age-friendliness of their district. Mr. Daring worked with a group of ten older people, aged 67–85, as co-researchers. Most of them felt part of the Baby Boom Generation, also called the Protest Generation. They all lived in the neighbourhood of Mr. Daring. The group was mixed in terms of gender, age, ethnic background and frailty. All were still living at home and were capable of traveling independently.

The PHR study was embedded in the World Health Organization (WHO) network of Age-Friendly Cities (World Health Organization 2007), of which the city of Amsterdam had become a member. The key strategy of Age-Friendly Cities is to facilitate the inclusion of older persons and to enhance participation in the community. This strategy fits the PHR approach in which 'equality and inclusion' is one of the seven main ethical principles of PHR (ICPHR 2013b).

Initially, a group of 15 professionals from seven different organizations were involved at the start of the Age-Friendly City PHR study in two neighbourhoods in Amsterdam. The occupations of these stakeholders were diverse, from academic researchers and teachers at the school for health professionals to various representatives of the municipality and the patient organization in the city. In short, the work began with a very large stakeholder group without any older citizen at the table from the neighbourhoods involved. Including those who are subject of the research right from the start of a PHR study can be challenging, especially in academic-led studies (Groot and Abma 2018). Therefore, the principles of PHR as 'participatory', 'inclusive' and 'collectively owned' (ICPHR 2013a) were from the very first moment of the study at stake.

We (BG amongst others) were involved in the second stage of the project as facilitators of a group of older persons in one of the two neighbourhoods. Our starting point was assembling a team of older citizens from the area as co-researchers, facilitating their research process by organizing a meeting twice a month over the course of a year in which we coached them in their role. The group of co-researchers generated 40 stories from older, mostly more vulnerable neighbours. The group creatively analysed the stories together and organized a validation session with the neighbours and multiple other stakeholders from the neighbourhood to inspire collective action. The group shared their findings in several meetings in the neighbourhood with a broad audience. During the period of working in partnership with the group, a few ethical principles of PHR such as 'mutual respect', 'inclusion' and 'democratic participation' were crucial to winning back the feeling of 'collectively owned' by the older co-researchers. This resulted in the announcement of the group that they wanted to continue in a partnership in the neighbourhood together with other stakeholders, with success. The project is continuing at the moment of writing.

A Change-Oriented Group: Driven by Action

Back to the start... Surprisingly, we gathered a group of co-researchers in a short period of time. All were living in the neighbourhood and were motivated to start inquiring into the age-friendliness of their district. Compared to our previous experiences with vulnerable older people, we were happy to find it was relatively easy to engage the co-researchers. From a historical point of view, it is understandable that baby boomers, with a lived history of creating change and more democratic structures, are eager to participate in such local action-oriented initiatives. Compared to other older generations, this group is the best-educated and has a history of effecting change (Haber 2009). They were raised in a period of great social and cultural changes, such as women's rights, the sexual revolution, flower power, the lifting of religious and socio-political barriers and putting environmental issues on the agenda (Fortuyn 1998). Mr. Daring can be seen as an example of this action-oriented generation.

In the introductory conversations with the group of co-researchers, the passion for change and collective action (Melucci 1996) was immediately clear. One co-researcher, for example, worked in the neighbourhood 30 years prior and had started feminist groups to empower women. She was glad that she could remain active in her neighbourhood after retirement. Another co-researcher noted that he was part of the student protests to claim a voice in the university in the 1960s. This energy and activism was still present for him at the age of 78.

Reflecting on the recruitment of co-researchers, we were not able to engage the most vulnerable older citizens directly in the design stage of the process, but chose to engage them via the older co-researchers who interviewed them. We felt that the more vital older people were intrinsically motivated, emphatic and able to get the viewpoints of older people in more vulnerable positions. Both perspectives were used as input for conversations with local policymakers.

Participation as 'Business'

The drive of the group to make a difference resulted in a meeting with city council members responsible for elderly policy. The meeting took place before the group had any findings. The group was eager to hear from an official that their contribution to Age Friendly Amsterdam was meaningful to people with power to make changes. Otherwise they might stop the process. The co-researchers told the city council member that they were investing their spare time in this initiative, wanting to hear from him if their effort would be taken seriously.

The moment after I (BG), as a facilitator, had arranged the meeting with the city council member, some stakeholders expressed wanting to benefit from the occasion. They wanted to be involved in the meeting, organizing a big event around it, including picture-taking and giving presents to the official. The group of co-researchers was surprised and stunned by this reaction. It looked to them like all stakeholders wanted profit from 'their' work and 'their' meeting. The group of co-researchers had initiated the meeting and therefore insisted that they were in charge of both content and process. The co-researchers expressed their concern and unease, deciding that they did not want the meeting to be open to other stakeholders. I remember a reaction of a co-researcher to my question if a stakeholder could take a picture of the group of elderly people together with an important official for the publicity of their organization: '*Well, okay, but I do not want to be used by the city council member and his neo-liberal party for election reasons*'. I took this as a warning to stay alert.

The meeting with the official had a very positive effect on the atmosphere in the group of co-researchers. They felt inspired and felt more ownership of the project than before. Yet, I (BG) was also in contact with the range of stakeholders who had not been invited to the meeting. The photograph taken at the meeting was sent out by someone to all stakeholders without the consent of the co-researchers. The message attached to the photograph stated: *'Attached we are sending a picture of the meeting. You can use this for marketing and sales purposes'*. This was precisely the result which the co-researcher quoted above had feared. The participation of the older people had become 'business'.

As the facilitator, I (BG) was very angry because I also felt that the stakeholder organizations could take advantage of the group and I was afraid it would affect the optimistic and productive working atmosphere. I stopped the process and asked to call back the photograph, explaining my action by referring to the basic principles of PHR, particularly the principle of 'ownership' (ICPHR 2013a). This would mean obtaining the permission of all partners regarding the dissemination of information on the project.

Lessons Learned

In the Netherlands, as in many European welfare states, participation is said to be a basic principle of public policy. Participation has been largely instrumentalized in the Dutch setting, while at the same time there is a growing interest in PHR. PHR initiatives have to deal with a highly politicized context. Politicians and others are eager to join in and learn from PHR projects. On the other hand, they are not used to working in partnership with people in more vulnerable situations. Another aspect is that PHR with older people is different now than 10 years ago, because the Baby Boom Generation is eager to work together in a participatory way in order to create social change. These political circumstances call for advanced stages of Developmental Action Logics (Torbert 2003, 2004; Torbert and Taylor 2008) from PHR facilitators. Developmental Action Logics help to interpret surroundings, reflect, learn and react in complex, chaotic settings and to move through these categories as abilities grow (Rooke and Torbert 1998).

In the case of the Taste Buddies, the older people became co-creators, and they developed shared ownership over the course of the research project. The residents who, like Mrs. Caring, had initially been cautious about expressing their experiences later considered it their responsibility to stand up for the other residents. This was new for a group of women from their generation who grew up as being seen but not heard, as 'grey-flannel conformists', accepting the institutional civic life and conventional culture (Howe and Strauss 2007). The sociality of the process was for them as important—or maybe even more important—than the political drive to change life within the institution, and finding 'a voice' and developing 'an agenda' were major achievements. This process towards mutually transforming power demonstrates that identities and relationships shifted and that the participants developed trust, openness and mutual understanding about common values. The Taste Buddies were therefore not only successful in terms of the concrete action they brought about but also in terms of bringing about a change in their own perceptions of self and how they were seen and approached in their immediate environment. The facilitator's focus was on fostering dialogue, action and empowerment, which included redefining the role of older people and developing a new, shared vision.

The case of the Age-Friendly City group shows that the younger generation of older people, like Mr. Daring, are perhaps more politically aware and eager to raise their voice and claim ownership. The current neo-liberal political climate promotes entrepreneurship and consumer action. This climate heightens the competition between organizations to work together with older people in service provision. As a PHR group who volunteered in their neighbourhood, the Age-Friendly City group wanted to take the credit for their success. Yet, as the old Dutch proverb says, success has many fathers. Participation and PHR is a serious 'business' in times of reform and the Dutch 'participation society'. Focusing on empowerment was not necessary in a project with people mostly from the Baby Boom Generation; rather, the facilitator emphasized personal and organizational transformation in a highly politicized context. Yet, to reach out to older people in a more vulnerable position and to include their experiences as well, the more vital elders actively approached these neighbours through interviews and thereby gave them a voice in the neighbourhood. Participation requires sometimes other modes of working to adjust to the needs and aspirations of various generations and personal biographies.

If we examine the required skill sets and abilities of a PHR facilitator from the Developmental Action Logics (Torbert 2003, 2004, 2013) perspective, we see that in both initiatives the facilitator shares transformational power with the group of older people. In facilitating the dialogue with other stakeholders in the Taste Buddies case, being a *diplomat* was enough (Baur and Abma 2012). The diplomat role of a facilitator promotes social cohesion in the group and ensures that attention is paid to the interests and needs of others. In the Age-Friendly City initiative, the power of politics and the goal of social transformation required more. Taking on the role of *expert* by bringing in knowledge of the principles underlying PHR was a start. It encouraged a collective learning process on the part of the stakeholders. To promote real change and effectively handle the kind of conflicts encountered here, a PHR facilitator needs to address the instinctive resistance of some stakeholders to change. In the case of the Age-Friendly City, this meant the resistance of stakeholders to sharing power. This role is called *strategist*. A facilitator who acts as a strategist is adept at helping groups to create a shared vision that encourages both personal and organizational transformations. In the eye of a strategist, change is an iterative process that requires close attention. The strategist masters second-order change regarding actions and agreements as well as the interplay of personal relationships, organizational relations and national and international developments (Rooke and Torbert 2005).

These were important lessons for us, but above all we have sensed how important it is for older people, from all generations, to have a meaningful role in determining important aspects of their lives and to connect with others.

Acknowledgements We thank all co-researchers and other stakeholders who participated in the initiatives. We would also like to thank our co-facilitators and colleagues Vivianne Baur, Elena Bendien and Maaike Muntinga.

References

Abma, T. A. (1998). Storytelling as inquiry in a mental hospital. *Qualitative Health Research, 8*(6), 821–838.

Abma, T. A. (2003). Learning by telling storytelling workshops as an organizational learning intervention. *Management Learning, 34*(2), 221–240.

Abma, T. A. (2005a). Responsive evaluation in health promotion: Its value for ambiguous contexts. *Health Promotion International, 20*(4), 391–397.

Abma, T. A. (2005b). Patient participation in health research: Research with and for people with spinal cord injuries. *Qualitative Health Research, 15*(10), 1310–1328.

Abma, T. A., & Broerse, J. E. (2010). Patient participation as dialogue: Setting research agendas. *Health Expectations, 13*(2), 160–173.

Abma, T. A., & Stake, R. E. (2001). Stake's responsive evaluation: Core ideas and evolution. *New Directions for Evaluation, 2001*(92), 7–22.

Abma, T. A., & Widdershoven, G. A. (2005). Sharing stories narrative and dialogue in responsive nursing evaluation. *Evaluation & the Health Professions, 28*(1), 90–109.

Abma, T. A., & Widdershoven, G. A. (2006). *Responsieve methodologie: Interactief onderzoek in de praktijk*. Amsterdam: Lemma.

Abma, T. A., Greene, J. C., Karlsson, O., et al. (2001). Dialogue on dialogue. *Evaluation, 7*(2), 164–180.

Baur, V. E. (2012). *Participation & partnership: Developing the influence of older people in residential care homes*. Doctoral dissertation, Free University.

Baur, V., & Abma, T. (2012). 'The Taste Buddies': Participation and empowerment in a residential home for older people. *Ageing and Society, 32*(06), 1055–1078.

Baur, V. E., Abma, T. A., & Widdershoven, G. A. (2010). Participation of marginalized groups in evaluation: Mission impossible? *Evaluation and Program Planning, 33*(3), 238–245.

Baur, V. E., Abma, T. A., Boelsma, F., & Woelders, S. (2013). Pioneering partnerships: Resident involvement from multiple perspectives. *Journal of Aging Studies, 27*(4), 358–367.

Becker, H. A. (1992). *Generaties en hun kansen*. Amsterdam: Meulenhoff.

Bindels, J., Baur, V., Cox, K., et al. (2014). Older people as co-researchers: A collaborative journey. *Ageing and Society, 34*(06), 951–973.

Boog, B. (2007). Handelingsonderzoek of action research. KWALON. *Tijdschrift voor Kwalitatief Onderzoek, 12*(1), 13–20.

Bos, G. F. (2016). *Antwoorden op andersheid: Over ontmoetingen tussen mensen met en zonder verstandelijke beperking in omgekeerde-integratiesettingen*. Doctoral dissertation, Free University.

Caron-Flinterman, J. F. (2005). *A new voice in science: Patient participation in decision-making on biomedical research*. Doctoral dissertation, Free University.

Cooperrider, D. L., & Srivastva, S. (1987). Appreciative inquiry in organizational life. *Research in Organizational Change and Development, 1*(1), 129–169.

Cooperrider, D., Whitney, D. D., & Stavros, J. M. (2008). *The appreciative inquiry handbook: For leaders of change*. Oakland: Berrett-Koehler Publishers.

Dedding, C. (2009). *Delen in mahct en onmacht, Kinderparticipatie in de (alledaagse) diabeteszorg*. Doctoral dissertation, Free University.

Diepstraten, I., Ester, P., & Vinken, H. (1999). Talkin'bout my generation. *Netherlands Journal of Social Sciences, 35*(2), 91–109.

Elberse, J. E. (2012). *Changing the health research system. Patient participation in health research*. Doctoral dissertation, Free University.

European Commission. (2014). *National reform programme 2014 the Netherlands*. Brussels: European Commission.

European Commission. (2016). *Stability programme of the Netherlands*. Brussels: European Commission.

Fortuyn, P. (1998). *Babyboomers Autobiografie van een generatie*. Houten: Bruna.

Fricker, M. (2013). Epistemic justice as a condition of political freedom? *Synthese 190*(7), 1317–1332.

Gergen, M. M., & Gergen, K. J. (2016). *Playing with purpose: Adventures in performative social science*. Abingdon: Routledge.

Groot, B. C. & Abma, T. A. (2018) Partnership, collaboration and power. In S. Banks & M. Brydon-Miller (2018) *Ethics in participatory research for health and social well-being*. Abingdon: Routledge.

Grootegoed, E. M. (2013). *Dignity of dependence: welfare state reform and the struggle for respect*. Doctoral dissertation, University of Amsterdam.

Guba, E. G., & Lincoln, Y. S. (1987) The countenances of fourth-generation evaluation: Description, judgment, and negotiation. In *The politics of program evaluation* (pp. 202–234) 15

Haber, D. (2009). Gerontology: Adding an empowerment paradigm. *Journal of Applied Gerontology, 28*(3), 283–297.

Howe, N., & Strauss, W. (2007). The next 20 years. *Harvard Business Review, 85*, 41–52.

International Collaboration for Participatory Health Research (ICPHR). (2013a). *Position paper 1: What is participatory health research? Version: May 2013*. Berlin: International Collaboration for Participatory Health Research.

International Collaboration for Participatory Health Research (ICPHR). (2013b). *Position paper 2: Participatory health research: A guide to ethical principals and practice, Version: October 2013*. Berlin: International Collaboration for Participatory Health Research.

Jacobs, G. C. (2001). *De paradox van kracht en kwetsbaarheid. Empowerment in feministische hulpverlening en humanistisch raadswerk*. Doctoral dissertation, University of Humanistic.

van Lieshout, F.. (2013). *Taking action for action: A study of the interplay between contextual and facilitator characteristics in developing an effective workplace culture in a Dutch hospital setting, through action research*. Doctoral dissertation, University of Ulster.

van Lieshout, F., & Cardiff, S. (2011). Innovative ways of analysing data with practitioners as co-researchers. In D. Bridges, D. Horsfall, Higgs, et al. (Eds.)., (2011) *Creative spaces for qualitative researching* (pp. 223–234). Dordrecht: Sense Publishers.

Maarse, J. H., & Jeurissen, P. P. (2016). The policy and politics of the 2015 long-term care reform in the Netherlands. *Health Policy, 120*(3), 241–245.

Melucci, A. (1996). *Challenging codes: Collective action in the information age*. New York: Cambridge University Press.

Nierse, C. J., & Abma, T. A. (2011). Developing voice and empowerment: The first step towards a broad consultation in research agenda setting. *Journal of Intellectual Disability Research, 55*(4), 411–421.

Oguz, N. B., Gulru, Z. G., & Erme, K. (2015). Symbiosis of action research and deliberative democracy in the context of participatory constitution making. In Bradbury (Ed.), *The SAGE handbook of action research*. Los Angeles: SAGE.

Rooke, D., & Torbert, W. R. (1998). Organizational transformation as a function of CEO's developmental stage. *Organization Development Journal, 16*(1), 11.

Rooke, D., & Torbert, W. R. (2005). Seven transformations of leadership. *Harvard Business Review, 83*(4), 66–76.

Schipper, K. (2012). *Patient participation & knowledge*. Doctoral dissertation, Free University.

Snoeren, M. (2015). *Working= learning*. Doctoral dissertation, Free University.

Stake, R. E. (1975). To evaluate an arts program. In R. E. Stake (Ed.), *Evaluating the arts in education: A responsive approach* (pp. 13–31). Columbus: Merrill.

Stake, R. E. (2004). *Standards-based and responsive evaluation*. Thousand Oaks: Sage.

Teunissen, G.J. (2014). *Values and criteria of people with a chronic illness or disability: Strengthening the voice of their representatives in the health debate and the decision making process*. Doctoral dissertation, Free University.

Torbert, W. R. (2003). *Personal and organisational transformations through action inquiry*. London: The Cromwell Press.

Torbert, W. R. (2004). *Action inquiry: The secret of timely and transforming leadership*. Oakland: Berrett-Koehler Publishers.

Torbert, W. R., & Taylor, S. S. (2008). Action inquiry: Interweaving multiple qualities of attention for timely action. In Reason, P., & Bradbury, H. (Eds.). Handbook of action research: Participative inquiry and practice. Second edition. Sage: London.

Torbert, W. R. (2013). Listening into the dark: An essay testing the validity and efficacy of collaborative developmental action inquiry for describing and encouraging transformations of self, society, and scientific inquiry. *Integral Review: A Transdisciplinary & Transcultural Journal for New Thought, Research, & Praxis, 9*(2).

Van der Donk, C., & Van Lanen, B. (2012). *Praktijkonderzoek in de school*. Bussum: Coutinho.

Vander Plaat, M. (1999). Locating the feminist scholar: Relational empowerment and social activism. *Qualitative Health Research, 9*(6), 773–785.

Weerman, A. (2016). *Ervaringsdeskundige zorg- en dienstverleners: Stigma, verslaving & existentiële transformatie*. Doctoral dissertation, Free University.

Widdershoven, G. A. (2001). Dialogue in evaluation: A hermeneutic perspective. *Evaluation, 7*(2), 253–263.

Wiles, J. L., Leibing, A., Guberman, N., et al. (2012). The meaning of "aging in place" to older people. *The Gerontologist, 52*(3), 357–366.

de Wit, M. P. T. (2014). *Patient participation in rheumatology research: A four level responsive evaluation*. Doctoral dissertation, Free University.

de Wit, M., Abma, T. A., & Koelewijn-van Loon, M. (2013). Involving patient research partners has a significant impact on outcomes research: A responsive evaluation of the international OMERACT conferences. *BMJ Open, 3*(5), e002241.

World Health Organization. (2007). *Global age-friendly cities: A guide*. Geneva: World Health Organization.

Chapter 12
Organizational Participatory Research in North America

Paula Louise Bush, Jeannie Haggerty, Carol Repchinsky, Michael T. Wright, Christine Loignon, Vera Granikov, Ann C. Macaulay, Jean-François Pelletier, Sharon Parry, Gillian Bartlett-Esquilant, and Pierre Pluye

Brief Overview of Participatory Health Research in Canada and the United States

Participatory health research (PHR) is informed by various works in community development, education, and organizational learning to name a few (Cargo and Mercer 2008; International Collaboration for Participatory Health Research (ICPHR) 2013a). Today, a host of terms are used to refer to various forms of participatory research in health and other domains creating confusion and debate around issues such as who participates in the research process, how, and when. Indeed,

P. L. Bush (✉) · J. Haggerty · C. Repchinsky · V. Granikov · G. Bartlett-Esquilant · P. Pluye
Department of Family Medicine, McGill University, Montreal, Quebec, Canada
e-mail: Paula.bush@mcgill.ca; jeannie.haggerty@mcgill.ca; Carol.repchinsky@bell.ca; Gillian.bartlett@mcgill.ca; pierre.pluye@mcgill.ca

M. T. Wright
Catholic University of Applied Sciences, Institute for Social Health, Berlin, Germany
e-mail: Michael.Wright@KHSB-Berlin.de

C. Loignon
Department of Family Medicine, Sherbrooke University, Longueuil, Quebec, Canada
e-mail: christine.loignon@usherbrooke.ca

A. C. Macaulay
Department of Family Medicine, McGill University, Montreal, Quebec, Canada

CIET/Participatory Research at McGill (PRAM), Montreal, Quebec, Canada
e-mail: Ann.macaulay@mcgill.ca

J.-F. Pelletier
University of Montreal Mental Health Research Institute, Montreal, Quebec, Canada
e-mail: Jean-Francois.Pelletier@yale.edu

S. Parry
Westmount YMCA, Westmount, Quebec, Canada
e-mail: sharon.parry@ymcaquebec.org

© Springer International Publishing AG, part of Springer Nature 2018
M. T. Wright, K. Kongats (eds.), *Participatory Health Research*,
https://doi.org/10.1007/978-3-319-92177-8_12

179

participatory health researchers in the North American Primary Care Research Group are currently grappling with clarifying the similarities and differences in their respective engaged research. It is beyond the scope of this chapter to delve into the multiple terms used and their varying definitions; we refer the reader to such works as Margaret Cargo and Shawna Mercer's critical review (2008) and those cited in an annotated bibliography of the Oxford University Press (Bush et al. 2018). In this chapter, PHR consists of the research process outlined in 1995 by Lawrence W. Green and colleagues in their publication *Study of Participatory Research in Health Promotion: Review and Recommendations for the Development of Participatory Research in Health Promotion in Canada* (Green et al. 1995). The authors wrote:

> Participatory research seeks to link the processes of research, by which data are systematically collected and analyzed, with the purpose of taking action or affecting social change. To link the two processes, participatory research demands a high level of participation by those most directly affected by the issue being studied, usually called the community. (p. 3)

The authors explain that a community is not necessarily geographic but is "any group of individuals sharing a given interest" (p. 4). Further, they describe the complementary nature of the university researchers and the community members' expertise as well as the bilateral nature of the learning that occurs through the process:

> Collaboration takes place between some people within the community whose interests lie in changing health status or conditions of living and one or more technically trained researchers whose interests lie in developing knowledge. The collaboration allows both to participate in new activities: researchers become highly involved in the change process, and community members become involved to varying degrees at each stage of the research process. The collaborative stages include: (a) identifying the problem and formulating the research questions; (b) selecting the research methods or instruments; (c) analyzing or interpreting the results; (d) applying results; and (e) disseminating results. (pp. 3–4)

Subsequent to these guidelines, Barbara A. Israel, in Detroit, USA, led a review that outlined eight key principles of partnering with communities for research (Israel et al. 1998). In the same year, the North American Primary Care Research Group (NAPCRG) accepted as a policy statement on PHR a document produced by a task force chaired by Ann C. Macaulay "Responsible Research with Communities: Participatory Research in Primary Care," an abridged version of which was subsequently published in the *British Medical Journal* (Macaulay et al. 1999). This policy statement was amended nearly two decades later (Allen et al. 2017) attesting to the strong and continued leadership of NAPCRG for PHR.

In their critical review regarding strategies to engage research partners for translating evidence into action in community health, Salsberg et al. (2015) used the keyword "participatory research" to identify the main authors with practical expertise in this area. The top four authors identified are North American (based on their CiteSpace centrality scores for literature published between 1995 and 2009), namely, Barbara A. Israel, Meredith Minkler, Nina Wallerstein, and Ann C. Macaulay. These women have co-edited important texts on PHR methods (Israel

2013; Israel et al. 2005; Minkler and Wallerstein 2008, 2003) and co-authored critical papers on the ethics and measurement of PHR (Minkler 2004; Oetzel et al. 2015; Wallerstein 2000; Wallerstein et al. 2008; Jones et al. 2014). Moreover, they are all strong advocates for PHR in their respective jurisdictions and universities. In 1995, Barbara A. Israel established the Detroit Community-Academic Urban Research Center which has been "fostering health equity through community-based participatory research (CBPR) for more than 20 years."[1] In the Southern United States, Nina Wallerstein is the director of the Center for Participatory Research, launched in 2009, which strives to, among other things, "co-create new knowledge and translate existing knowledge to improve quality of life among New Mexico's diverse populations."[2] For her part, Meredith Minkler served on the advisory board of the Center for Collaborative Research for an Equitable California which was in operation from 2009 to 2015 when funding ended.[3] In Canada, Dr. Ann C. Macaulay is the inaugural director of Participatory Research at McGill, which was merged with CIET in 2015.[4] She has co-authored literature reviews that have helped to advance the science of PHR (Bush et al. 2017; Jagosh et al. 2012; Macaulay et al. 1999) and three editions of an annotated bibliography for PHR in public health published by the Oxford University Press (Macaulay et al. 2011, 2015; Bush et al. 2018) and is a leader for PHR among indigenous populations in Canada helping to produce, for instance, a chapter on the matter in the *Tri-Council Policy Statement: Ethical Conduct for Research Involving Humans* (TCPS).[5]

Additional noteworthy PHR work in North America includes some long-standing community-university partnerships that have developed sustainable infrastructure and have published extensively on their work. For instance, in 1986, the Vietnamese Community Health Promotion Project[6] was founded as a community-academic research unit at the University of California, San Francisco, with the mission of improving the health of Vietnamese living in the United States. In Quebec, Canada, the Kahnawake Schools Diabetes Prevention Project (KSDPP)[7] began in August 1994 with the goal of decreasing the onset of type 2 diabetes among present and future generations. One of the notable achievements of this partnership is the code of research ethics (available on the website). For its part, the Native Hawaiian Cancer Network, 'Imi Hale,[8] began in 2000 and has since leveraged considerable capacity for cancer research in Hawaii.

---

[1] https://www.detroiturc.org.

[2] https://cpr.unm.edu/about/index.html.

[3] https://ccrec.ucsc.edu/.

[4] http://pram.mcgill.ca/.

[5] http://www.pre.ethics.gc.ca/eng/index/).

[6] http://www.suckhoelavang.org/sklvweb/en/.

[7] https://www.ksdpp.org/index.php.

[8] http://www.imihale.org/.

Participatory Health Research with Organizations

The preceding examples all include communities of place partnering with academic researchers and seek to improve healthy lifestyle behaviors of populations. Yet, as specified by the ICPHR, "in PHR, those engaged in the research as active partners may be patients or users of services, members of health-related interest groups or other communities of identity or place, health care or related practitioners, managers and policy-makers" (International Collaboration for Participatory Health Research (ICPHR) 2013b, p. 4). This chapter discusses PHR carried out with health practitioners and other staff working in health organizations, such as hospitals or primary care clinics, to ultimately benefit the patients for whom they care. PHR in the organizational context (compared to the community one) is a strategy for organizational change and requires that some additional aspects be considered. For instance, when conducting PHR within a health organization, its hierarchy, policies, and routines need to be known and understood by the outside researchers to enable the integration of the PHR into the organization. Together, university and organization stakeholders blend quantitative, qualitative, or mixed methods research with action, to evaluate and improve healthcare practices, services, and policies (Argyris et al. 1985; Lewin 1946; Munn-Giddings et al. 2008; Munten et al. 2010; Soh 2011; Waterman et al. 2001). In particular, organization stakeholders also develop research capacity and increase reflective practice, e.g., practitioners not only collect facts regarding their practice but reflect on their practice to uncover and understand tacit knowledge (i.e., knowledge that is not explicitly articulated (Lam 2000)).

Four literature reviews have examined what the authors refer to as "action research" carried out with and within health organizations (Munn-Giddings et al. 2008; Munten et al. 2010; Soh et al. 2011; Waterman et al. 2001) with the purpose of organizational change (e.g., improvement of care practices or policies). While the reviewed studies illustrate academics working with organizations through the action research cycle outlined by Kurt Lewin (1946), not all of them illustrate research co-governance. In our systematic review, we included 83 studies that represent research that was co-governed between academic and health organization stakeholders. That is, organization stakeholders and "outsider" university researcher stakeholders co-constructed the research, making decisions jointly regarding at least three phases: (a) identifying the research question(s); (b) setting the methodology, collecting and/ or analyzing the data, or interpreting the findings/results; and (c) implementing or disseminating the research findings (Bush et al. 2017). This description of co-governance in research is in line with other typologies of PHR across community and organizational settings (Cornwall and Jewkes 1995; Hart and Bond 1995; Holter and Schwartz-Barcott 1993; Jagosh et al. 2012). Hereafter, we refer to this particular type of PHR as Organizational Participatory Research (OPR).

In our review of OPR, the comprehensive and systematic search of bibliographic and gray literature databases led to the retrieval of over 8000 records. Based on the above definition of OPR, two independent reviewers screened the records and read the subsequently selected full text publications to include 83 studies in the review (see Bush et al. 2017 for a detailed description). Sixteen of these were conducted in Canada or the United States. Drawing on these 16 studies, together with some examples from our own OPR, we will describe how this type of research has been conducted in North American contexts and with what effects. To this end, we provide examples of participatory processes in the key research phases and the outcomes associated with these processes. For the most part, we provide examples of OPR successes as these are the stories currently available in the empirical OPR literature. It is important to note that while the examples provided may help mitigate challenges, OPR requires effort, patience, perseverance, and resolve. We conclude the chapter with a discussion of some challenges North American OPR partnerships have faced and how they addressed them. Finally, to offer an integral perspective of the processes and outcomes of OPR, four vignettes are included, focusing on communication, research initiation, participatory data analysis, and challenges.

Organizational Participatory Research in North America

This chapter cites examples from 16 OPR studies conducted in Canada and the United States (Table 12.1). These studies are variously referred to by their authors as CBPR, PAR, participatory research, action research, and community-based action research, which emphasizes the need to better define the terminology in all forms of partnership research. Table 12.1 indicates the terms each study uses together with the literature authors cite as the basis for their participatory studies. For the most part, OPR in Canada and the United States has taken place in hospitals (e.g., emergency room, operating room, psychiatric ward, etc.). In five studies, the organization partners were all nurses (Smith 1995; Breda et al. 1997; Jones-Baucke 1997; Senesac 2004; Lausten 2005), whereas other studies illustrate multidisciplinary partnerships. Only three included patients or service users on the research team (Mirza et al. 2008; Williams 2009; Malus et al. 2011). This is striking and represents an area of development for future OPR. Patients and the public are affected by organization practices, and have experience receiving health and social services and navigating the system. They possess a wealth of insider knowledge that could be integrated into OPR to help improve the relevance of the practice changes sought. Perhaps in the coming years, more OPR studies will engage patients and the public in the research process given the current trend toward patient engagement in the United States with the Patient-Centered Research Outcomes Institute (PCORI)[9] and in Canada with the Strategy for Patient-Oriented Research (SPOR).[10] Working with patients may carry additional challenges. For instance, Ann Sawyer Williams (2009) discusses issues regarding adapting to the visual impairments of the patient partners. Examples of how to adapt to the needs of stakeholders are included in a practice guide for OPR (Bush et al. 2017) that is freely available from the

---

[9] https://www.pcori.org/.

[10] http://www.cihr-irsc.gc.ca/e/41204.html.

Table 12.1 Description of OPR studies included in the systematic review by Bush et al. (2017)

First author[a] (year)	City, province/ state, country	Organization(s)	Organization stakeholders (as described in the publication)	Research objective(s) (as described in the publication)	Method(s)	Duration (months)[b]	OPR label (authors cited)
Barker & Barker (1994)	Richmond, Virginia, USA	Substance abuse inpatient unit in a large university teaching hospital	Key staff members including managers	To manage change in an interdisciplinary substance abuse inpatient unit	Qualitative	36[b]	AR (Lewin 1946; French 1969)
Smith (1995)	Alberta, Canada	Urban public health unit	Public health nurses	To explore to what extent and how is PAR a form of collective, self-reflective inquiry that supports the implementation of democratic, empowering healthcare practices	Qualitative	15	PAR (Freire 1970)
Breda et al. (1997)[a]	Waterloo, Ontario, Canada	A small, private psychiatric hospital in rural New England	Nurses	To increase nurses' autonomy by implementing changes	Qualitative	12	PAR (Freire 1996; Reason 1994)
Jones-Baucke (1997)	Washington, DC, USA	A large, urban, nonprofit, 477-bed hospital	Nurses	To increase nurses' use of standardized nursing languages	Mixed	Unknown	AR (Argyris & Shon (1991); Holter and Schwartz-Barcott 1993) and PAR (Elden and Levin 1991)
Mason (2003)	Toronto, Ontario, Canada	Sunnybrook and Women's College hospital community	Social workers, nurses, psychologists, and physicians	To influence the medical system to respond better to the needs of abused women	Qualitative	12[b]	AR (Carr and Kemmis 1986) and Community development (Labonte 1997)

Senesac (2004)	Northeast USA	295-bed community hospital	Nurses	To implement a pain resource nurse role in a community hospital	Qualitative	12	AR (Lewin 1946)
Lausten (2005)	Western USA	Hospital-based, operating room and post-anesthesia care unit in an urban, western, Veterans Administration hospital	Nurses	To address nursing behaviors with negative environmental consequences	Qualitative	8	CBAR (cites traditions from Freire to McTaggert; Reason to Minkler, Wallerstein, and Israel)
Williams et al. (2005)[a]	New Haven, Connecticut, USA	Leeway, Inc. (a 40-bed nonprofit, nursing facility dedicated to community-based AIDS care)	Staff	To test a randomized controlled trial of metta meditation and massage for adults with AIDS at the end of life	Quantitative	22	CBPR (Israel et al. 1998)
Eisenberg et al. (2006)	USA	An urban community hospital, emergency room	Emergency room managers	To gain a better understanding of the challenges facing emergency departments in a local context and to use these insights to help this particular department develop more effective responses	Qualitative	6	AR (Argyris 1995; Elden and Levin 1991; Greenwood and Levin 1998)

(continued)

Table 12.1 (continued)

First author[a] (year)	City, province/ state, country	Organization(s)	Organization stakeholders (as described in the publication)	Research objective(s) (as described in the publication)	Method(s)	Duration (months)[b]	OPR label (authors cited)
Hamelin et al. (2007)[a]	Montreal, Quebec, Canada	Montreal area hospital	Head nurse, nurses and assistant nurses, head of service, project coordinator, attendants, support staff, and others with direct contact with patients, union representatives	To create an optimal psychosocial environment in the workplace	Qualitative	12	PAR (Green et al. 1995)
Mirza et al. (2008)[a]	Chicago, Illinois, USA	Centers for Independent Living (for people living with psychiatric disability)	Program directors	To gain a better understanding of the experiences of people with psychiatric disabilities within the program; to explore better ways of supporting them during the move into the community and during long-term community living and participation	Qualitative	15	PAR (Freire 1970; Selener 1997)

Williams (2009)	Cleveland, Ohio, USA	Diabetes Association of Greater Cleveland (DAGC)	Staff and patients	To identify changes needed to make the diabetes education materials and programs of the DAGC accessible for people who have visual impairment and diabetes	Qualitative	12	PAR (Coughlin and Brannick 2001; Stringer 1999; Greenwood and Levin 1998)
Dobransky-Fasiska et al. (2010)[a]	Pittsburgh, Pennsylvania, USA	Three community organizations committed to evidence-based care for minority elderly	Diverse blend of community partners from family health centers; social service and mental health consumer advocacy agencies; and a pharmacy services network	To create a depression care model for disadvantaged adults utilizing service agencies, through a community-academic partnership	Qualitative	60[b]	Cargo and Mercer (2008), Jones and Wells (2007), Minkler and Wallerstein (2003), and Israel et al. (1998)
Chen et al. (2011)[a]	Los Angeles, California, USA	The West Los Angeles Veterans Affairs Medical Center	Emergency department staff	To examine the implementation of nontargeted opt-in HIV rapid testing in an urban hospital emergency department	Mixed	4	CBPR (Israel et al. 1998)
Malus et al. (2011)	Montreal, Quebec, Canada	Primary care teaching clinic	Staff and patients	To adapt and implement a patient satisfaction questionnaire	Mixed	24	PR (Macaulay et al. 1999; Cargo and Mercer 2008)

(continued)

Table 12.1 (continued)

First author[a] (year)	City, province/ state, country	Organization(s)	Organization stakeholders (as described in the publication)	Research objective(s) (as described in the publication)	Method(s)	Duration (months)[b]	OPR label (authors cited)
Cashman et al. (2012)[a]	Worcester, Massachusetts, USA	Community health center and YWCA	Staff	To describe partnership approach taken by 2 CBOs, determine staffs' views of this partnership, highlight aspects of the partnership that contributed to its success, identify challenges and mechanisms for overcoming them, and note lessons learned	Qualitative	36	CBPR (Minkler and Wallerstein 2008; www.ccph. info)

AR action research, *CBO* community-based organization, *CBPR* community-based participatory research, *CBAR* community-based action research, *PAR* participatory action research, *PR* participatory research

[a]Organization members are co-authors

[b]Duration of partnership at the time of publication, i.e., ongoing partnership work

Quebec-SPOR unit for the Support for People and Patient-Oriented Research and Trials (SUPPORT).[11] Additional lessons can be drawn from the patient engagement literature (see, e.g., https://ceppp.ca/en/).

Relationships

The relationships that develop among all stakeholders, including the university researchers, influence the OPR and the success and sustainability of their achievements and their partnership, making positive relationships the most important ingredient in OPR. It is common practice for university and organization stakeholders to form a working group and hold regular meetings. Working group members may not know one another at the outset or may even have strained relationships; regular meetings provide a structure to develop relationships while working collaboratively toward a common goal (Breda et al. 1997; Lausten 2005; Hamelin Brabant et al. 2007; Dobransky-Fasiska et al. 2009; Barker and Barker 1994; Smith 1995; Williams 2009; Senesac 2004). Moreover, meetings provide opportunities for communication among working group members, and between the working group and the rest of the organization, that may not exist without the research. Ideally, meetings are run by a member who can foster an environment where stakeholders can openly discuss and debate the research and related decisions, voice their thoughts and fears, and be heard and understood by others (Eisenberg et al. 2006). Speaking and listening are vital. For instance, clarifying goals and parameters, recognizing and respecting the complementary skills and knowledge of all partners, and commending achievements are all crucial to help build and nurture fruitful relationships (Dobransky-Fasiska et al. 2009; Williams 2009), work through challenges, remain motivated, and sustain the partnership (Bush and García Bengoechea 2016; Dobransky-Fasiska et al. 2009; Smith 1995). Barker and Barker (1994) wrote:

> In contrast to the initial assessment period, staff members were now openly supporting each other, asking for assistance from staff members in other disciplines and collaborating on problem solving. The sarcasm and blaming readily observed in meetings prior to the project were seen less often, with good-natured teasing and humor displayed more frequently. (p. 89)

The composition of the working group can impact the relationships and, ultimately, the research. Multidisciplinary working groups are common; the research and its outcomes are infused with the voices of a variety of stakeholders leading to research products and activities that are tailored to their context and needs (Barker and Barker 1994; Bush and García Bengoechea 2016; Malus et al. 2011).

Regarding the participation of management, in her dissertation, Smith (1995) mentions that the presence of managers at working group meetings led to health professionals holding back and adversely affected group dynamics. On the other

---

[11] http://unitesoutiensrapqc.ca/.

hand, others underscore the importance of management being part of the working group because they can support the work by allocating resources and bypassing red tape, for instance (Barker and Barker 1994; Hamelin Brabant et al. 2007; Lausten 2005; Mason 2003; Malus et al. 2011). Ultimately, working group membership should be discussed and debated in relation to the actors and context involved. The working group may decide that while including managers may hold challenges, implementing communication and other group processes may help to overcome the challenges and enable the OPR to benefit from the input of multiple stakeholder groups. Vignette 1 provides an illustration of some benefits of extensive interaction via regular meetings.

Vignette 1: Communication

In Cleveland, Ohio, USA, a researcher sought to make the patient education materials and programs of the Diabetes Association of Greater Cleveland (DAGC) accessible to people with visual impairment. A working group of people with visual impairment and diabetes (PVID), DAGC staff members, and the researcher met regularly. To adapt to the needs of the PVID, meeting notes were provided in their preferred format (large print or audio) and were read aloud at the beginning and end of each meeting. Meetings provided a setting for extended direct contact and cooperation between the working group members, enhancing both the products of this project and the process of discovering ways to meet the needs of PVID.

PVID had felt anger and suspicion of the DAGC staff members at the beginning of the project, but those feelings changed as the DAGC staff members demonstrated their willingness to listen and change. In particular, the process gave the PVID an opportunity to communicate their own experiences of living with diabetes and visual impairment and to be heard by a group of professionals. Some PVID felt that participation in this project increased their skills for expressing themselves and confidence in doing so. One explained: "Medical professionals are a mixed bag. They don't all know how to serve everyone. We often have to teach them how to serve us." Another had a hospitalization following the project and later expressed that her recent experience with DAGC had prepared her to explain her needs clearly to healthcare professionals in the hospital. Furthermore, the PVID members' communicating aspects of their experience that were unknown to the sighted participants gave the DAGC staff a deeper, more authentic understanding of accessibility needs. Notably, PVID mentioned the importance of opportunities for socializing, especially around meals.

Summary developed from excerpts from

Williams, A. S. (2002). A focus group study of accessibility and related psychosocial issues in diabetes education for people with visual impairment. *The Diabetes Educator, 28*(6), 999–1008. https://doi.org/10.1177/01457217 0202800614

Williams, A. S. (2005). Using participatory action research to make diabetes education accessible for people with visual impairment. *Dissertation Abstracts International: Section B: The Sciences and Engineering, 66*(5-B), 2883.

Williams, A. S. (2009). Making Diabetes Education Accessible for People with Visual Impairment. *The Diabetes educator, 35*(4), 612–621. https://doi.org/10.1177/0145721709335005

Initiation and Focus of the Research

OPR begins in a variety of ways. In some studies, organizations may seek out academics with whom to partner to help them address an issue they have identified. Cashman et al. (2012) provide an explicit example in their health promotion study conducted with community health organizations. Other times, the idea for the focus of the research is proposed by the academics, and the organization stakeholders agree with the importance of the issue and choose to partner to address it. This is the model described in a study between university researchers and nurses in a public health unit in Alberta, Canada (Smith 1995). Finally, the research focus can be determined jointly among all partners. Lausten (2005) provides such an example in his study with nurses to improve ecological practices in a hospital. Agreeing on the focus of the research may not be simple. Sometimes, the various stakeholders each have their respective priorities and discussion and negotiations are needed to come to consensus on the issue to address through the OPR. Ultimately, addressing an issue which is important to the organization and that may be usefully addressed through research is paramount and contributes to the success of the OPR (Bush et al. 2017). A study that took place in Pittsburgh, USA, provides an example of researchers deferring to the organization's interest. Academics and leaders of 11 community organizations formed the Research Network Development Core to improve depression care. The authors write:

> Before the [Research Network Development Core] was created the academics had research goals of reducing depression among African-American and White older adults. However, the public organizations serve people of all ages and all racial and ethnic groups. Thus, the researchers shifted focus to include disadvantaged adults of any age in order to be aligned with the community partners. (Dobransky-Fasiska et al. 2010, p. 2)

Others illustrate some benefits of focusing on organization priorities. Lausten (2005) asked nurses participating in his dissertation work what they thought about being active participants in research, one said: "I think it's important because I think when you give people a choice to be involved in what their ideas are they're more apt to work harder on it" (p. 54). This is further underscored by Hamelin Brabant et al. (2007) who write: "the results revealed that the organizational changes are seen as less threatening when suggestions come from colleagues rather than from managers, who are often seen as less adept than the employees at solving the internal problems of a care unit or service unit" (p. 319).

It should be underscored that reaching consensus on a research focus that is beneficial to all working group members can be challenging. Developing a shared understanding of each other's needs and expectations, as well as feasible contributions of all working group members, may require multiple lengthy conversations and can be complex and even frustrating. The process will benefit from stakeholders' ability to express where they are and are not prepared to compromise as well as a willingness to understand and to learn from one another and to help achieve their respective needs. Other important qualities for working group members are patience and perseverance, together with group facilitation skills. These initial negotiations help set the foundation for the relationships among the working group members that are needed to conduct the OPR. Vignette 2 describes how one study was initiated, how ideas for action were generated by stakeholders, and the potentially sustainable effects of the OPR processes.

Vignette 2: Research Initiated by Organization Stakeholders
Seeking a better understanding of how to serve people with psychiatric disabilities in the community reintegration program, the program directors at two Centers for Independent Living (CIL) serving a large metropolitan region in the United States met with three researchers from the University of Illinois at Chicago, to discuss a research partnership. Together, they developed the project's aims: (1) to gain a better understanding of the experiences of people with psychiatric disabilities within the community reintegration program and (2) to explore better ways of supporting them in community reintegration. To begin the data collection process, they decided to hold a focus group, co-led by a researcher and a community partner, the content of which was determined with the community partners. Results revealed a need for increased communication between various organizations that provide services for people with psychiatric disabilities in the community.
   To initiate a dialogue between the various entities involved in the provision and use of psychiatric disability services, a community resource meeting was planned. Meeting participants unanimously agreed that opening up lines of communication between the various stakeholders was the next step in the process of promoting community integration of people with psychiatric disabilities. It was decided that this process could be initiated through the creation of an email listserv, where individuals could post information on advocacy efforts and other local and statewide initiatives that they were undertaking to promote community services for people with psychiatric disabilities. Two of the participants, one of whom was a person with a psychiatric disability and CIL representative and the other a service provider, volunteered to take the lead in developing the listserv. This listserv is currently active and continues to be a forum where participants communicate and share ideas on an ongoing basis. Other steps recommended for developing a seamless service system included the creation of a clearinghouse of information and a toll-free number

for service providers and consumers. While these latter steps have not come to fruition as yet, they are under consideration and being collaboratively worked upon. This project has laid the foundations for future bridge building between people with psychiatric disabilities and the broader disability community, particularly in the area of promoting community integration.

Summary developed from excerpts from

Mirza, M., Gossett, A., Chan, N. K., Burford, L., & Hammel, J. (2008). Community reintegration for people with psychiatric disabilities: challenging systemic barriers to service provision and public policy through participatory action research. *Disability & Society, 23*(4), 323–336.

Participatory Data Analysis

Given the inclusion of the varied and complementary knowledge and expertise of all partners, a participatory data analysis process can enhance the work. For instance, organization stakeholders provide the necessary insider's lens to heighten the contextual relevance of the results, whereas the academic stakeholders contribute the research expertise needed to not compromise the scientific rigor. Again, lengthy discussions and negotiation are often involved and compromises required. Participatory analysis of data can take many forms. Although organization stakeholders may not have the expertise, time, or interest to complete the technical work of quantitative and/or qualitative analyses, their input in this research phase is possible and valuable. For instance, in Montreal, Quebec, Canada, Bush and García Bengoechea (2016) worked with a YMCA to evaluate their adolescent program. While the academic partners carried out the statistical analyses, decisions regarding how to analyze the quantitative program data were made together with YMCA partners. For example, partners had multiple discussions pertaining to questions and hypotheses and feasible analyses given the sample and the nature of the data. Similarly, the university partners coded the qualitative data, but the deductive coding framework was developed with the academic and YMCA partners and based on the peer-reviewed and gray literature as well as YMCA partners' knowledge. In other studies, the working group does the technical work of the analysis, working together to code qualitative data and develop themes as described in one article co-written by all stakeholders.

> All [working group]nurses met six times for 3 hours to analyze the research findings and to develop categories, or themes, of analysis. Breda [the first author] recorded each session on tape, listened repeatedly to the recordings, and pulled out salient topics for discussion at the following meeting. We spent the subsequent meeting reflecting on these topics and adding new input from events that had transpired in the interim. We continued this process until all components of the project were analyzed. All working group nurses were active in the dialogue and decided together on the meaning of experiences. In the end, we easily reached consensus on three themes that we believed reflected the major changes that were experienced in our collective inquiry. (Breda et al. 1997, p. 79)

Other studies follow this model, but only some members of the working group carry out the analysis. This is illustrated in a study led by one of our co-authors (Pluye). University and organization partners describe how they worked together, as co-researchers, iteratively coding qualitative data, discussing their codes, and inductively developing new codes to produce a reliable coding manual (El Sherif et al. 2015). Finally, others opt to have the researcher do some initial analysis and return preliminary results to the group for discussion as depicted in Vignette 3.

Vignette 3: Collective Data Analysis

In a primary care clinic in Montreal, Quebec, Canada, an interdisciplinary committee (patients, manager, psychologist, administrators, support staff, nurse, physicians, and researchers) evaluated a patient satisfaction questionnaire (PSQ) for its suitability in the clinic. The committee, chaired by the research coordinator, met monthly from 2007 to 2009.

The qualitative researcher completed semi-structured interviews with other clinic staff and patients regarding their perspectives of the relevance of each item in the original PSQ. She analyzed these interviews and presented the results to the committee. The content, wording, and appropriateness/relevance of each question were discussed until a consensus was reached, as follows. The chair ensured every member had a chance to express and explain his or her opinion, preventing any committee member from dominating the discussion and asking quieter members for their views. The chair continuously summarized the points of view, identifying similarities and differences. In one instance, voting was required to reach consensus. The committee divided into two groups and each group discussed and nominated a representative, who then presented their view to the full committee. Committee members then voted on the issue anonymously. This time-consuming, but enriching, process led to rewording, eliminating, or adding new items to the PSQ. This adapted PSQ was tested in three 1 h focus groups where patients were asked to complete the adapted PSQ and discuss their overall impressions of it as well as any issues with specific items. Again, the qualitative researcher completed the analysis of the focus group transcripts and presented the results to the committee for discussion. Finally, minor changes to the questionnaire were made.

Summary developed from excerpts from

Malus, M., Shulha, M., Granikov, V., Johnson-Lafleur, J., d'Souza, V., Knot, M., Holcroft, C., Hung, K., Pereira, I., Ricciuto, C., Salsberg, J., & Macaulay, A. C. (2011). A participatory approach to understanding and measuring patient satisfaction in a primary care teaching setting. *Progress in community health partnerships: research, education, and action, 5*(4), 417–424.

Returning Results

The research results, including preliminary ones, can have a profound effect on organization members, and the organization as a whole, and must be communicated to the working group and the broader organization throughout the study process. This allows for results to be put into practice, as noted by Eisenberg et al. (2006): "Our observations were used by a newly formed interdisciplinary organizational development team seeking to create baseline measures and begin a number of targeted interventions. Some of the changes that occurred were a direct result of this study" (p. 204). Beyond achieving their planned objectives, Canadian and American examples describe how research results can surprise organization stakeholders or confirm their perceptions, both of which motivate them to enact changes, even without the help of the academic partners (Smith 1995; Bush and García Bengoechea 2016; Mason 2003). Moreover, this process can help to keep partners engaged and even motivate stakeholders to continue the partnership work (Bush and García Bengoechea 2016). The following excerpt from Dobransky-Fasiska et al. (2010) illustrates this.

> Because of the time required for the participatory research process, success depends on both intangible and tangible benefits that the partners consider to be significant enough to sustain their effort. Both the process and the results of the needs assessment were early benefits. (p. 4)

Returning OPR results to the organization can be done in many ways. In Canadian and American examples of OPR, some have provided research results to staff and management both orally and in writing during their regular meetings (Eisenberg et al. 2006; Barker and Barker 1994; Bush and García Bengoechea 2016; Mason 2003) and with poster displays in key areas of the organization (Lausten 2005). Working with the organization partners at this stage is paramount to ensure the language, tables, and figures used to communicate the results are appropriate. In her dissertation, Bush (2014) cites an organization partner who alludes to some challenges and benefits of speaking different languages (i.e., research language vs. organization language).

> It kind of surprised me when I saw the [teenagers'] names [in your report of results]. So, it was little bit of a gasp reaction. It took me a while to get used to that. But, after a while it occurred to me that it's a very interesting way of looking at things. (p. 124)

Similarly, this organization partner found it challenging to translate the organization language to the university partners: "we don't always have those words because the things that are obvious to us we think are obvious to everyone" (p. 143). We suggest that additional insight for how to proceed may be gained from existing knowledge translation frameworks (Grimshaw et al. 2012; Lavis et al. 2003; Straus et al. 2009).

Changes in Knowledge, Attitudes, and Behaviors

The increased awareness and knowledge that all working group members gain through OPR should not be underestimated. Organization stakeholders, for instance, not only learn about research and the issue they are addressing through the study (Dobransky-Fasiska et al. 2010; Lausten 2005), but they also gain an understanding of each other and their needs and constraints regarding their respective roles in the organization. Some report how staff gained an understanding of and increased sensitivity to patients' needs (Dobransky-Fasiska et al. 2010; Williams 2009). Working group members also acquire or improve upon such skills as problem identification and solving, decision making, cooperation, leadership, and communication (Barker and Barker 1994; Williams 2009). In one study, a working group member said: "There were two benefits—first, we have a stronger working relationship with you folks [academics] and second, at least an understanding, if not a working relationship with the other partners that we probably would not have developed alone … It increased our awareness of the other agencies and what they do" (Dobransky-Fasiska et al. 2009, p. 959). In the few studies including patients in the working group, benefits for them are also apparent. For example, Ann Sawyer Williams (2009) writes about how the people with visual impairment and diabetes with whom she conducted the OPR described the benefit of learning more about diabetes, quoting two partners: "It made us a lot more conscious of what we're doing when we go into the store to buy food. Now, before I buy something new, I get someone to read the labels to me, so I know what is in the food" (p. 84). Regarding university partners, while we know from our own experiences that, as part of the working group, university researchers learn, for instance, about group processes, develop group facilitation skills, and gain awareness of organizational cultures and how to navigate them, such learnings are rarely documented in peer-reviewed journal articles. Indeed, only 6% of the studies in our systematic review of OPR documented such benefits for the university partners (Bush et al. 2017), one of which was North American (Williams 2005).

As a result of the OPR approach, authors report observing reduced resistance to change and greater acceptance for change (Mason 2003; Hamelin Brabant et al. 2007; Lausten 2005; Barker and Barker 1994). For instance, Mason (2003) noted that the approach "supported broad-based acceptance of the violence initiative at a time when other imposed changes were resisted" (p. 22). Many observed changes in culture, diffusion of change to other organization members or to the organization as a whole, and continued collaboration to improve practices (Mason 2003; Dobransky-Fasiska et al. 2009, 2010, 2012; Lausten 2005; Breda et al. 1997; Barker and Barker 1994). OPR authors have also found that the participatory research approach contributes to improved relationships and teamwork (Senesac 2004), increased professional satisfaction and excitement, and increased commitment to and responsibility for actions (Williams 2005).

Organizations and their stakeholders have used results for such things as informing modifications to work processes and practices (e.g., improve triage, implement staff meetings to clarify expectations, and improve support) (Barker and Barker 1994; Eisenberg et al. 2006; Dobransky-Fasiska et al. 2010; Lausten 2005; Mason 2003; Mirza et al. 2008; Jones-Baucke 1997), improving their programming (Mirza et al. 2008), informing their strategic planning and changing policies (Dobransky-Fasiska et al. 2009, 2010, 2012; Lausten 2005), improving the workplace psychosocial environment (Hamelin Brabant et al. 2007), and communicating with board members and funding agencies about their work (Bush and García Bengoechea 2016; Dobransky-Fasiska et al. 2010). Some authors write explicitly that the OPR approach produced research activities and products that were more acceptable and relevant to the stakeholders and were more sustainable than what the academic researchers could have produced alone (Malus et al. 2011; Williams et al. 2005; Dobransky-Fasiska et al. 2010; Chen et al. 2011; Williams 2009).

Challenges

Academic and health organization contexts and purposes are very different and this can translate into challenges for the working group members. For example, the organizational context influences all aspects of the research. Budget constraints, staff reduction and turnover, and broad organizational change and restructuring are all issues that have been faced in the North American context. As illustrated in Vignette 4, understanding each other's language can be time-consuming and challenging. The same is true for managing stakeholders' varying expectations (e.g., regarding the pace of the project (Bush and García Bengoechea 2016; Lausten 2005)). Moreover, the time investment required to build a common understanding and relationships, define mutual objectives, and work through the phases of the study together can be frustrating and, in some instances, may not be feasible for some of the partners. Ann Sawyer Williams (2009) provides an example:

> The major disadvantage of the [OPR] process for [Diabetes Association of Greater Cleveland] staff was the necessary amount of staff time spent in meetings. Generally, two or three staff members were present at the monthly meetings, for about three hours a month for 10 months. In addition, two staff members spent about three hours each making recordings, and the entire staff attended the in-service program. Therefore, the estimated total amount of staff time spent on this project was approximately 106–136 hours total. (p. 92)

Another example concerns randomized controlled trials where control group participants may feel denied the opportunity to benefit from an intervention. This was the case with a randomized controlled trial of metta meditation and massage for adults with AIDS at the end of life (Williams et al. 2005). The authors write about one of the most difficult challenges they faced in their OPR, explaining that "Once the initial cohort had a favorable study experience, they provided informal endorsement via the "grapevine" among the community, further fueling the sense of injustice among those who were ineligible or in the control group" (p. 99). While all the partners met to discuss possibilities to resolve the issue, the authors write: "it became clear that addressing the residents' perceived needs would involve a compromise of the randomized controlled methodology or a need for additional funding support. The former was not acceptable to the research partners, and the latter option was pursued unsuccessfully" (p. 99). In community contexts, some PHR researchers have dealt this issue by using a delayed intervention design, but this precludes long-term follow-up (Stein et al. 2003; Macaulay et al. 2013).

Although OPR can increase buy-in, implementing changes in a health organization with this approach is not always a seamless process. In a hospital in Montreal, Quebec, Canada, one working group sought to reorganize care to create an optimal psychosocial environment in the workplace. They obtained commitment from management and healthcare workers, collected their perceived work constraints, and implemented action plans to address them. Yet, the authors found that some employees were indifferent to or actively resisted changes. Reasons included failure of past projects, fear of losing privileges, and the need to acquire new technical skills. The authors write that establishing opportunities for discussion contributed to the involvement of staff in the change as they were able to share fears and feelings associated with the change (Hamelin Brabant et al. 2007). Another strategy to help mitigate potential challenges is for partners to agree on a set of guiding principles or terms of reference that make the needs and responsibilities of all partners explicit and details a process for dealing with disagreements. Such documents are rarely described in OPR publications. In Table 3.1 of her dissertation, Pamela Senesac (2004) provides one example where she outlines issues for which explicit clarification was required. These issues included the scope of the project, to whom the researcher and team were responsible, the process of reaching consensus, confidentiality, and the development of a 'parking lot' of future issues requiring attention.

Vignette 4: Working Through Challenges
In Allegheny County, Pennsylvania, USA, researchers from Western Psychiatric Institute and Clinic and leaders of community organizations formed the Research Network Development Core (RNDC) to create new research projects to pursue mutual concerns stemming from mental health disparities. The community/academic partnership was established slowly over a 3-year period and evolved through ongoing discussions and iterative review of ideas that eventually led to consensus at monthly meetings. Differences of opinion were discussed openly, and decisions were made through consensus. For the community partners, the challenges began with communications and developing an understanding of the mission of the partnership. One felt overwhelmed initially: "I'm going to be working with all these academics, who are all into research. I'm never going to be able to understand them, or to understand research." Another expressed, "I noticed that we speak different languages … It took time for both groups to develop an understanding of the languages." The problem with the languages was resolved over time through interacting, especially as the RNDC investigators spent considerable time at the community partners' sites. One partner commented, "The more you came here and got to know about what we did and

how we worked helped us to trust you more. You were not just trying to get funding for yourself." The distinguishable gap between research and practice was another challenge for community partners. One said: "I think the major problem is with academics understanding the practical ... It is frustrating. We function on two entirely different levels. We do not know academia, and academics do not know the day-to-day practice."

An essential part of developing and maintaining enduring relationships with the partners was to clarify goals and parameters that would facilitate the development of a constructive working framework. The principal investigator led discussions and facilitated input from all partners. The mechanisms of discussing issues were perceived by partners as follows: "Many ideas have been discussed around the table each month. Typically, we discuss ideas during a meeting ... then present interpretation of ideas at later meetings, and discuss plans for moving forward." Another stated:

> It is an opportunity to keep on pursuing an issue until it is satisfactory to you and to us. It sometimes seems like it is too much, but you have to do it. You think there has got to be an easier way, but there is not. The variety of agencies involved is spectacular. It makes it harder to get a common understanding.

Although it has been challenging to find common ground, the diversity within the partnership provided an opportunity to develop a unique synergy to better serve economically disadvantaged adults. One partner stated, "The partnership allows us to have a voice and transform that research into practice. Often with researchers they come and do the research and then you never hear from them again. You come back and explain what you found." From this study's perspective, the participatory aspect is the essential element in this work, unifying the partnership and serving as a catalyst for designing and testing new models.

Summary developed from excerpts from

Dobransky-Fasiska, D., Brown, C., Pincus, H. A., Nowalk, M. P., Wieland, M., Parker, L. S., Cruz, M., McMurray, M. L., Mulsant, B., & Reynolds, C. F. (2009). Developing a community-academic partnership to improve recognition and treatment of depression in underserved african american and white elders. *American Journal of Geriatric Psychiatry, 17*(11), 953–964. https://doi.org/10.1097/JGP.0b013e31818f3a7e.

Dobransky-Fasiska, D., Nowalk, M. P., Pincus, H. A., Castillo, E., Lee, B. E., Walnoha, A. L., Reynolds, C. F., 3rd, & Brown, C. (2010). Public-academic partnerships: improving depression care for disadvantaged adults by partnering with non-mental health agencies. *Psychiatr Serv, 61*(2), 110–112. https://doi.org/10.1176/appi.ps.61.2.110.

Dobransky-Fasiska, D., Nowalk, M. P., Cruz, M., McMurray, M. L., Castillo, E., Begley, A. E., Pyle, P., Partners, R. N.-C., Pincus, H. A., Reynolds 3rd, C. F., & Brown, C. (2012). A community-academic partnership develops a more responsive model to providing depression care to disadvantaged adults in the US. *The International journal of social psychiatry, 58*(3), 295–305.

Summary

This chapter has provided an overview of organizational participatory health research in North America. Specific examples, taken from 16 studies identified through a rigorous systematic search, have been used to describe how this type of research has been carried out in North America, with what types of stakeholders, in what contexts, and with what types of effects. In summary, in OPR, academic researchers partner with organization stakeholders in a working group to co-construct research-related decisions throughout the study. This allows organization stakeholders to shape the OPR according to their perceived needs. Moreover, the challenges and barriers to change that all stakeholders experience can be brought to the fore and taken into account. The result is a practice change or improvement initiative likely to be acceptable, feasible, pertinent, and sustainable. In short, OPR is a research approach that facilitates the identification, evaluation, and implementation of health practitioner and health organization practice improvements.

References

Allen, M. L., Salsberg, J., Knot, M., LeMaster, J. W., Felzien, M., Westfall, J. M., et al. (2017). Engaging with communities, engaging with patients: Amendment to the NAPCRG 1998 policy statement on responsible research with communities. *Family Practice, 34*(3), 313–321. https://doi.org/10.1093/fampra/cmw074.

Argyris, C., Putnam, R., & Smith, D. M. (1985). *Action science: Concepts, methods, and skills for research and intervention*. San Francisco, CA: Jossey-Bass.

Argyris, C. (1995). Action science and organizational learning. *Journal of Managerial Psychology, 10*(6), 20–26.

Argyris, C., & Schön, D. (1991). Participatory action research and action science compared. In W. F. Whyte (Ed.), Participatory action research (pp. 85–96). Newbury Park: Sage.

Barker, S. B., & Barker, R. T. (1994). Managing change in an interdisciplinary inpatient unit: An action research approach. *Journal of Mental Health Administration, 21*(1), 80–91.

Breda, K. L., Anderson, M. A., Hansen, L., Hayes, D., Pillion, C., & Lyon, P. (1997). Enhanced nursing autonomy through participatory action research. *Nursing Outlook, 45*(2), 76–81.

Bush, P. L. (2014). *Building on a YMCA's health and physical activity promotion capacities: A case study of a researcher-organization partnership to optimize adolescent programming*. (PhD), McGill University, Montreal

Bush, P. L., & García Bengoechea, E. (2016). Building on a YMCA's health and physical activity promotion capacities: A case study of a researcher-organization partnership to optimize adolescent programming. *Evaluation and Program Planning, 57*, 30–38. https://doi.org/10.1016/j.evalprogplan.2016.02.005.

Bush, P. L., Hamzeh, J., & Macaulay, A. C. (2018). Community-Based Participatory Research Oxford Bibliographies Online: Public Health (3rd ed.): Oxford University Press.

Bush, P. L., Hamzeh, J., & Macaulay, A. C. (2018). *Community-based participatory research, Oxford Bibliographies Online: Public Health*. Oxford: Oxford University Press. https://doi.org/10.1093/obo/9780199756797-0126.

Cargo, M., & Mercer, S. L. (2008). The value and challenges of participatory research: Strengthening its practice. *Annual Review of Public Health, 29*, 325–350. https://doi.org/10.1146/annurev.publhealth.29.091307.083824.

Carr, W., & Kemmis, S. (1986). Becoming critical: education, knowledge, and action research. Philadelphia (PA): Falmer Press.

Cashman, S. B., Flanagan, P., Silva, M. A., & Candib, L. M. (2012). Partnering for health: Collaborative leadership between a community health center and the YWCA central Massachusetts. *Journal of Public Health Management and Practice: JPHMP, 18*(3), 279–287.

Chen, J. C., Goetz, M. B., Feld, J. E., Taylor, A., Anaya, H., Burgess, J., et al. (2011). A provider participatory implementation model for HIV testing in an ED. *American Journal of Emergency Medicine, 29*(4), 418–426.

Cornwall, A., & Jewkes, R. (1995). What is participatory research? *Social Science & Medicine, 41*(12), 1667–1676. https://doi.org/10.1016/0277-9536(95)00127-s.

Coughlin, D., & Brannick, T. (2001). Doing action research in your own organization. Thousand Oaks, CA: Sage.

Dobransky-Fasiska, D., Brown, C., Pincus, H. A., Nowalk, M. P., Wieland, M., Parker, L. S., et al. (2009). Developing a community-academic partnership to improve recognition and treatment of depression in underserved African American and white elders. *American Journal of Geriatric Psychiatry, 17*(11), 953–964. https://doi.org/10.1097/JGP.0b013e31818f3a7e.

Dobransky-Fasiska, D., Nowalk, M. P., Pincus, H. A., Castillo, E., Lee, B. E., Walnoha, A. L., et al. (2010). Public-academic partnerships: Improving depression care for disadvantaged adults by partnering with non-mental health agencies. *Psychiatric Services, 61*(2), 110–112. https://doi.org/10.1176/appi.ps.61.2.110.

Dobransky-Fasiska, D., Nowalk, M. P., Cruz, M., McMurray, M. L., Castillo, E., Begley, A. E., et al. (2012). A community-academic partnership develops a more responsive model to providing depression care to disadvantaged adults in the US. *The International Journal of Social Psychiatry, 58*(3), 295–305.

Eisenberg, E. M., Baglia, J., & Pynes, J. E. (2006). Transforming emergency medicine through narrative: Qualitative action research at a community hospital. *Health Communication, 19*(3), 197–208.

El Sherif, R., Roy, P., Tang, D. L., Pluye, P., Bush, P., Doray, G., et al. (2015). Toward an information management system for handling parenting information users' comments. *Proceedings of the Association for Information Science and Technology, 52*(1), 1–3. https://doi.org/10.1002/pra2.2015.145052010076.

Elden, M., & Levin, M. (1991). Cogenerative learning: Bringing participation into action research. In W. F. Whyte (Ed.), Participatory action research (pp. 127–142). Newbury Park, CA: Sage.

French, W. (1969). Organization development objectives, assumptions, and strategies. *California Management Review, 12*(2), 23–34.

Freire, P. (1970). *Pedagogy of the oppressed* (M. B. Ramos, Trans.). New York: Herder and Herder.

Freire, P. (1996) Pedagogy of the opressed. NewYork: Continuum.

Green, L. W., George, M. A., Daniel, M., Frankish, C. J., Herbert, C. J., Bowie, W. R., et al. (1995). *Study of participatory research in health promotion: Review and recommendations for the development of participatory research in health promotion in Canada*. Ottawa: The Royal Society of Canada.

Greenwood, D., & Levin, M. (1998). Introduction to action research. Thousand Oaks, CA: Sage.

Grimshaw, J., Eccles, M., Lavis, J., Hill, S., Squires, J. (2012). Knowledge translation of research.

Hamelin Brabant, L., Lavoie-Tremblay, M., Viens, C., & Lefrancois, L. (2007). Engaging health care workers in improving their work environment. *Journal of Nursing Management, 15*(3), 313–320.

Hart, E. O., & Bond, M. (1995). *Action research for health and social care: A guide to practice*. Buckingham: Open University Press.

Holter, I. M., & Schwartz-Barcott, D. (1993). Action research: What is it? How has it been used and how can it be used in nursing? *Journal of Advanced Aging, 18*, 298–304.

International Collaboration for Participatory Health Research (ICPHR). (2013). *'Position Paper 1: What is Participatory Health Research?' Version: May 2013*. Berlin: International Collaboration for Participatory Health Research (Accessed: 2 Nov 2017).

International Collaboration for Participatory Health Research (ICPHR). (2013b). *'Position Paper No. 2: Participatory Health Research: A Guide to Ethical Principles and Practice' Version: October 2013*. Berlin: International Collaboration for Participatory Health Research.

Israel, B. A. (2013). *Methods for community-based participatory research for health*. San Francisco: Jossey-Bass.

Israel, B. A., Schulz, A. J., Parker, E. A., & Becker, A. B. (1998). Review of community-based research: Assessing partnership approaches to improve public health. *Annual Review of Public Health, 19*, 173–202. https://doi.org/10.1146/annurev.publhealth.19.1.173.

Israel, B. A., Eng, E., Schulz, A. J., & Parker, E. A. (2005). *Methods in community-based participatory research for health*. San Francisco: Jossey-Bass.

Jagosh, J., Macaulay, A. C., Pluye, P., Salsberg, J., Bush, P. L., Henderson, J., et al. (2012). Uncovering the benefits of participatory research: Implications of a realist review for health research and practice. *The Milbank Quarterly, 90*(2), 311–346. https://doi.org/10.1111/j.1468-0009.2012.00665.x.

Jones, D. J., Bush, P. L. and Macaulay, A. C. (2014). Beyond Consent: Respect for Community in Genetic Research. In eLS, John Wiley & Sons, Ltd (Ed.). https://doi.org/10.1002/9780470015902.a0005179.pub2

Jones-Baucke, D. L. (1997). *A qualitative study of the implementation of a system to increase nurses' use of standardized nursing languages*. (Ph.D.), UNIVERSITY OF WASHINGTON, Seattle (WA).

Jones, L. and Wells, K. (2007) 'Strategies for Academic and Cli- nician Engagement in Community–Participatory Partnered Research.' Journal of the American Medical Association 297: 407–410.

Labonte, R. (1997). Community, community development, and the forming of authentic partnerships: Some critical reflections. In: M. Minkler (Ed.), Community organizing and community building for health. New Brunswick: Rutgers University Press.

Lam, A. (2000). Tacit knowledge, organizational learning and societal institutions: An integrated framework. *Organization Studies, 21*(3), 487–513. https://doi.org/10.1177/0170840600213001.

Lausten, G. R. (2005). *Promoting ecological behavior in nurses through action research*. Denver: Univesity of Colorado.

Lavis, J., Robertson, D., Woodside, J., McLeod, C. B., & Abelson, J. (2003). How can research organizations more effectively transfer research knowledge to decision-makers. *The Millbank Quarterly, 8*(2), 221–248.

Lewin, K. (1946). Action research and minority problems. *Journal of Social Issues, 2*, 34–46.

Macaulay, A. C., Commanda, L. E., Freeman, W. L., Gibson, N., McCabe, M. L., Robbins, C. M., et al. (1999). Participatory research maximises community and lay involvement (Research Support, Non-U.S. Gov't Review). *British Medical Journal, 319*(7212), 774–778. http://www.bmj.com/cgi/reprint/319/7212/774.pdf; expanded version at http://www.napcrg.org/responsibleresearch.pdf.

Macaulay, A. C., Sirett, E., Bush, P. L. (2011). *Community-based participatory research*. Oxford Bibliographies Online: Public Health. Oxford University Press. https://doi.org/10.1093/obo/9780199756797-0126.

Macaulay, A., Jagosh, J., Pluye, P., Bush, P. L., & Salsberg, J. (2013). Quantitative methods in participatory research: Being sensitive to issues of scientific validity, community safety, and the academic-community relationship. *Revue Nouvelle Practiques Society, 25*, 159–172.

Macaulay, A. C., Sirett, E., Bush, P. L., (2015). *Community-based participatory research*. Oxford Bibliographies Online: Public Health (2nd edition): Oxford University Press. https://doi.org/10.1093/obo/9780199756797-0126.

Malus, M., Shulha, M., Granikov, V., Johnson-Lafleur, J., d'Souza, V., Knot, M., et al. (2011). A participatory approach to understanding and measuring patient satisfaction in a primary care teaching setting. *Progress in Community Health Partnerships: Research, Education, and Action, 5*(4), 417–424.

Mason, R. A. (2003). Action research: A hospital responds to domestic violence. *Healthcare Management Forum/Canadian College of Health Service Executives Forum Gestion des soins de sante/College Canadien des directeurs de services de sante, 16*(3), 18–22.

Minkler, M. (2004). Ethical challenges for the "Outside" researcher in community-based participatory research. *Health Education & Behavior, 31*(6), 684–697. https://doi.org/10.1177/1090198104269566.

Minkler, M., & Wallerstein, N. (Eds.). (2003). *Community-based participatory research for health.* San Francisco: Jossey-Bass.

Minkler, M., & Wallerstein, N. (2008). *Community-based participatory research for health: From process to outcomes.* San Francisco: Jossey-Bass.

Mirza, M., Gossett, A., Chan, N. K. C., Burford, L., & Hammel, J. (2008). Community reintegration for people with psychiatric disabilities: Challenging systemic barriers to service provision and public policy through participatory action research. *Disability & Society, 23*(4), 323–336.

Munn-Giddings, C., McVicar, A., & Smith, L. (2008). Systematic review of the uptake and design of action research in published nursing research, 2000–2005. *Journal of Research in Nursing, 13*(6), 465–477. https://doi.org/10.1177/1744987108090297.

Munten, G., Van Den Bogaard, J., Cox, K., Garretsen, H., & Bongers, I. (2010). Implementation of evidence-based practice in nursing using action research: A review. *Worldviews on Evidence-Based Nursing, 7*(3), 135–157. https://doi.org/10.1111/j.1741-6787.2009.00168.x.

Oetzel, J., Zhou, C., Duran, B., Pearson, C., Magarati, M., Lucero, J., et al. (2015). Establishing the psychometric properties of constructs in a community-based participatory research conceptual model. *American Journal of Health Promotion, 29*(5), e188–e202. https://doi.org/10.4278/ajhp.130731-QUAN-398.

Reason, P. (1994). Three approaches to Participative Inquiry. In N. Denzin & Y. Lincoln (Eds.), Handbook of Qualitative Research (pp. 324–329). Thousand Oaks (CA): Sage.

Salsberg, J., Parry, D., Pluye, P., Macridis, S., Herbert, C. P., & Macaulay, A. C. (2015). Successful strategies to engage research partners for translating evidence into action in community health: A critical review. *Journal of Environmental and Public Health, 2015*, 191856. https://doi.org/10.1155/2015/191856.

Senesac, P. M. (2004). *The roy adaptation model: An action research approach to the implementation of a pain management organizational change project.* (Ph.D.), Boston College, William F. Connell Graduate School of Nursing. Chestnut Hill, MA

Selener, D. (1997). Participatory action research and social change. Ithaca, NY: Cornell Participatory Action Research Network.

Smith, S. E. (1995). *Dancing with conflict: Public health nurses in participatory action-research.* Canada: University of Calgary.

Soh, K. L. (2011). Action research studies in the intensive care setting: A systematic review. *International Journal of Nursing Studies, 48*, 258–268. https://doi.org/10.1016/j.ijnurstu.2010.09.014.

Soh, K. L., Davidson, P. M., Leslie, G., & Rahman, A. B. A. (2011). Action research studies in the intensive care setting: A systematic review. *International Journal of Nursing Studies, 48*(2), 258–268. https://doi.org/10.1016/j.ijnurstu.2010.09.014.

Stein, B. D., Jaycox, L. H., Kataoka, S. H., et al. (2003). A mental health intervention for school-children exposed to violence: A randomized controlled trial. *JAMA, 290*(5), 603–611. https://doi.org/10.1001/jama.290.5.603.

Straus, S. E., Tetroe, J., & Graham, I. D. (Eds.). (2009). *Knowledge translation in health care: Moving from evidence to practice.* Oxford: Wiley-Blackwell.

Stringer, E. T. (1999). Action research. 2nd ed., Thousand Oaks, CA: Sage.

Wallerstein, N. (2000). A participatory evaluation model for healthier communities: Developing indicators for New Mexico. *Public Health Report.* US Department of Health and Human Services, *115*, 199–204.

Wallerstein, N., Oetzel, J., Duran, B., Tafoya, G., Belone, L., & Rae, R. (2008). What predicts outcomes in CBPR? In M. Minkler & N. Wallerstein (Eds.), *Community-based participatory research for health: From process to outcomes* (pp. 371–392). San Francisco: Jossey-Bass.

Waterman, H., Tillen, D., Dickson, R., & de Koning, K. (2001). Action research: A systematic review and guidance for assessment. *Health Technology Assessment, 5*(23), 1–166 http://www. hta.ac.uk/execsumm/summ523.shtml.

Williams, A. S. (2005). *Using participatory action research to make diabetes education accessible for people with visual impairment.* San Francisco: Saybrook Graduate School and Research Center.

Williams, A. S. (2009). Making Diabetes Education Accessible For People With Visual Impairment. *The Diabetes Educator, 34*(4), 612–621. https://doi.org/10.1177/0145721709335005.

Williams, A. L., Selwyn, P. A., McCorkle, R., Molde, S., Liberti, L., & Katz, D. L. (2005). Application of community-based participatory research methods to a study of complementary medicine interventions at end of life. *Complementary Health Practice Review, 10*(2), 91–104.

Chapter 13
Participatory Health Research in North America: From Community Engagement to Evidence-Informed Practice

Jon Salsberg and Nickoo Merati

Participatory Health Research: History and Application

Participatory health research (PHR) is the systematic co-creation of new knowledge by researchers working in equitable partnerships with those affected by the issue under study or those who will benefit from or ultimately act on its results (Green et al. 1995; Israel et al. 1998; Macaulay et al. 1999). These include, among others, communities, organizations, patients, or practitioners. PHR has been shown to benefit all those involved, including the research itself. Taking a PHR approach is shown to ensure cultural and logistical appropriateness of research, enhance recruitment capacity, result in productive conflicts followed by useful negotiation, increase the quality of outputs and outcomes over time, increase the sustainability of project goals beyond funded time frames and during gaps in external funding, and create system changes and new unanticipated projects and activities (Jagosh et al. 2012). For health intervention research, proponents also argue that PHR strengthens academic-community relations; ensures relevancy of research questions; increases capacity of data collection, analysis, and interpretation; and minimizes negative stigma associated with research (Israel et al. 1998, 2005; Macaulay et al. 1998, 1999; O'Fallon and Dearry 2002; Cargo and Mercer 2008; Cargo et al. 2008). PHR is also believed to increase communities' capacity to identify and solve their problems (Macaulay et al. 1999; Gaventa and Cornwall 2006) and decision-makers' and service providers' ability to mobilize resources, improve policies, and enhance professional capacity and practices (Minkler and Wallerstein 2008a). PHR furthermore

J. Salsberg (✉)
Graduate Entry Medical School and Health Research Institute (HRI), University of Limerick, Limerick, Ireland
e-mail: jon.salsberg@ul.ie

N. Merati
Department of Family Medicine, McGill University, Montreal, Canada
e-mail: nickoo.merati@mail.mcgill.ca

© Springer International Publishing AG, part of Springer Nature 2018
M. T. Wright, K. Kongats (eds.), *Participatory Health Research*,
https://doi.org/10.1007/978-3-319-92177-8_13

integrates knowledge translation into the knowledge creation process, by assuring that the appropriate end users of the results are implicated throughout all key phases of the research. Importantly, from a PHR perspective, end users should be involved in (at least) the research phases of identifying needs, setting research questions, interpreting results, and disseminating and applying findings (Macaulay et al. 1999; Minkler and Wallerstein 2008a; Parry et al. 2009; Salsberg et al. 2014).

Participatory health research finds its origins in both social action research and emancipatory philosophy, or as has been suggested, from northern and southern traditions, respectively (Wallerstein and Duran 2008). Kurt Lewin's action research framework (Lewin and Lewin 1948), often referred to as the northern heritage of PHR, proposed a cycle of continuous inquiry, action, and evaluation, undertaken with or by – as opposed to *for* or *on* – society's marginalized or disenfranchised. The aim of Lewin's action research framework was to empower mainly urban-dwelling ethnic minorities to create social equity in overcoming racial and class disparities. This framework has been expanded and developed over the ensuing decades, most notably by Argyris and others (Argyris and Schön 1978; Argyris et al. 1985) who applied it as a means of promoting improvement in organizational efficiency.

Paulo Freire's emancipatory theory in *Pedagogy of the Oppressed* (Freire 1970), often referred to as the southern heritage of PHR, questioned the value of both knowledge and education by critically examining their products in relation to political power and oppression. Freire posited individuals not as empty vessels but as potential masters of their own future, able to best determine their own needs to improve their lives. Agendas for both education and research should hence serve their self-defined needs; furthermore, people, and indeed communities, should no longer be seen as objects of study but instead as full participants in inquiry (Wallerstein and Duran 2008; Freire 1970). Freire's work has been particularly influential for action in developing area studies: researchers and international organizations such as UNESCO and the World Bank have used Freire's framework toward empowering marginalized and disenfranchised communities to generate the evidence they needed in order to force local or national policy changes, which grant them hitherto denied rights and resources (Rahman 1993). Freire's *conscientização* ran parallel with the critical consciousness of emerging feminist perspective in North America and was a philosophical building block for the Indigenous and decolonizing methodologies to come (Denzin et al. 2008; Chavez et al. 2008; Duran and Duran 1995).

In both emancipatory and action-oriented work, social change and access to often life-sustaining resources were paramount, often devaluing the need or desire to apply "rigorous" research methods (Rahman 1993). From an epistemological – and indeed *Freirean* – perspective, if PHR knowledge is to motivate an individual's behavior or action for change (Semali and Kincheloe 1999; Bradbury and Reason 2008), then the knowledge products of people's own self-research, as well as the methods that produced them, are the most valid and rigorous so long as they foment desired social change. This methodological consideration later became a point of contention, as participatory methods were seen by some as "soft" when applied to topics and areas where other scientific methods were the norm (Minkler and Baden 2008).

Shift from Methodology to Approach

For a long time, participatory health research was seen explicitly as a qualitative methodology: a branch of qualitative enquiry where people could come together, usually with outside support, to inquire into their own social issues (Patton 1990; Schwandt 2007). This qualitative trend is indeed congruent with the methodological realities of the PHR approach: if the knowledge created through the PHR process is to benefit a more-or-less homogeneous group of people, then how that knowledge is defined and understood (epistemology) and the means of apprehending it (research methods) must match (Patton 1990; McIntyre 2008; Kirby et al. 2006). For most groups or societies in which the PHR process was being applied, people were not placed in an objective, positivist paradigm that is congruent with more quantitative methods; instead, people were concerned with the need for action in their particular context and practicable by themselves, which is shown to be more congruent with qualitative methods (Fine et al. 2008). Hence, PHR knowledge creation typically resembled more qualitative inquiry. It is also possible that this association between PHR and qualitative methods was a reflection of which outside academics or activists were involved.

In the 1980s, as participatory methods were beginning to be applied to health promotion, two things changed. First, many practitioners involved in public health and equity research had epidemiological training; they were interested in addressing the disproportionate burden of ill-health experienced by marginalized or underserved communities. Focus thus began to shift from the developing world to include industrialized nations where these communities existed, with new studies appearing in North America (Epp 1986; Labonte 1986). Second, because the health promotion framework addresses social determinants of health, many projects began to include more diverse stakeholders that were needed to address system and policy change (Robertson and Minkler 1994). This meant that not only were local populations participating but also program planners, policy-makers, and service providers – anyone whose behavior, opinion, or practice needed to change to create the intended social or health change. In this new multi-stakeholder, multi-perspective context, a single PHR project likely represents multiple epistemologies. As such, from this point forward, it became impossible to see participatory health research solely as a methodology or a set of methods congruent with a single epistemology – but rather an approach where multiple stakeholders could negotiate and align their action needs around a particular issue and develop new knowledge products that were necessary from their own perspectives to address it. The fundamental principal of PHR thus became equitable co-ownership of knowledge (Israel et al. 1998; Macaulay et al. 1999; Minkler and Baden 2008). Hereafter, participatory "methods" no longer referred to methods of data collection and analysis; instead, participatory "methods" now referred to methods of partner engagement, methods of locating power, and methods of ownership at every stage of the research process (Minkler and Baden 2008). In addition, "research *on* the PHR process" henceforth became research on how best to create and maintain engagement among project stakeholders with meaningful and sustained ownership over the research and action process (Cargo et al. 2008, 2011).

1980s, 1990s, and Beyond: Participatory Health Research and Health Promotion

As early as 1984, one development researcher recognized:

> What is needed is a research process which incorporates both qualitative and quantitative methods adapted to field conditions. Such a process would include… a preliminary qualitative stage…, a quantitative stage…, a follow-up qualitative stage to investigate inconsistencies between initial qualitative and quantitative data which might indicate compounding or unidentified variables, representative in-depth case studies, [and] periodic follow-up research to account for social change. (Nichter 1984)

Nichter immediately follows this statement with a question: "But who is there to conduct such research?" (Nichter 1984). It is argued that this call was answered by the burgeoning field of health promotion: with its focus on the health equity, the social determinants of health, and, importantly, the primacy of the community in setting its own policy research and intervention agenda (Epp 1986; Labonte 1986; Robertson and Minkler 1994).

This expanded view of health to include health promotion was embodied in the *Ottawa Charter of Health Promotion*, which defined health promotion as "the process of enabling people to increase control over, and improve, their health" (WHO 1986). Robertson and Minkler (1994) saw "the new public health" as a social movement, including (1) a broader definition of health to include the social determinants of health, (2) emphasis on social and political intervention strategies over individual ones, (3) the centrality of individual and community empowerment, and (4) meaningful participation. Moreover, Robertson and Minkler used Arnstein's ladder of participation to critique the then-current notions of true participation (Arnstein 1969).

Those involved in health promotion planning looked to PHR as a process for communities to organically determine their own health priorities by accounting for the various ecological spheres that encapsulate and constrain healthy behavior. Green and Kreuter (2005) took participatory processes as central to their PRECEDE-PROCEED model of health promotion planning and evaluation (Green and Kreuter 2005); this has been the most robustly applied model of community intervention planning and evaluation since its initial introduction in the early 1990s. Other health promotion practitioners and evaluators also turned to PHR as an appropriate approach to community-university partnerships for change, highlighting that communities must have the self-determination to identify and redress their own health issues (Minkler 2000; Israel et al. 1998; Macaulay et al. 1999).

From Health Promotion to Health Services Research and Integrated Knowledge Translation

At this point, PHR had entered the health research literature largely through its usefulness as an approach to community-based health promotion. Leading health promotion researchers such as Meredith Minkler, Barbara Israel, and Nina Wallerstein were early to recognize the value of this approach for other health research areas (Minkler and Wallerstein 2008b; Israel 2005). By the early 2000s, PHR once again experienced a push as health service researchers and evaluators began to grapple with the limitations of evidence-based practice in both health care and in public health policy.

Despite industrialized nations' significant investment in developing evidence-based practice for the improvement of health, health services, and systems, there has been recognition over the last two decades that, despite significant gains, the evidence created is not necessarily applied in practice (Straus et al. 2009, 2011; Graham et al. 2002; Graham and Tetroe 2007). As researchers, practitioners, and educators began to turn their attention to this *know-do* gap, it was estimated to take on average 17 years for just 14% of all primary research conducted to make it into practice (Weingarten et al. 2000; Green 2008). In addition, many viewed the progress of knowledge into practice as if moving through a pipeline: vast amounts of knowledge derived from primary research are increasingly synthesized, refined, and tailored to eventually be put into use (Green 2008). While this process is important to assure only high quality and efficacious findings are applied – especially in the biomedical clinical setting – it can also limit or unduly delay the application of beneficial findings into practice to finally affect individuals' health outcomes. Furthermore, it is not always clear what these "beneficial" findings are: beneficial to whom? Is beneficial to the patient the same as beneficial to the service provider or other health stakeholders? Is there a way we can better understand this process of moving knowledge into action, to accelerate the identification, uptake, and use of beneficial knowledge? This query has led directly to the study and practice of bridging these implementation gaps: knowledge translation.

Knowledge Translation and Integrated Knowledge Translation

Knowledge translation (KT) begins from a different premise: the movement of knowledge into action is not viewed as a linear pipeline but rather a cycle of interaction (Graham et al. 2006; Armstrong et al. 2006; Greenhalgh et al. 2004; Green et al. 2009). From this view, the needs of "end users" including practitioners, interveners, policy-makers, communities, and individuals drive primary research as much as the latter constrains practice. Knowledge translation has thus been defined by the Canadian Institutes of Health Research (CIHR) as a dynamic and iterative process that includes synthesis, dissemination, exchange, and ethically sound application of knowledge to improve and provide more effective health services (Graham et al. 2006). This complex system of interactions may vary in intensity, complexity, and level of engagement, depending on the nature of the research as well as the needs of the particular knowledge user, i.e., those who must ultimately act on the results of the research, or for whom the outcome benefits are intended (Graham et al. 2006). The Canadian view of KT is an attempt to define an overarching conceptual framework that includes all stages of discovery: from basic science, through clinical application, to health of populations. However, its applicability to public health often has been applied or received coolly. In the USA, for example, the National Institutes of Health (NIH) have clearly differentiated between "Translational Research 1," bench to preclinical and clinical usage, and "Translational Research 2," basic, clinical, and intervention research to community and population health (NIH Roadmap 2012). Until the recent advent of the large NIH Clinical and Translational Science Awards, these two areas of KT were seen as distinct, and the majority of resources were dedicated to the first.

As dynamic, multidirectional, and complex as KT can be from the bench to the clinic, it can be argued that its complexity compounds when translating research results into effective outcomes at the public health level (Green and Glasgow 2006). While there are certainly added levels of complexity in public health, many of the encountered issues are fundamentally the same. These issues are still founded on the mismatch between the context in which knowledge is produced and the context in which end users (clinical practitioners, policy-makers, patients, and people at large) need to put this knowledge to use (Bradbury and Reason 2008; Green and Glasgow 2006).

Graham et al. (2006) outline a broad typology of definitions of KT, which vary mainly on the directionality of flow, end user audience, and level of engagement between different stakeholders in the translation process. They eventually built the *knowledge-to-action* (KTA) model (which underlies the CIHR definition of KT), based on a synthesis of 31 identified theoretical or logic models of knowledge implementation, mobilization, exchange, transfer, utilization, and usage (Graham and Tetroe 2007). Although their model acknowledges that knowledge producers can tailor activities to potential users' needs at any phase, the KTA model as originally presented seemed to describe the activities of knowledge creation and knowledge translation as structurally distinct: beginning with the creation and refinement of new knowledge, followed by a cyclical process of needs assessment, knowledge adaptation, implementation, evaluation, and sustaining (Graham and Tetroe 2007).

Integrated KT reconceptualizes KT from a corollary of knowledge production to a fundamental part of it (Bowen and Graham 2013; Salsberg et al. 2014; Salsberg and Macaulay 2013) and embraces the Canadian Health Services Research Foundation (CHSRF)'s definition of knowledge exchange:

> ...collaborative problem-solving between researchers and decision makers that happens through linkages and exchange. Effective knowledge exchange involves interactions between decision makers and researchers and results in mutual learning through the process of planning, producing, disseminating and applying existing or new research in decision-making. (Graham et al. 2006)

Integrated KT is hence a dynamic, multidirectional process (Ward et al. 2009) where researchers and appropriate knowledge users are meaningfully and equitably involved in *all appropriate stages of the research*: from identification of the need, through interpretation of results, to dissemination and application of the findings (Parry et al. 2009; Salsberg et al. 2014). It is precisely the *participation* of all stakeholders at all appropriate stages that ultimately allows KT to address any epistemological and contextual divides as they arise; integrated KT ultimately ensures that the co-created knowledge is applicable to the knowledge users in the community and population settings.

In his review of CIHR's KT programs, McLean et al. (2013) note: "researchers and [knowledge users] describe building meaningful collaboration as key to research project success and impact, however, the term 'meaningful' is quite nuanced and contextually-bound" (McLean et al. 2013). In describing the dimensions of *meaningful engagement*, he concludes that:

- Meaningful partnerships are characterized by mutual learning, mutual respect, mutually agreed upon roles and responsibilities, mutual recognition of efforts, and mutual exchange of information.
- Mutual does not necessarily denote that partners give and receive equally but that all parties play a role in negotiating roles and expectations.
- Researchers and knowledge users have different understandings of the roles and responsibilities required of each team member in order to make collaboration meaningful.
- Meaningful partnerships are negotiated based on many factors including, but not limited to, resources, external commitments, technical skills, and epistemology (McLean et al. 2013).

Knowledge Translation and Evidence-Based Practice

Historically, there exists a link between the emergence of KT as a field and the growth of *evidence-based practice*. Evidence-based practice (EBP) first emerged in the early 1990s (Sackett et al. 1996; Sackett 2000) in response to a need for health intervention and practice based on clearer and more rigorous scientific "evidence." Over the ensuing years, EBP has become the predominant paradigm for training health professionals and for designing and delivering public health policy initiatives. The EBP process proceeds along the following steps (as summarized by Kohatsu et al. 2004): (1) state the scientific question of interest; (2) identify the relevant evidence; (3) determine what evidence is relevant to answering the scientific question of interest; (4) determine the best course of action considering the patient or population; and (5) evaluate process and outcome. It is at stage four, determining the best course of action, that the effectiveness of EBP as a guide to action tends to break down, as we will demonstrate below.

Many criticisms of EBP have been put forward. Kohatsu et al. (2004) summarize the issues of EBP through its de-emphasis of patients' [or community's] values, perspectives, and choices, its failure to account for individual social and biological variation, its de-emphasis of clinicians' insights, and the lack of a model to inform how these all could be combined to choose the optimal course of action. In essence, EBP falls short due to its relative failure to address both context and differing constructions of evidence (i.e., epistemologies). One facet of EBP's failure in addressing context is that "rigorous" scientific evidence is subject to the limitations of publication bias: where negative results do not get published or even submitted as frequently as positive results. However, negative results are certainly of interest because:

> they often tell the practitioner about the intervention's misfit with populations or conditions other than those in which the original research leading to guidelines was conducted. (Green et al. 2009)

Thus, excluding negative results fails practitioners because:

> The literature on which the [evidence-based] guidelines are based constitutes an unrepresentative sample of the varied circumstances and populations in which the interventions might be usable or unusable. (Green et al. 2009)

Furthermore, there is a fundamental contradiction between the basis for EBP and the way it is acted upon. Clinicians operate in a world that is epistemologically distinct from that in which the knowledge they must act on was produced. Evidence-based clinical practice guidelines (CPGs) are (at their "highest level of rigor") derived from a synthesis of controlled, decontextualized experimentation. Whereas clinicians generally rely heavily on experiential evidence accumulated over the course of their practice, novice clinicians such as medical residents are much more likely to adhere closely to CPGs than senior clinicians, who rely more on the context before them when deciding on a course of action (Greenhalgh 2012). This is doubly confounded by the fact that multiple, often conflicting, CPGs can exist for any single given issue. For this reason, we witness a tendency for clinicians to disregard CPGs and instead fall back on experience when faced with complex decisions for action (Greenhalgh 2012).

Green (2008), Greenhalgh (Greenhalgh et al. 2004), and others have proposed that the solution to these problems is not to dilute the rigors of scientific evidence but rather to recontextualize the impetus for the creation of action-oriented knowledge in the first place. As Green (2008) succinctly puts it: "if it is an evidence-based practice, where's the practice-based evidence?" Both Green and Greenhalgh call for knowledge that is co-created with the full participation of those who must ultimately apply it (i.e., *integrated KT* with end users); they call for the creation of knowledge that is necessarily imbued with the contextual imperatives to render knowledge useful to the setting in which it needs to be applied. In other words, they are recommending *participatory health research*. Furthermore, knowledge creation should focus on process (i.e., why the intervention is appropriate for the context, rather than is it effective), be ecological (i.e., explore the relationship between the intervention and the context in which it took place), and be theory-driven (i.e., based on a theoretical understanding of the mechanism for action or change) (Greenhalgh et al. 2004).

Knowledge Translation and Public Health

In the preceding sections, we have discussed the overall issues at stake in KT when translating knowledge to action, especially when applied to the complex public health sphere. Furthermore, KT in public health is taking place within a broader set of stakeholders; at any given point in the translation process, any or all of these stakeholders' interests may conflict, leading to a breakdown of implementation. Moreover, stakeholder groups (e.g., *all* policy-makers or *all* community members) are certainly not monolithic and can experience dissent from within. It is also worthwhile to note that stakeholders in public health policy often come with political, bureaucratic, or social agendas that may compete with strict health-related goals. As such, the formulation of evidence-based public health policy and programing by policy-makers and practitioners comes up against several particular barriers. These include an absence of personal contact between researchers, policy-makers, and practitioners; lack of timeliness of research; mutual mistrust between stakeholders; power and budget struggles within or between agencies; poor quality of research, from an evidence-based perspective; political instability; and a debate over what constitutes evidence (Armstrong et al. 2006). Furthermore, the timing of policy planning and budgetary cycles is such that it is often impossible to act on new significant evidence once policy-makers have already begun implementing a program. Thus, action on the new knowledge is often delayed for years or even relegated to obscurity (Parry et al. 2009).

Public health interventions are by nature complex; hence evidence for their efficacy or effectiveness is notoriously difficult to come by (Pawson 2006). The link between cause, effect, and solution is practically impossible to establish for these complex interventions. Public health interventions must also serve a large heterogeneous population whose health is constrained by myriad upstream social and environmental determinants. However, as stated above (Green 2008; Greenhalgh et al. 2004), an integrated KT approach helps address all of these issues by ensuring that those whose health is being benefitted are implicated in identifying the need, designing the means of filling it, applying the results, helping to decide whether it was successful, and sustaining the effort (Salsberg et al. 2014; Parry et al. 2009). Most importantly for public health, the participatory nature of integrated KT directly addresses the social determinants of health by building community capacity in terms of human, social, and environmental capital, addressing both community and organizational readiness, and fostering a sense of community ownership and empowerment that leads to the sustainability of both programs and health outcomes (Jagosh et al. 2012; Labonte 1986; Salsberg et al. 2017b).

Future Directions of Participatory Health Research for Policy and Practice

Research on the process and outcomes of PHR is still growing. With each new study, we learn a bit more about what works, for whom, and in what contexts. This contextual condition of PHR in itself points to the difficulty in locating an overarching framework for PHR. In any event, after more than a decade and a half of evidence-based practice, the tides seem to be shifting once more toward less linear, more contextualized approaches to practice change. While public health intervention research is still firmly rooted in evidence-based models, the broad shift in clinical care to reemphasize the primary care setting, patient-oriented or managed care, and the "medical home" has resituated evidence-based practice as evidence-*informed* practice (Davies et al. 2000). This much more nuanced approach explicitly places equal if not greater weight on external validity, the clinical experience, and the individual needs of patients, their lived lives, and their families. In public health, this can be reflected in Kohatsu et al.'s (2004) definition of EBPH as "the process of integrating science-based interventions with community preferences to improve the health of populations." In general, a continued emphasis on PHR as the preferred means of co-creating action-oriented knowledge in both the clinical and population spheres will assure that contextual and epistemological factors are always at the core of knowledge translation – thus improving relevance, uptake, and sustainability of knowledge use.

Key Limitations and Knowledge Gaps

The gaps and limitations in our understanding of the process and outcomes of participatory health research fall mainly into two categories. Firstly, does, and if so then how does taking a PHR approach lead to better research outcomes than taking a conventional, research-led approach? Relatedly, what do we mean by better (Macaulay et al. 2011; Glasgow et al. 1999; Jagosh et al. 2011)? Secondly, what is the evidence supporting the various aspects or stages to a PHR conceptual model? Several PHR conceptual models have been suggested, most recent and notable being those proposed by Cargo and Mercer (2008) and by Wallerstein and colleagues (Cacari-Stone et al. 2014; Sanchez et al. 2011; Oetzel et al. 2014). Wallerstein's team is currently undertaking a program of research to delve into the stages of their conceptual model. In the knowledge translation world, Graham and colleagues are similarly engaged in a program of study to investigate the processes and impacts of stakeholder involvement in improving both research and health system outcomes (Kothari et al. 2017; Gagliardi et al. 2017). The results of both of these programs will significantly further our understanding of participatory processes. In addition, a new line of inquiry using social network analysis is attempting to demonstrate how PHR processes shift ownership and self-determination over knowledge production from academic to community stakeholders (Salsberg et al. 2017a, b).

Conclusion

Participatory health research has come to be recognized as an approach that enhances the quality of the research process and its outcomes, including the relevance and uptake of its products (Jagosh et al. 2012; Macaulay et al. 1999). At the same time, PHR builds community capacity and self-determination while addressing issues of equity and social and environmental justice (Cargo and Mercer 2008; Israel et al. 1998). Gaps remain, however, in our understanding of these strategies, processes, and mechanisms to support these benefits. Bridging these knowledge gaps will benefit all research aimed at empowering community members and organizations, patients, caregivers, service providers, and other decision-makers and end users in creating the knowledge they need for action on wellness, empowerment, and sustained change.

References

Argyris, C., & Schön, D. A. (1978). *Organizational learning*. Reading: Addison-Wesley.

Argyris, C., Putnam, R., & Smith, D. M. (1985). *Action science*. San Francisco: Jossey-Bass.

Armstrong, R., Waters, E., Roberts, H., Oliver, S., & Popay, J. (2006). The role and theoretical evolution of knowledge translation and exchange in public health. *Journal of Public Health, 28*(4), 384–389.

Arnstein, S. R. (1969). A ladder of citizen participation. *Journal of the American Institute of Planners, 35*(4), 216–224.

Bowen, S., & Graham, I. D. (2013). Integrated knowledge translation. In E. Straus, J. Tetroe, & I. D. Graham (Eds.), *Knowledge Translation in Healthcare: Moving from Evidence to Practice* (pp. 14–23). Oxford: Wiley/BMJ Books.

Bradbury, H., & Reason, P. (2008). Issues and choice points for improving the quality of action research. In M. Minkler & N. Wallerstein (Eds.), *Community based participatory research for health* (2nd ed., pp. 225–242). San Francisco: Jossey-Bass.

Cacari-Stone, L., Wallerstein, N., Garcia, A. P., & Minkler, M. (2014). The promise of community-based participatory research for health equity: A conceptual model for bridging evidence with policy (research support, non-U.S. gov't). *American Journal of Public Health, 104*(9), 1615–1623. https://doi.org/10.2105/AJPH.2014.301961.

Cargo, M., & Mercer, S. L. (2008). The value and challenges of participatory research: Strengthening its practice. *Annual Review of Public Health, 29*, 325–350. https://doi.org/10.1146/annurev.publhealth.29.091307.083824.

Cargo, M., Delormier, T., Levesque, L., Horn-Miller, K., McComber, A., & Macaulay, A. C. (2008). Can the democratic ideal of participatory research be achieved? An inside look at an academic indigenous community partnership. *Health Education Research, 23*, 904–914 doi:cym077 [pii] 91093/her/cym077.

Cargo, M., Delormier, T., Levesque, L., McComber, A., & Macaulay, A. (2011). Community capacity as an "inside job": Evolution of perceived ownership of a university-aboriginal community partnership. *American Journal of Health Promotion, 26*(2), 96–100 http://ajhpcontents.org/toc/hepr/26/2.

Chavez, V., Duran, B., Baker, Q. E., Avila, M. M., & Wallerstein, N. (2008). The dance of race and privilege in CBPR. In Minkler, M., & Wallerstein, N. (Eds.), *Community-based participatory research for health: From process to outcomes*. San Francisco: Jossey-Bass.

Davies, H. T., Nutley, S. M., & Smith, P. C. (2000). *What works?: Evidence-based policy and practice in public services*. Boston: MIT Press.

Denzin, N. K., Lincoln, Y. S., & Smith, L. T. (2008). *Handbook of critical and indigenous methodologies*. Los Angeles: Sage.

Duran, E., & Duran, B. (1995). *Native American postcolonial psychology*. Albany: SUNY Press.

Epp, J. (1986). Achieving health for all: A framework for health promotion. *Health Promotion, 1*(4), 419–428.

Fine, M., Tuck, E., & Zeller-Berkman, S. (2008). Do you believe in Geneva? In Denzin, N. K., Lincoln, Y. S. & Smith, L. T. (Eds), *Handbook of critical and indigenous methodologies*. Thousand Oaks, CA: SAGE Publications Ltd. https://doi.org/10.4135/9781483385686

Freire, P. (1970). *Pedagogy of the oppressed*. New York: Herder and Herder.

Gagliardi, A. R., Kothari, A., & Graham, I. D. (2017). Research agenda for integrated knowledge translation (IKT) in healthcare: What we know and do not yet know (editorial). *Journal of Epidemiology and Community Health, 71*(2), 105–106. https://doi.org/10.1136/jech-2016-207743.

Gaventa, J., & Cornwall, A. (2006). Challenging the boundaries of the possible: Participation, knowledge and power. *IDS Bulletin, 37*(6), 122–128.

Glasgow, R. E., Vogt, T. M., & Boles, S. M. (1999). Evaluating the public health impact of health promotion interventions: The RE-AIM framework. *American Journal of Public Health, 89*(9), 1322–1327.

Graham, I. D., & Tetroe, J. (2007). How to translate health research knowledge into effective healthcare action. *Healthcare Quarterly, 10*(3), 20–22 http://www.ncbi.nlm.nih.gov/entrez/query.fcgi?cmd=Retrieve&db=PubMed&dopt=Citation&list_uids=17632905.

Graham, I. D., Harrison, M. B., Brouwers, M., Davies, B. L., & Dunn, S. (2002). Facilitating the use of evidence in practice: Evaluating and adapting clinical practice guidelines for local use by health care organizations. *Journal of Obstetric, Gynecologic, and Neonatal Nursing, 31*(5), 599–611 http://www.ncbi.nlm.nih.gov/entrez/query.fcgi?cmd=Retrieve&db=PubMed&dopt=Citation&list_uids=12353740.

Graham, I. D., Logan, J., Harrison, M. B., Straus, S. E., Tetroe, J., Caswell, W., et al. (2006). Lost in knowledge translation: Time for a map? *The Journal of Continuing Education in the Health Professions, 26*(1), 13–24. https://doi.org/10.1002/chp.47.

Green, L. W. (2008). Making research relevant: If it is an evidence-based practice, where's the practice-based evidence? *Family Practice, 25*(Suppl 1), i20–i24 doi:cmn055 [pii] 271093/fampra/cmn055.

Green, L. W., & Glasgow, R. E. (2006). Evaluating the relevance, generalization, and applicability of research issues in external validation and translation methodology. *Evaluation & the Health Professions, 29*(1), 126–153.

Green, L. W., & Kreuter, M. W. (2005). *Health program planning : An educational and ecological approach*. New York: McGraw-Hill.

Green, L. W., George, A., Daniel, M., Frankish, C. J., Herbert, C. P., Bowie, W. R., et al. (1995). *Study of participatory research in health promotion: Review and recommendations for the development of participatory research in health promotion in Canada*. Ottawa: Royal Society of Canada.

Green, L., Ottoson, J., García, C., & Robert, H. (2009). Diffusion theory and knowledge dissemination, utilization, and integration in public health. *Annual Review of Public Health, 30*, 151.

Greenhalgh, T. (2012). Why do we always end up here? Evidence-based medicine's conceptual cul-de-sacs and some off-road alternative routes. *Journal of Primary Health Care, 4*(2), 92–97 http://www.ncbi.nlm.nih.gov/pubmed/22675691.

Greenhalgh, T., Robert, G., Macfarlane, F., Bate, P., & Kyriakidou, O. (2004). Diffusion of innovations in service organizations: Systematic review and recommendations. *The Milbank Quarterly, 82*(4), 581–629. https://doi.org/10.1111/j.0887-378X.2004.00325.x.

Israel, B. A. (2005). *Methods in community-based participatory research for health*. San Francisco: Jossey-Bass.

Israel, B. A., Schulz, A. J., Parker, E. A., & Becker, A. B. (1998). Review of community-based research: Assessing partnership approaches to improve public health. *Annual Review of Public Health, 19*, 173–202.

Israel, B. A., Parker, E. A., Rowe, Z., Salvatore, A., Minkler, M., Lopez, J., et al. (2005). Community-based participatory research: Lessons learned from the centers for children's environmental health and disease prevention research. *Environmental Health Perspectives, 113*(10), 1463–1471 http://www.ncbi.nlm.nih.gov/entrez/query.fcgi?cmd=Retrieve&db=PubMed&dopt=Citation&list_uids=16203263.

Jagosh, J., Pluye, P., Macaulay, A. C., Salsberg, J., Henderson, J., Sirett, E., et al. (2011). Assessing the outcomes of participatory research: Protocol for identifying, selecting, appraising and synthesizing the literature for realist review. *Implementation Science, 6*, 24 doi:1748-5908-6-24 [pii] 10.1186/1748-5908-6-24.

Jagosh, J., Macaulay, A. C., Pluye, P., Salsberg, J., Bush, P. L., Henderson, J., et al. (2012). Uncovering the benefits of participatory research: Implications of a realist review for health research and practice. *The Milbank Quarterly, 90*(2), 311–346. https://doi.org/10.1111/j.1468-0009.2012.00665.x.

Kirby, S. L., Greaves, L., & Reid, C. (2006). *Experience research social change: Methods beyond the mainstream.* Toronto: University of Toronto Press.

Kohatsu, N. D., Robinson, J. G., & Torner, J. C. (2004). Evidence-based public health: An evolving concept. *American Journal of Preventive Medicine, 27*(5), 417–421.

Kothari, A., McCutcheon, C., & Graham, I. D. (2017). Defining integrated knowledge translation and moving forward: A response to recent commentaries. *International Jouranl of Health Policy Management, 6*(5), 299–300. https://doi.org/10.15171/ijhpm.2017.15.

Labonte, R. (1986). Social inequality and healthy public policy. *Health Promotion, 1*(3), 341–351.

Lewin, K., & Lewin, G. W. (1948). *Resolving social conflicts, selected papers on group dynamics [1935–1946].* New York: Harper.

Macaulay, A., Paradis, G., Potvin, L., Cross, E., Saad-Haddad, C., McComber, A., et al. (1998). Primary prevention of diabetes type II in first nations: Experiences of the Kahnawake Schools Diabetes Prevention Project. *Canadian Journal of Diabetes Care, 22*, 44–49 Link unavailable.

Macaulay, A. C., Commanda, L. E., Freeman, W. L., Gibson, N., McCabe, M. L., Robbins, C. M., et al. (1999). Participatory research maximises community and lay involvement. North American Primary Care Research Group. *BMJ, 319*(7212), 774–778 http://www.bmj.com/cgi/reprint/319/7212/774?maxtoshow=&HITS=10&hits=10&RESULTFORMAT=&fulltext=Participatory+research+maximises+community&searchid=1&FIRSTINDEX=0&resourcetype=HWCIT.

Macaulay, A. C., Jagosh, J., Seller, R., Henderson, J., Cargo, M., Greenhalgh, T., et al. (2011). Assessing the benefits of participatory research: A rationale for a realist review. *Global Health Promotion, 18*(2), 45–48 http://www.ncbi.nlm.nih.gov/pubmed/21744664.

McIntyre, A. (2008). *Participatory action research.* Los Angeles: Sage Publications.

McLean, R. K., Tucker, J., Graham, I., Macleod, M., Tetroe, J., Manuel, C., et al. (2013). *Evaluation of CIHR's knowledge translation funding program.* Ottawa: Canadian Institutes of Health Research.

Minkler, M. (2000). Using participatory action research to build healthy communities. *Public Health Reports, 115*(2–3), 191–197.

Minkler, M., & Baden, A. C. (2008). Impacts of CBPR on academic researchers, research quality and methodology, and power relations. In M. Minkler & N. Wallerstein (Eds.), *Community-based participatory research for health: From process to outcomes* (2nd ed., pp. 243–262). San Francisco: Jossey-Bass.

Minkler, M., & Wallerstein, N. (2008a). *Community-based participatory research for health: From process to outcomes.* San Francisco: Jossey-Bass.

Minkler, M., & Wallerstein, N. (Eds.). (2008b). *Community-based participatory research for health: From process to outcome* (2nd ed.). San Francisco: Jossey-Bass.

National Institutes of Health. (2012). NIH Roadmap for Medical Research. US Department of Health and Human Services. URL: https://pubs.niaaa.nih.gov/publications/arh311/12-13.pdf. Accessed: 18 May, 2018.

Nichter, M. (1984). Project community diagnosis: Participatory research as a first step toward community involvement in primary health care (research support, non-U.S. gov't). *Social Science & Medicine, 19*(3), 237–252 http://www.ncbi.nlm.nih.gov/pubmed/6484613.

O'Fallon, L. R., & Dearry, A. (2002). Community-based participatory research as a tool to advance environmental health sciences. *Environmental Health Perspectives, 110*(Suppl 2), 155–159 doi:sc271_5_1835 [pii].

Oetzel, J. G., Zhou, C., Duran, B., Pearson, C., Magarati, M., Lucero, J., et al. (2014). Establishing the psychometric properties of constructs in a community-based participatory research conceptual model. *American Journal of Health Promotion: AJHP.* https://doi.org/10.4278/ajhp.130731-QUAN-398.

Parry, D., Salsberg, J., & Macaulay, A. C. (2009). *A guide to researcher and knowledge-user collaboration in health research.* Ottawa: Canadian Institutes of Health Research Available at: http://www.cihr-irsc.gc.ca/e/44954.html. Accessed: 1 Oct 2009).

Patton, M. (1990). *Qualitative evaluation and research methods.* Newbury Park: Sage Publications.

Pawson, R. (2006). *Evidence-based policy: A realist perspective.* London: Sage.

Rahman, A. (1993). *People's self-development: Perspectives on participatory action research – a journey through experience.* Dhaka: Zed Books.

Robertson, A., & Minkler, M. (1994). New health promotion movement: A critical examination. *Health Education Quarterly, 21*(3), 295–312 http://www.ncbi.nlm.nih.gov/pubmed/8002355.

Sackett, D. L. (2000). *Evidence-based medicine.* Wiley Online Library.

Sackett DL, Rosenberg WMC, Gray JAM, Haynes RB, Richardson W. (1996). Evidence based medicine: what it is and what it isn't BMJ 1996; 312 :71.

Salsberg, J., & Macaulay, A. (2013). Linkage and exchange interventions. In S. E. Straus, J. Tetroe, & I. D. Graham (Eds.), *Knowledge translation in health care: Moving from evidence to practice* (pp. 176–182). Oxford: Wiley-Blackwell/BMJ Books.

Salsberg, J., Macaulay, A. C., & Parry, D. (2014). Guide to integrated knowledge translation research. In I. D. Graham, J. Tetroe, & A. Pearson (Eds.), *Turning knowledge into action: Practical guidance on how to do integrated knowledge translation research* (pp. 176–182). Adelaide: Wolters Kluwer-Lippincott-JBI.

Salsberg, J., Macridis, S., Garcia Bengoechea, E., Macaulay, A. C., Moore, S., & Committee, K. S. T. P. (2017a). Engagement strategies that foster community self-determination in participatory research: Insider ownership through outsider championship. *Family Practice, 34*, 336–340. https://doi.org/10.1093/fampra/cmx001.

Salsberg, J., Macridis, S., Garcia Bengoechea, E., Macaulay, A. C., Moore, S., & Committee, K. S. T. P. (2017b). The shifting dynamics of social roles and project ownership over lifecycle of a community-based participatory research project. *Family Practice, 34*, 305–312. https://doi.org/10.1093/fampra/cmx006.

Sanchez, V., Carrillo, C., & Wallerstein, N. (2011). From the ground up: Building a participatory evaluation model. *Progress in Community Health Partnerships, 5*(1), 45–52. https://doi.org/10.1353/cpr.2011.0007.

Schwandt, T. A. (2007). *The SAGE dictionary of qualitative inquiry.* Los Angeles: Sage Publications.

Semali, L., & Kincheloe, J. L. (1999). *What is indigenous knowledge?: Voices from the academy.* London: Taylor & Francis.

Straus, S. E., Tetroe, J., & Graham, I. (2009). Defining knowledge translation (review). *Canadian Medical Association Journal, 181*(3–4), 165–168. https://doi.org/10.1503/cmaj.081229.

Straus, S. E., Tetroe, J. M., & Graham, I. D. (2011). Knowledge translation is the use of knowledge in health care decision making (review). *Journal of Clinical Epidemiology, 64*(1), 6–10. https://doi.org/10.1016/j.jclinepi.2009.08.016.

Wallerstein, N., & Duran, B. (2008). The theoretical, historical, and practical roots of CBPR. In M. Minkler & N. Wallerstein (Eds.), *Community-based participatory research for health: From process to outcomes.* San Francisco: Jossey-Bass.

Ward, V., House, A., & Hamer, S. (2009). Developing a framework for transferring knowledge into action: A thematic analysis of the literature. *Journal of Health Services Research & Policy, 14*(3), 156–164.

Weingarten, S., Garb, C. T., Blumenthal, D., Boren, S. A., & Brown, G. D. (2000). Improving preventive care by prompting physicians. *Archives of Internal Medicine, 160*, 301–308.

WHO. (1986). Ottawa charter of health promotion. *Canadian Journal of Public Health. Revue Canadienne de Sante Publique, 139*, 425–430.

Chapter 14
Participatory Health Research International Experience from Four Portuguese-Speaking Countries

Irma Brito, Donizete Daher, Crystiane Ribas, Fernanda Príncipe, Fernando Mendes, Filipa Homem, Hayda Alves, Lina Berardinelli, Maria do Céu Barbieri-Figueiredo, Maria da Conceição Martins Silva, Maria Elisabete da Costa Martins, Nathalia Miranda, Sonia Acioli, Vanessa Correa, Vera Saboia, and Verónica Pinheiro

Participatory Health Research: International Context

With a long and diversified history, participatory health research (PHR) is used across multiple disciplines and countries, each one developing its own vision of research practices. While most PHR guidelines tend to have a procedural focus, often only addressing PHR core values and principles, other guidelines focus on developing a memorandum of understanding, in which values and principles are locally unveiled and act as a local standard to guide research (Ledwith and Springett 2010). The International Collaboration for Participatory Health Research (2013a) is

I. Brito (✉) · F. Homem · M. E. da Costa Martins
Nursing School of Coimbra & UICISA:e, Coimbra, Portugal
e-mail: irmabrito@esenfc.pt

D. Daher · C. Ribas · V. Saboia
Aurora de Afonso Costa Nursing School, Fluminense Federal University, Niterói, Brazil
e-mail: donizete@predialnet.com.br; verasaboia@uol.com.br

F. Príncipe
Red Cross Portuguese Health School of Oliveira Azeméis, Oliveira de Azeméis, Portugal
e-mail: fernandaprincipe@esenfcvpoa.eu

F. Mendes
IREFREA, Coimbra, Portugal

H. Alves
Rio das Ostras Faculty, Fluminense Federal University, Niterói, Brazil

L. Berardinelli · N. Miranda · S. Acioli · V. Pinheiro
Nursing Faculty, Rio de Janeiro State University, Rio de Janeiro, Brazil
e-mail: l.m.b@uol.com.br; veronica.pinheiro@bol.com.br

© Springer International Publishing AG, part of Springer Nature 2018
M. T. Wright, K. Kongats (eds.), *Participatory Health Research*,
https://doi.org/10.1007/978-3-319-92177-8_14

in line with the latter, as well as the Portuguese researchers who report their experiences here.

In 2009, the ICPHR started to build an international consensus on PHR principles, and its first position paper was to recognize PHR as a research approach, rather than a technique or research method. Many researchers argue that PHR accepts eclectic methodologies and as a result are reluctant to impose rigid standards on a still-emerging complex, context-bound process that depends on a particular set of relationships. In 2013, the ICPHR developed a set of PHR ethical and practice principles (ICPHR 2013a, b), from the consensus of international researchers (the so-called champions in this specific field). Several researchers from various countries were contacted with the purpose of compiling the multiple definitions of PHR and building the 11 core characteristics presented in the first ICPHR Position Paper (ICPHR 2013a) reported in Chap. 1 which include: PHR is participatory (research is not done on people but with them); PHR is locally situated; PHR is a collective research process; PHR projects are collectively owned; PHR aims for transformation through human agency; PHR promotes critical reflexivity; PHR produces knowledge that is local, collective, co-created, dialogical, and diverse (it incorporates multiple perspectives and types of knowledge); PHR strives for a broad impact; PHR produces local evidence based on a broad understanding of generalizability; PHR follows specific validity criteria; and, finally, PHR is a dialectical process characterized by messiness (confusion and difficulties).

The validity of the PHR approach stems from the authentic participation of non-expert actors in the project, as well as from the project's potential to create and support conditions for action. The participatory research methods chosen depend on the research focus and type of data required, which often means a deviation from the methodological standards of nonparticipatory health research. According to the ICPHR (2013a, pp. 20), validity in PHR is conceptualized as:

- *Participatory validity:* The extent to which all stakeholders are able to take an active part in the research process to the full extent possible
- *Intersubjective validity:* The extent to which the research is viewed as being credible and meaningful by the stakeholders from a variety of perspectives
- *Contextual validity:* The extent to which the research relates to the local situation

M. do Céu Barbieri-Figueiredo
Nursing School of Porto & CINTESIS-UP, Porto, Portugal
e-mail: ceu@esenf.pt

M. da Conceição Martins Silva
Institute of Health Sciences, University of Angola, Luanda, Angola

V. Correa
UNIRIO-Rio de Janeiro State University, Rio de Janeiro, Brazil
e-mail: vanessa.correa@unirio.br

- *Catalytic validity:* The extent to which the research is useful in presenting new possibilities for social action
- *Ethical validity:* The extent to which the research outcomes and the changes exerted on people by the research are sound and just
- *Empathic validity:* The extent to which the research has increased empathy among the participants

The knowledge and action strategies generated by PHR result from a collective research process that is characterized by a dialogue among participants with different perspectives on the research subject. This dialogue does not necessarily result in a consensual view; it can reveal and promote different points of view, which result in different ways of addressing a health issue. Therefore, knowledge is a dialogical co-creation that incorporates multiple perspectives, which, from a conventional point of view, would seem extremely complex and difficult to describe.

Searching for PHR Projects in Portuguese-Speaking Countries

Thinking about participatory health research in Portuguese implies diversity and specifically cultural diversity. While participatory research builds on co-created knowledge by doing research with people not on them, it becomes challenging to reflect on the singularities of this approach among Portuguese-speaking projects.

Portuguese-speaking countries have significant global reach: there are nine states spread across four continents (Europe, America, Africa, and Asia, but mostly in the southern hemisphere), about 7.2% of the planet's land; there are more than 280 million Portuguese speakers in the world, the fifth most spoken language in the world, the third most spoken in the Western Hemisphere, and the first most spoken in the Southern Hemisphere (CPLP 2017). In addition to its economic importance (Oliveira 2013), the greatness of this language is revealed in its diplomatic potential, since the Portuguese is a language with official status or special status in 26 international organizations, among them in 5 of the 17 regional economic blocs that exist today in the world, including the European Union and Mercosur countries. Contrary to Spanish-speaking or German-speaking countries, there are no Portuguese-speaking countries that share borders with another country of the same language. Therefore, instead of leading to linguistic insulation, what has resulted is a diverse cross-cultural country amalgam (Oliveira 2013).

As most of the Portuguese-speaking countries were colonized, they are multicultural. Starting from an analogy between imperialism as a "center" and colonialism as a "periphery," Boaventura de Souza-Santos (2007) discusses the marginal place for epistemologies produced outside "the center," where such knowledge is not considered relevant or understandable because it is external to "the center" and considered as the "other" (Souza-Santos 2007). This monopoly of truth that is held at "the center" gives validity to knowledge while disqualifying others at the "periphery" and determines who produces this knowledge. However, this same process of colonization was also the engine of a necessary insurgence leading to the creation of new participatory epistemologies. This has been the case with participatory research in Latin America: first, the Brazilian educator Paulo Freire was one of the pioneers of working with communities in a participatory perspective, and he was committed to supporting communities in leading the construction of a pedagogy against oppression and exploitation; and second, Orlando Fals Borda, a Colombian, also denounced social inequality and claimed popular power through what he had called participatory action research. Both have had an important influence on PHR as pioneers in the heart of social change.

Since 2009, the co-authors on this chapter became members of the ICPHR (2009) and noticed an underrepresentation of PHR studies conducted in Portuguese. As a result of the underrepresentation of PHR studies conducted in Portuguese-speaking countries within the ICPHR, in 2013, Martins and Brito (2013) conducted a literature review to identify Portuguese studies that used a PHR approach. In total, 1704 studies were identified through several databases including Biblioteca do Conhecimento Online (B-ON), Repositório Científico de Acesso Aberto de Portugal (RCAAP), Scientific Electronic Library Online (SciELO), and Virtual Health Library (VHL) using the following keywords: *assessoria popular* (popular directive counseling); *círculos de cultura* (culture circles); *estudos de intervenção* (intervention studies); *intervenção comunitária* (community intervention); *investigação ação, investigação-acção, investigação acção, pesquisa ação, pesquisa acção, pesquisa-ação, pesquisa-acção* (action research – Brazilian and Portuguese words); *investigação participativa*; *pesquisa participativa* (participatory research); *melhoria contínua* (continuous improvement); *pesquisa colaborativa* (collaborative research); and *pesquisa participativa baseada na comunidade* (community-based participatory research). A total of 177 primary full-text studies (scientific articles or academic papers), written in Portuguese and published between 1990 and 2012, were selected. Brito and Martins (2013) used the four categories of participation defined by Cornwall and Jewkes (1995) to assess participation: contractual, consultative, collaborative, or collegiate. Of the 177 papers included, 81 studies used a participatory research approach, 49 were considered to be collaborative (e.g., researchers and local people worked together on designing, initiating, and managing projects by researchers), and 32 were labeled as collegiate (e.g., researchers and local people worked together as colleagues, combining their different skills in a process of mutual learning).

Martins and Brito (2013) concluded that, although researchers in Portuguese-speaking countries were engaging with participatory health research, several so-called PHR studies had participation levels that were more tokenistic (e.g., where people are contracted into the projects of researchers and people act as informants or doers), thus departing from fundamental principles and philosophical assumptions, motivations, expectations, and practices that characterize PHR. This is problematic, as other authors have emphasized that when research does not comply with ethical principles, participatory research can cause distrust and distress for the community and those involved (ICPHR 2013b).

Based on these findings from the literature review conducted by Martins and Brito (2013), the Portuguese-speaking members of ICPHR (many who are co-authors on this paper) proposed that *Pesquisa-ação Participativa em Saúde*

(PaPS) (participatory action research in health) should be used instead of *Pesquisa Participativa em Saúde* (participatory health research). The new expression would highlight the role of action and participation in research to denote PHR, which goes beyond a merely contractual or consultative contribution found in 54.2% of the 177 studies that were denominated *Pesquisa Participativa* (participatory research) in the previous review (Martins and Brito 2013).

PHR Case Studies in Portuguese-Speaking Countries

After this initial review by Martins and Brito (2013), Portuguese-speaking members of the ICPHR had a goal to work to improve the quality of PHR in Portuguese-speaking countries. Co-authors on this chapter started to disseminate the PHR approach through workshops and strived to improve its use in academia. Four years after their integration into the ICPHR network, the co-authors decided to reflect on the question of how PHR is emerging in Portuguese-speaking countries. They started to reflect on case studies to address previous challenges and planned to conduct a synthesis of case studies (Popay et al. 2010; Cruzes et al. 2015) conducted by Portuguese-speaking researchers from Angola, Brazil, Cape Verde, and Portugal (Portuguese-speaking countries were PHR was already ongoing).

Selection Process and Criteria

The selection criteria of case studies were participative research in the field of health, native Portuguese-speaking researchers, research developed in their countries of origin, and projects created or further developed during the two editions of the international course on participatory health research led by Brito and Mendes (2015) in Coimbra, Portugal. Researcher coordinators were invited to reflect on PHR principles and give examples of PHR best practices that had already been published (as peer-reviewed papers, oral/poster presentations, reports). Although researchers from diverse disciplinary areas had attended the course led by Brito and Mendes (2015), only nurse-led projects were more fully developed. This may be due to the fact that the majority of ICPHR Portuguese members come from a nursing background and have created a strong network that had helped to facilitate further research projects and action.

Analysis and Frameworks Used

PHR coordinators were asked to contribute a research narrative and then used a specific template (Appendix 1) to synthesize the PHR projects. Narratives are important for personal and social change and can be understood by examining specific aspects of projects and sharing stories of struggles, dreams, and expectations, thereby leading to changes in research practice. According to Cruzes et al. (2015), the synthesis of case studies must take into account the flexible nature of the cases, the mixed qualitative and quantitative characteristic of the data, and the type of cases being studied. The flexibility in the choice of methods for performing a case study is one of the characteristics that lead to challenges in conducting the synthesis of case studies. Despite any potential bias, a narrative-based strategy allowed the research team to gather more information beyond the analysis of existing scientific publications.

Evidence from each PHR project was summarized (narrative) and then coded under broad thematic headings (i.e., based on the presence/absence of variables and outcomes in each PHR study). Units of analysis and categories were developed according to ICPHR principles (2013a) and split in three subcategories: objective, relevance, and context of the research, target group and participation type, and data collection/analysis methods and dissemination. Next, the data was summarized within themes across studies with a brief citation of primary evidence. Commonalities and differences between the studies were noted. Finally, the co-authors on this chapter did a cross-case analysis of the findings, which contributed to providing different views of each PHR case synthesis.

Findings and Discussion

In total, nine PHR projects developed in Portuguese-speaking countries (Appendix 2) were compared based on the ICPHR categories (2013a) summarized in Table 14.1. Research coordinators classified data according to defined parameters and pre-established concepts (Bardin 2006); therefore, data were analyzed using an a priori thematic analysis process. Researchers categorized their project's activities based on a concordance or discordance analysis against each PHR principle, filling the template in Appendix 1. Next, the researchers identified key aspects regarding how the project could be improved and, last, synthesized the project's impact on the corresponding context. Each project had different levels of complexity; hence, the analysis focused on the project's research process and adequacy to PHR principles and values. Findings, discussed in the following section, are presented by comparing the following aspects: research design and validity, participation, impact of research, and dissemination.

These nine nurse-led projects developed in Angola (A1), Brazil (B2, B3, B4, and B5), Cape Verde (C6), and Portugal (P7, P8, and P9) all used a PHR approach (i.e., ethical actions, participatory techniques of data production, and reproducibility of scientific knowledge) to address relevant problems in their target community, namely, improving the health status of groups or communities. All nine projects were community health-oriented practices, which take into account the practical knowledge and the need for health professionals to incorporate different perspectives and lay knowledge (Acioli 2006).

Table 14.1   Units of content analysis and thematic categories

Content analysis units	Thematic categories
A. Research design (ICPHR 2013a)	A1. Objective, relevance, and context of the research
	A2. Target group
	A3. Methods and techniques of data collection
	A4. Outcome
	A5. Types of validity (A5.1, participatory, A5.2, intersubjective, A5.3 contextual, A5.4, catalytic, A5.5, ethics, A5.6, empathic)
B. Participation (Cornwall and Jewkes 1995: 1669)	B1. Contractual. People are contracted into the projects of researchers to take part in their enquiries or experiments
	B2. Consultative. People are asked for their opinions and consulted by researchers before interventions are made
	B3. Collaborative. Researchers and local people work together on projects designed, initiated, and managed by researchers
	B4. Collegiate. Researchers and local people work together as colleagues with different skills to offer, in a process of mutual learning where local people have control over the process
C. Impact of research (ICPHR 2013a)	C1. Increased knowledge and performance
	C2. Establishment of partnerships with other community members
	C3. Positive contributions to the community
	C4. Financial contribution
	C5. Increased demand for services that are difficult to deliver

About Research Design and Validity

The objectives of the analyzed research projects were relevant to the target community and related to health status improvement: addressing health problems, namely, adolescent pregnancy (B2) and fishermen wounds (B5); reducing youth violence (C6); identifying problems in nightlife settings and creating public safety policies (P9); improving adherence to health programs, namely, cancer screening (A1); chronic disease management (B3 and P7); creating health promotion settings (P8); and improving best practices in health services (B4). In all projects, the researchers engaged the target subjects/groups using participatory practices aimed at greater empowerment and autonomy. The research questions were formulated based on the local context where the research outcomes would be later applied.

The projects were developed in community-based settings (A1, B2, B5, C6, P8, P9), outside the hospital environment (B3), or in health-care centers (B4, P7). The participants/groups (e.g., young people, female market vendors, fishermen, students, "partygoers," people living with chronic diseases, vulnerable communities, and health professionals) were involved in the research projects using a variety of different methods, including culture circles, peer education, popular education, mapping, interviews, focus groups, world café, participatory observations, interactive games, and talk circles. In view of the above, PHR data collection tools should be applied in different settings, thus allowing for the production of collective knowledge among people who have different perspectives but common objectives (Loewenson et al. 2014).

The outcomes reported by these PHR projects were extremely relevant, such as improved health literacy and management of health and disease. All case studies incorporated the knowledge co-created by all participants into practice, (see case example B3: people living with chronic illness who changed their lifestyle by engaging family and friends).

Despite similarities between the case examples, there were significant differences between the projects due to the different settings where they took place. For example, both case studies B3 (Brazil) and P7 (Portugal) aimed to empower people living with chronic diseases, but the different cultures and health services/structures of each country led to the development of distinct PHR projects. For example, in Brazil most of the group activities took place in the hospital, while in Portugal most took place in health-care centers. However, these two projects had a very similar impact: greater levels of engagement, satisfaction, and well-being among participants and the co-creation of useful knowledge. We found that all nine projects included in the synthesis confirmed previously identified international criteria that the PHR process is characterized by the dialogue among participants with different perspectives on the topic under study, which can result in different ways of addressing the issue. For example, the project PEER-IESS (P8) aimed to engage higher education institutions with the goal of promoting healthy settings through participatory action research based on different student community groups, which led to different outcomes (i.e., health promotion projects) due to the different organizations involved. In another example, four of the nine PHR projects (A1, B2, B3, B5) started with a conventional approach to involve people and communities and then moved from conventional professional nursing guidelines to a completely different research design such as peer education and popular education processes. In these projects, knowledge was co-created dialogically and incorporated multiple perspectives, revealing the micro-politics of everyday life, allowing new connections between theory and practice, and laying the groundwork for change at the individual, family, community, and organizational levels. For example, the project to prevent cervical cancer in Angola (A1) aimed to increase knowledge and compliance for the purpose of preventing cervical cancer among women market vendors (mostly illiterate), in an innovative way using peer educators. A similar strategy was used with the project "Environmental impact, work and health of Guanabara Bay fishers - RJ, Brazil: Peer Education as a prevention strategy."

With regard to validity, not all narratives included in the multi-case study synthesis complied with these criteria. The PHR projects analyzed used both qualitative and quantitative methods depending on the type of data required. Some studies deviated from the methodological standards of traditional research, namely, by using a quantitative approach with non-randomized samples (A1, B2, P8, P9) and focus groups in which participants summarized their views on wall murals (B3, B5, P7). This deviation may have been due to the fact that project coordinators experienced difficulties in publishing scientific articles and had to adapt the report of PHR study to journals' criteria.

Overall, we found that the nine projects reported on the five PHR validity criteria (ICPHR 2013a): participatory, intersubjective, contextual, ethical, and empathic validity. However, despite the social relevance of the research, seven projects showed no evidence of catalytic validity, probably due to the fact these studies were mostly academic projects (collaborative), which may have hindered proposing new intervention possibilities. In our synthesis, we found that almost all studies were developed by academic research teams, in which the researchers' main role was to facilitate a shared decision-making process after data collection and analysis. However, even in the project "Before You get Burned: health and safety in nightlife settings" (P9), which was first initiated in 2007 (Brito 2009), student mobilization has not yet translated into public policies like providing outreach service in every university city during academic festivities. Co-author Brito found that the nightlife industry (alcohol and drug selling, festivals, and local accommodation) is hardly influenced by collective empowerment movements of students to improve health and safety. The other studies included in the case study analysis also faced constraints, namely, the ownership of studies, which seemed to hamper the catalytic process (B4, B5); financial constraints, which prevented replication in other settings (A1, C6); neoliberalism, which is hardly influenced by collective empowerment movements (P8, P9); and health-care routines, which are a barrier to innovation (B3, P7). ICPHR networking is one way to help PHR projects overcome some of these constraints and catalytic challenges.

Another important aspect that was found in this case analysis was that scientific publications do not always reflect collaborative work. An example of this is that while all projects had related papers, such as Miranda, N., et al. (2016), Silva et al. (2016) and Alves et al. (2017), these papers did not reflect all the work developed. One reason for this being that popular scientific journals use a conventional methodology that is not suitable for conducting research studies with people and communities. Cartography could be an innovative alternative to conventional knowledge creation methods (Passos et al. 2010); however, journal publishers have some ways to go to better reflect the work of PHR researchers.

About Participation

The purpose of PHR is to maximize the participation of the target individuals/ groups at all stages of the research process, including in the formulation of the research question and objectives, the development of the research design, the selection of data collection and analysis methods, the implementation of the research, and the interpretation and dissemination of the results (ICPHR 2013a). All nine projects showed evidence of the four different modes of participation, as defined by Cornwall and Jewkes (1995:1669):

> *Contractual: People are contracted into the projects of researchers to take part in their enquiries or experiments; Consultative: People are asked for their opinions and consulted by researchers before interventions are made; Collaborative: Researchers and local people*

work together on projects designed, initiated and managed by researchers; Collegiate: Researchers and local people work together as colleagues with different skills to offer, in a process of mutual learning where local people have control over the process.

During the research process, almost all projects (except for P7 and P9) showed an evolution from "contractual" to "collaborative" participation. In these PHR projects, participants were initially selected for the project to act as "informants." However, as the project evolved, they were invited to give their opinion before the interventions were designed, thus acting as "consultants." When interventions began, researchers and non-experts worked together in the activities, as part of a collaborative process. However, one of the most significant gaps identified in the case study analysis was that there is lack of participant involvement in data reporting or project dissemination, which may be explained by conventional academic values. Both PEER-IESS (P8) and Before You get Burned (P9) are examples of "collegiate" participation in that both studies engaged the target students in the research (peer educational and peer research). This higher level of participation may be due to the fact that higher education students are seen as academic researchers and not lay people.

The nine PHR projects in this synthesis demonstrated citizen mobilization, by engaging people whose problem or condition was the focus of the PHR study, members of civil society (through non-governmental organizations), health and social welfare professionals, health organizations, academic researchers, and policymakers. However, not all projects were explicit that the collective process allowed participants to become co-owners of the project by gaining control over the research, which limits the evidence base linking participation and impact in PHR. There is also limited evidence on decision-making processes regarding the best way to report research findings and achieve collective goals. Further, scientific publications often do not reveal the actual research process (i.e., they miss out on reporting much of the collaborative process) and do not refer to all researchers as co-authors.

PHR projects have the potential for collegiate participation due to their nature and focus and because they are developed with community partners. Both researchers and citizens work together as colleagues (peer researchers), combining their different skills within a mutual learning process. The academy can develop relevant PHR projects if it is accepted and/or adopted in formal health education.

About Impact of Research and Dissemination

The impact of PHR in each context should also be highlighted. According to Cook et al. (2017), the impact in all forms of research has become an important focus with many funding bodies demanding that researchers define what kind of evidence will be proffered to demonstrate that impact. This has raised questions for researchers about what form that impact takes and how it is recognized and by whom. The case study analysis discussions in this project revealed not only that researchers had difficulties in clarifying the participatory dimension of their research but also that while authors were able to discuss the particular impact of their work, the evidence of that impact was often absent from their published papers or scientific presentations. The researchers of the nine PHR projects included in this study were asked to reflect on the following aspects in their projects: increased knowledge and performance, establishment of partnerships with other community members, positive contributions to the community, financial contribution, and increased demand for services that are difficult to deliver. All PHR participants reported co-creation and increased knowledge, such as new ways of dealing with daily life or illness incidents and peer practices. Only five projects had their research reported in the media (B2, C6, P7, P8, P9), and five projects had a financial budget (B2, B3, B4, B5, C6).

In terms of positive contributions to the community, all projects in the case analysis can be included in the following categories, as defined by WHO (2015) as good practices in nursing and midwifery toward Health 2020 goals: promotion of healthy lifestyles and life changes among school-aged children (B2) and college students (P8, P9); counseling to young people and their families (C6); support and early care based on an integrated multiagency service model (A1, B3, P7); creation of support groups to promote healthy lifestyles and decision-making (B5, P8); and contribution to an empowered and health literate population (B5) and community-engaged health workforce (B4). In fact, the World Health Organization (2015a) considered that two of the projects (P8 and P9) represented best practices for creating resilient communities and supportive environments. Several PHR narratives included in the analysis focused on positive contributions, such as the involvement of people helped to improve health literacy and prevent harmful behavior (Smith et al. 2013; Brito 2014), using peer education with young people as a way of mobilizing communities and creating healthy settings (Shannon et al. 2016), and the engagement of families for the promotion of home care by strengthening knowledge and developing family members and caregivers' skills (WHO 2015).

Examples of other impacts include projects receiving financial contributions from partners and stakeholders (A1, B2, P9); increased demand for services that are difficult to provide, namely, cervical cancer screening (A1); support for people living with chronic illness (B3, B5, P7); risk reduction in recreational settings (P9); health promotion in school settings (B2, P8); and excellence in care (B4). For being a research approach that is based on people's daily lives and work, PHR produces positive social changes and promotes citizens' mobilization, making them more capable of acting upon the co-created knowledge. Through critical reflexivity, participants can recognize their current situation and the sociopolitical causes of health and disease processes. This aspect is particularly relevant concerning the dynamics related to social exclusion and the search for community health solutions. Based on the PHR case study analysis, we found that interventions that produced social changes are both part of the process and research subject: African women, fishermen, and students reflect about their own vulnerability and fight for adequate health services; people living with chronic diseases become engaged beyond attending scheduled meetings; and health professionals integrate lay knowledge into their clinical practice and disseminate the project.

PHR projects show that learning, research, and action are not separate entities, as advocated by traditional research, and the use of mixed methods helps to strengthen the process for individual and social change (Loewenson et al. 2014). Social learning is a key dimension of PHR, whose dynamics is rooted in the continuous cycle of "looking, reflecting, acting." People who are engaged in transformative learning change their perceptions about themselves and the world through interactive processes that influence both the personal and the collective domains. In many of these projects (A1, B2, B3, B4, P7, P8, P9), the collective efforts are never completed, to the extent that the group seeks to act based on the research findings and have a wider impact, which goes beyond the production of scientific knowledge.

The primacy of the local context in PHR studies has implications for the generalization of the results. Researchers want to replicate interventions and disseminate the context-centered, co-created knowledge, which requires the processes and methods to be considered. For example, the same study was replicated in two PHR projects which were conducted in different contexts: Brazil (B3) and Portugal (P7). The outcomes were two completely different interventions, both focused on the person living with chronic illness. In addition, P9 attempted to replicate the same project in several Portuguese universities, but all interventions were distinct due to different cultural aspects and contexts.

In PHR, it is not possible to generate representational knowledge which can be used to develop standardized interventions aimed at similar local settings. However, the diversity of the responses obtained when replicating similar interventions enriches the knowledge produced, as shown by the research network created by Portuguese-speaking researchers.

How PHR Is Emerging in Portuguese-Speaking Countries

The nine PHR projects developed in Portuguese-speaking countries resulted in significant outcomes for participants, namely, increased health literacy and autonomy in the management of health/disease transition, improved understanding of illness processes, and increased potential for sociocultural changes. The research settings where the PHR project took place were predominantly community-based (primary health-care centers) and go beyond institutional health-care settings. Different methods were used (culture circles, peer education, popular education, mapping, interviews, focus groups, world café, participatory observation, interactive games, talk circles) to engage different types of project members (young people, female vendors in an African market, fishermen, students, people living with chronic diseases, vulnerable communities, and health professionals). The project researchers aimed to develop participatory practices with the purpose of empowering and developing the autonomy of the participants and groups involved. The research questions were directed at the social system which is likely to implement the changes as a result of the research process. In all projects, knowledge was co-created by all participants; however it still remains closely linked to the academy, since projects often depended on research funding and community support services. Project researchers focused on the primacy of the (local) community context to obtain practical, relational (process), credible, and valid results. The key aspect of the PHR projects conducted in Portuguese-speaking countries is that the collaborative process is conducted by a group representing several partners. However, these projects can hardly benefit from what Cornwall and Jewkes (1995) call the collegiate domain of participation due to their relationship with the academy. PHR allows for a participation that goes beyond the simple interaction, and the created groups are often defined as a therapeutic setting aimed at meaningful learning. There is an initial feeling of distrust within the group, then participants are positively surprised with the research, and finally, they become completely engaged and predisposed to collaborate. The democratization of knowledge is a key aspect of PHR, to the extent that scientific and lay knowledge are brought together to form new knowledge, which in turn will allow reshaping ways of living/dealing with health problems and social change.

The co-creation of knowledge is based on reflexive and explicit values such as authenticity, transparency, and transferability. The barrier between scientific and lay knowledge must be overcome so that proposals can generate organizational or public policies, by emphasizing the impact of powerlessness in people's daily lives and activities and developing critical awareness among participants. Community health professionals must develop interventions targeted at specific time and place, giving priority to the local context and generating local evidence that accumulates over time in order to strengthen participants' capacity to take effective action on health issues. Therefore, this is about promoting collective empowerment (Brito 2014), which means assuming that the impact goes beyond the production of academic knowledge. Positive changes translate into the engagement of research participants, researchers, the community in general, and community organizations. Ultimately, it means that the academy must invest more in PHR approaches.

In Portuguese-speaking countries, PHR must be developed on the basis that learning and research are not separate entities. These gaps relate to the power held by the academy over scientific research and translate into low participation in data analysis, dissemination of results, and, consequently, research ownership. The consolidation of the existing knowledge and the consensus on a common PHR terminology and principles can strengthen the role of PHR in intervention design and decision-making on health issues and health education. To this end, guidelines should be elaborated in Portuguese for conducting and evaluating PHR in Portuguese-speaking settings. It would also be important to describe the theories and evidence produced by this approach and define a systematic literature review process in the context of PHR in order to contribute to the development of an international database on PHR knowledge.

According to Fals Borda and Rahman (1991), PHR goes beyond the institutional boundaries and attempt to actively involve the people in the production of knowledge about their own condition and associated changes. PHR requires social scientists' strong commitment to de-professionalize their expertise and share it with the people while recognizing that the communities directly involved have the critical voice in determining the direction and goals of change as subjects rather than objects.

The authors of this chapter stand for this transformation in their own academy by promoting and supporting an increasing number of PHR projects that have the potential to support social change through people-/community-centered services and increased responsiveness/inclusion in health-care systems. The authors also hope to improve the quality of PHR in Portuguese-speaking countries and continue to disseminate PHR approaches through workshops, as well as increase Portuguese-speaking researcher's integration into the ICPHR network.

Appendix 1. Template to Synthesize PHR Projects

	Units of analysis and categories, according to ICPHR (2013)	A1	B2	B3	B4	B5	C6	P7	P8	P9
Objective, relevance, and context of the research	Relevance of the research:									
	Academic interest (professional skills)	x	x	x	x	x				x
	Magnitude of the problem	x	x	x	x	x	x	x	x	x
	Mobilization of groups/ community			x	x	x		x	x	x
	Context of the research:									
	Health/social services		x	x	x			x		
	Community institutions				x	x				
	Community	x		x		x		x		
	Higher education institutions		x	x	x	x		x	x	x
	Objective of the research:									
	Improve health literacy and personal/social skills	x	x	x	x	x	x	x	x	x
	Improve health indicators	x	x	x	x	x	x	x	x	x
	Reduce social determinants of health problems		x	x		x	x	x		x
	Promote healthy contexts			x	x	x		x	x	x
	Produce health/social policies				x		x		x	x

	Units of analysis and categories, according to ICPHR (2013)	A1	B2	B3	B4	B5	C6	P7	P8	P9
Target group and participation mode	What were the modes of participation of people whose life, health/illness, or work is the focus of the research?									
	Contractual	x	x	x	x	x	x	x	x	x
	Consultative	x	x	x	x	x	x	x	x	x
	Collaborative	x	x	x	x	x	x	x	x	x
	Collegiate							x	x	x
	How was the community (or group) contacted:									
	Researcher	x	x	x	x	x		x		x
	Person appointed by the group/community	x		x			x	x	x	x
	Health/social services		x	x	x		x	x		
Data collection and analysis methods and dissemination	Elaboration of the research question:									
	Researchers	x	x	x	x	x				x
	People whose life, health/illness, or work is the focus of the research			x	x	x	x	x	x	x
	Local structures and partners	x	x	x		x	x	x	x	x
	Selection of data collection methods:									
	Researchers	x	x	x	x	x	x	x	x	x
	People whose life, health/illness, or work is the focus of the research	x		x	x	x		x	x	x
	Local structures and partners		x			x	x	x	x	x
	Data analysis and discussion of results:									
	Researchers	x	x	x	x	x	x	x	x	x
	People whose life, health/illness, or work is the focus of the research			x	x	x	x	x	x	x
	Local structures and partners		x			x	x	x	x	x
	Dissemination of results:									
	Researchers	x	x	x	x	x	x	x	x	x
	People whose life, health/illness, or work is the focus of the research			x	x	x			x	x
	Local structures and partners	x	x	x		x	x		x	x

Appendix 2. Summary of PHR Projects Under Review

Principal investigator(s)	Authors	Title (in Portuguese and translation into English)	N
Maria da Conceição Martins da Silva	Maria da Conceição Martins da Silva, Irma da Silva Brito, Maria Adriana Pereira Henriques, Bebiana Calisto Bernardo, Eurica da Natividade Sinclética Graça Neves da Rocha, Ana Maria Pascoal, Judith Arminda Venâncio Candeias	Cancro do colo do útero: conhecimento e prática sobre a prevenção do cancro do colo do útero de mulheres vendedoras de um mercado do município de Luanda-Angola	A1
		Cervical cancer: knowledge and practices on the prevention of cervical cancer in women market vendors in the municipality of Luanda-Angola	
Hayda Alves	Hayda Alves, Andréa de Araújo Viana, Bruno Ferreira Teixeira, Cláudia Pontes Braz, Irma Brito, Lidia Santos Soares, Michella Florência Câmara, Paula Martins Sirelli, Rafaela Cristina de Andrade Santos, Thamires Rodrigues da Silva	(Des) embarazo: pesquisa-ação participante com adolescentes para prevenção da gravidez (RO, RJ, Brasil)	B2
		(Des) embarazo: participatory action research with adolescents for pregnancy prevention (RO, RJ, Brazil)	
Lina Marcia Berardinelli	Lina Berardinelli, Nathália Aparecida Costa Guedes Miranda, Louise Theresa de Araújo Abreu, Larissa Pereira Costa	Produção de cuidado participativo com pessoas que vivenciam a fibromialgia	B3
		Production of participatory care with patients with fibromyalgia	
Vanessa Corrêa	Vanessa Corrêa, Sonia Acioli	Projetos terapêuticos: uma construção coletiva para a prática do enfermeiro na estratégia saúde da família	B4
		Therapeutic projects: a collective construction for nurses' practice in the family health strategy	
Crystiane Ribas Ribeiro	Crystiane Ribas Ribeiro, Vera Maria Sabóia	Impacto ambiental, trabalho e saúde de pescadores da Baía de Guanabara – RJ, Brasil: A Educação pelos Pares como estratégia de prevenção	B5
		Environmental impact, work and health of Guanabara Bay fishers – RJ, Brazil: peer education as a prevention strategy	

Principal investigator(s)	Authors	Title (in Portuguese and translation into English)	N
Fernando Mendes and Irma Brito	Fernando Mendes, Irma Brito, Suzana Delgado, Filipa Homem, Maria do Rosário Mendes, and Cape Verde Ministry of Youth	*Bo Ki Ta Disidi*. Educação, apoio e aconselhamento para reduzir a violência juvenil nas cidades de Cabo Verde	C6
		Bo Ki Ta Disidi. Education, support, and counseling to reduce youth violence in the cities of Cape Verde	
Donizete Vago Daher and Irma Brito	Irma Brito, Donizete Daher, Ana Pedro Costa, Maria de Fátima Cravo, Ana Filipa Cardoso, António Fernandes, Cristina Neves, Janete Ferreira, Sónia Ribeiro, Catarina Simões, Cristina Ventura	Reconstruindo o viver com diabetes	P7
		Rebuilding life with diabetes	
Fernanda Príncipe and Irma Brito	Fernanda Príncipe, Irma Brito, António Ferreira, Henrique Pereira, Maribel Carvalhais, Manuela Ferreira, Ana Torres, Sónia Novais, Liliana Mota, Alexandra Brandão, Fernando Mendes	PEER-IESS. Ativar instituições de ensino superior na promoção de contextos salutogénicos, através da pesquisa-ação participativa baseada na comunidade estudantil	P8
		PEER-IESS. Activate higher education institutions for the promotion of healthy settings through participatory action research based on the student community	
Irma Brito and Fernando Mendes	Irma Brito, Fernando Mendes, Filipa Homem, Verónica Coutinho, Paulo Anjos, Armando Silva, Maria da Alegria Simões, Luís Paiva, Maria do Rosário Mendes, Lucília Rodrigues	Antes que te Queimes: saúde e segurança em contextos recreativos	P9
		Before you get burned: health and safety in nightlife settings	

References

Acioli, S. (2006). Sentidos e práticas de saúde em grupos populares e a enfermagem em saúde pública. *Revista Enfermagem UERJ, 14*, 21–26 Available via http://www.facenf.uerj.br/v14n1/v14n1a03.pdf. Accessed 06 Jan 2017.

Alves, H., et al. (2017). Adolescent pregnancy and local co-planning: A diagnostic approach based on the PRECEDE-PROCEED model. *Revista de Enfermagem Referência, IV*, (12), 35–44. doi:https://doi.org/10.12707/RIV16058.

Bardin, L. (2006). *Análise de conteúdo*. Edições 70. Lisboa.

Brito, I. (2009). PEER – peer education engagement and evaluation research. In *Escola Superior de Enfermagem de Coimbra*. ESEnfC, Coimbra. Available via ESEnfC/UICISA-E http://web.esenfc.pt/public/index.php?module=ui&target=outreach-projects&id_projecto=54&id_linha_investigacao=1&tipo=UI. Accessed 03 Jan 2017.

Brito, I. (2014). Um modelo de planeamento da promoção da saúde: Modelo PRECEDE-PROCEED. In R. R. Pedroso, I. Brito (Eds.), *Saúde dos estudantes do ensino superior de enfermagem: Estudo de contexto na Escola Superior de Enfermagem de Coimbra: Unidade de Investigação em Ciências da Saúde: Enfermagem* (pp. 33–83). Escola Superior de Enfermagem de Coimbra.

Brito, I., & Mendes, F. (2015). *Curso Internacional de Pesquisa-ação Participativa em Saúde em português (CIPaPS)*. Coimbra: Escola Superior de Enfermagem de Coimbra, ESEnfC, Coimbra Available via ESEnfC/UICISA-E. http://www.esenfc.pt/event/3cipapes. Accessed 06 Jan 2017.

Cook, T., et al. (2017). Accessing participatory research impact and legacy: Developing the evidence base for participatory approaches in health research. *Educational Action Research, 25*(4), 473–488. https://doi.org/10.1080/09650792.2017.1326964.

Cornwall, A., & Jewkes, R. (1995). What is participatory research? *Social Science and Medicine, 41,* 1667–1676.

CPLP. (2017). Comunidade dos Países de Língua Portuguesa. Available via https://www.cplp.org/. Accessed 06 Jan 2017.

Cruzes, D., et al. (2015). Case studies synthesis: A thematic, cross-case, and narrative synthesis worked example. *Empirical Software Engineering, 20*(6), 1634–1665.

Fals-Borda, O., & Rahman, M. (1991). *Action and knowledge: Breaking the monopoly with participatory action research*. Michigan: Apex Press.

ICPHR. (2009). International collaboration on participatory health research. Available via www.icphr.org. Accessed 06 Jan 2017.

ICPHR. (2013a). What is participatory health research? Position paper 1. Available via International Collaboration for Participatory Health Research: http://www.icphr.org/position-papers/position-paper-no-1. Accessed 06 Jan 2017.

ICPHR. (2013b). Participatory health research: A guide to ethical principals and practice. Position paper 2. Available via International Collaboration for Participatory Health Research: http://www.icphr.org/uploads/2/0/3/9/20399575/ichpr_position_paper_2_ethics_-_version_october_2013.pdf. Accessed 06 Jan 2017.

Ledwith, M., & Springett, J. (2010). Participatory practice, community based action for transformative change. doi:https://doi.org/10.1080/01609513.2010.490897.

Loewenson, et al. (2014). *Investigación-acción participativa en sistemas de salud: una guía de métodos*. Harare: TARSC, AHPSR, WHO, IDRC Canada, EQUINET.

Martins, E., & Brito, I. (2013). Investigação-acção participativa em saúde: revisão integrativa da literatura em língua portuguesa. Coimbra: ESEnfC. Retrieved from http://repositorio.esenfc.pt/private/index.php?process=download&id=27076&code=480

Miranda, N., et al. (2016). Práxis interdisciplinar de cuidado em grupo de pessoas que vivem com fibromialgia. *Revista Brasileira de Enfermagem, [en linea], 69*(6), 1115–1123 Available via Redalyc http://www.redalyc.org/html/2670/267048565015/ Accessed 06 Jan 2017.

Oliveira, G. M. (2013). Política linguística e internacionalização: a língua portuguesa no mundo globalizado do século XXI. *Trabalhos em Linguística Aplicada, 52*(2), 409–433. https://doi.org/10.1590/S0103-18132013000200010.

Passos, E., Kastrup, V., & Escóssia, L. (2010). *Pistas do método da cartografia: pesquisa intervenção e produção de subjetividade* (1st ed.). Porto Alegre: Editora Sulina.

Popay, J., et al. (2010). Developing methods for the narrative synthesis of quantitative and qualitative data in systematic reviews of effects. Available via Centre for Review and Dissemination http://www.york.ac.uk/inst/crd/projects/narrative_synthesis.htm. Accessed in 06 Jan 2018.

Shannon, A., et al. (2016). Peer health educators can promote worksite and community health. SPE International Conference and Exhibition on Health, Safety, Security, Environment, and Social Responsibility. Available via Society of Petroleum Engineers. https://www.onepetro.org/conference-paper/SPE-179496-MS. Accessed 06 Jan 2017.

Silva, M., et al. (2016). *Prevenção do cancro do colo do útero: capacitação de mulheres de uma comunidade de Luanda* (pp. 2183–4008). Omnia, Lisboa. Available via http://omnia.grei.pt/n05201610240915/[0507].pdf. Accessed 06 Jan 2017.

Smith, S., Nutbeam, D., & McCaffery, K. (2013). Insights into the concept and measurement of health literacy from a study of shared decision-making in a low literacy population. *Journal of Health Psychology, 8*, 1011–1022.

Souza-Santos, B. (2007). Para além do pensamento abissal: das linhas globais a uma ecologia de saberes. *Novos Estudos CEBRAP, 79*, 71–94 Available via http://www.scielo.br/pdf/nec/n79/04.pdf Accessed 06 Jan 2017.

WHO. (2015). *European compendium of good practices in nursing and midwifery towards health 2020 goals*. Copenhagen: WHO Regional Office for Europe.

Chapter 15
Participatory Health Research in South Africa

Maghboeba Mosavel, Jodi Winship, and Rashid Ahmed

Introduction

In this chapter, we will explore participatory health research (PHR) in social and behavioural health within the South African context and, in particular, how participation is operationalized in PHR in South Africa. Especially important to consider is that PHR is implemented within a particular historical and community context that necessarily will determine how participation is operationalized. In South Africa, the most defining contextual factor that permeates all praxis is still the legacy of apartheid. In the present context, this emerges as an enormous gap between the rich (still largely White) and the poor (still largely People of Colour), as South Africa remains one of the most unequal societies in the world (Chitiga et al. 2015). Regarding health issues, this appears as a bifurcated health system: one for the rich and another for the poor. While 1994 marked the official end of institutionalized apartheid rule in South Africa and the adoption of one of the most progressive constitutions in the world (Worden 2011), the effects of decades of racism and economic disparity continue to reverberate to this day.

Health disparities are inextricably linked to equity and social justice, especially with regard to the fair distribution of resources and availability of care and treatment. Highly affected by the social determinants of health, and specifically the powerful remnants of apartheid—including inequitable, highly discriminatory political, economic and health systems—the burden of disease in South Africa is concentrated amongst poor Blacks (Coovadia et al. 2009). Chronic disease rates—

M. Mosavel (✉) · J. Winship
Department of Health Behavior and Policy, Virginia Commonwealth University, School of Medicine, Richmond, VA, USA
e-mail: maghboeba.mosavel@vcuhealth.org

R. Ahmed
Department of Psychology, University of the Western Cape, Bellville, Republic of South Africa

© Springer International Publishing AG, part of Springer Nature 2018
M. T. Wright, K. Kongats (eds.), *Participatory Health Research*,
https://doi.org/10.1007/978-3-319-92177-8_15

especially hypertension, diabetes and cancer—have alarmingly increased in South Africa (Steyn et al. 2006), and the country continues to battle some of the highest rates of HIV/AIDS in Africa (Gouws and Karim 2010). Furthermore, while there have been various progressive policies adopted in relation to health, it is not surprising that the implementation of these policies has been challenging, especially given the limited and compromised infrastructure, including severe fragmentation of the overall healthcare system (Coovadia et al. 2009). Thus, access to care and treatment is a still huge concern as most South Africans do not have private health insurance and mainly use public health services, which generally offer excellent care, but are hugely overburdened and infinitely under-resourced (Coovadia et al. 2009).

Unsurprisingly, apartheid policies directly impacted health research. Historically, medical and behavioural research in South Africa was seen as the domain of the ruling class, steeped in power dynamics and reflective of the limited voice of the marginalized majority (Deacon 2000). Furthermore, poverty accompanied by alarming rates of violence, specifically gender-based violence, and the biggest HIV epidemic on the African continent (Gouws and Karim 2010) greatly influences research foci.

Highly relevant to PHR is that apartheid was dismantled largely because of a strong, participatory movement, which highlights the significance of grassroots engagement in determining outcomes, including health outcomes (Coovadia et al. 2009). Building local capacity and partnerships was another defining feature of the anti-apartheid movement, as well as the core understanding that local insiders are critical agents of social change. Furthermore, South Africa's global importance propelled by its past inglorious human rights abuses and its rather exemplary (not perfect) transition to democracy has itself garnered considerable outsider interest and support as demonstrated by various international partnerships and financial aid (Habib and Taylor 1999). These research partnerships are of particular relevance to a discussion of PHR, as some of these partnerships may inadvertently perpetuate the power dynamics of the financially powerful North and the pigeonholed "needy" South (Tomlinson et al. 2006). The emancipatory, equalizing philosophy of PHR not only has an intuitive resonance with South Africans, but these values are at the core of its own social and political endeavours.

While context and level of engagement are important in determining participatory frameworks, participation in health research is dependent on various facilitating factors which include trust, community entrée and access, funding, community partners and opportunities for mutual benefit. If not present, these factors can just as easily serve to impede participatory efforts. Specifically, power imbalances and inability to share power through the distribution of resources and building local capacity can severely interfere with participatory health efforts. PHR, at best, is necessarily time consuming as the relational elements required for the successful conduct and dissemination of research are being tended to. The next sections will discuss PHR in the South African context with specific reference to the following elements: participation, formative research, partnerships, community advisory boards and building capacity. We acknowledge that there are numerous other central features of PHR; however, in this chapter we focus on key aspects most relevant in South Africa.

PHR in the South African Context

Participation

Meaningful participation is the overarching principle in participatory health research (Cornwall and Jewkes 1995; International Collaboration for Participatory Health Research 2013), and the importance of participatory health approaches to tackle issues of health disparity has been recognized by the World Health Organization (WHO). In its strategy for national health in the twenty-first century, the WHO acknowledged the essential role of all stakeholders, from the government to community members themselves, to be included in all phases of healthcare design: from planning to implementation and follow-up (Rohrer and Rajan 2016). Therefore, it may be no surprise that operationalizing participation is one of the most vexing questions to PHR and critics alike. In social and behavioural research, participation occurs on a continuum. Ideally, in PHR the participation of stakeholders is included at the design, data collection, analysis and dissemination phases.

There are many different forms of participation in South African research. Musesengwa and Chimbari (2017) provide an important overview of community engagement practices in Southern Africa. Community members frequently provide input on the design of intervention materials and on the development of culturally appropriate intervention protocols (Mabunda et al. 2016; Mosavel et al. 2005; Remien et al. 2013; Wechsberg et al. 2015; Woodsong et al. 2014). Specific strategies for seeking community feedback to inform the research design include broad stakeholder meetings with the research team, healthcare providers and community members. Several of these strategies are also accompanied by the integration of laypersons in the role of community researchers. In these cases, community members are trained to conduct interviews and collect data (Bradley and Puoane 2007; Mosavel et al. 2005) or to facilitate the actual intervention (Batist et al. 2013).

Who Is the Community?

PHR is largely conducted in location-based, marginalized communities and/or communities who are experiencing a major health disparity. International media accounts of South Africa simplistically portray the country's population as Black or White. In reality, South Africa's population is made up of a number of racial and ethnic communities which have their own cultural and linguistic traditions. Post-apartheid, South Africans continue to grapple with apartheid era racial classifications; however, there is a strong recognition at the societal level of the social construction of race and the continued barriers and privileges associated with race and ethnicity.

However, PHR is not only confined to racial/ethnic communities but also includes any group that may be bound by commonalities including geography (urban vs. rural), identity, illness (such as cancer, diabetes, etc.) or a health need. Because PHR is conducted with communities that are often in dire need of services, and the research process can often be long and laborious, communities and researchers alike struggle with the "service delivery versus research dilemma" even as they commit to the relationship-building principles of PHR (Simon et al. 2007). Some communities may find the time spent on conducting formative research as frustrating, given that they would rather that the researchers focus on the intervention, while other communities may welcome researcher efforts to understand the community's experiences and perspectives. In our own research in South Africa, we found that utilizing the principles of PHR allowed us to provide an early "deliverable" to the community in the form of training and capacity building which helped to mediate, if only slightly, the inevitable tension that arises from a community's immediate needs for change (Mosavel et al. 2005).

Who Are the Researchers?

In addition to assessing the degree of participation, identifying the role of the researcher in this process is also critical. In participatory research there is a required acknowledgement of the identity and positionality of the researcher (Maxwell et al. 2016; Simon and Mosavel 2011) as this element influences the dynamics relevant to PHR. Researchers who are perceived as similar to the community in terms of race, language or culture may experience more initial implicit trust than researchers who are perceived as outsiders (Richman et al. 2012; Simon and Mosavel 2011). The implicit trust and insider-outsider dichotomy are also an issue for international researchers; one can argue that, depending on positionality, there are varying degrees of distance between researcher and community (Tomlinson et al. 2006).

Participation in health research is rooted in a community's history and their relationship with researchers. Since the transition to democracy in 1994, there is an emerging, highly educated, Black workforce, and this includes academics with research careers. Prior to 1994, most researchers were middle-class Whites. Due to apartheid era constraints, there were fewer Black and Coloured individuals able to receive formal research training; thus they were frequently excluded from this specialization (Tomlinson et al. 2006). More recently, local South African universities are graduating thousands of Black researchers (South Africa Department of Higher Education and Training 2014), and there are many Black academics who are conducting social and behavioural research which is inevitably informed by their own lived experiences. While these are important shifts that may facilitate greater participation, further research is needed to assess whether these shifts have made a difference. As highlighted earlier, given the dominance of the Northern agenda, there is a concern that Black researchers may still be reproducing that agenda and ways of doing research that impede participation or the production of local knowledge (Daniels 2011).

Who Are the Participants?

Who is participating and why are also questions that must be critically analysed, as its answer(s) may provide guidance about key stakeholders who may be absent (Cornwall and Jewkes 1995). While participation by the intended community of focus is critical, there are various other stakeholders who are not usually included, such as the private sector and stakeholders who may not be comfortable with the usual participatory structures.

Participation is often an outcome of the relationship with community, the use of effective outreach strategies and the use of trusted community members as frontline workers (Kingori 2013). Often not discussed is that effective participation presupposes a belief in an outcome that will be of benefit to the community. A scepticism about social change or even more intermediary change is a key reason why broad-based participation may be challenging. This is of central importance in the South African context. The vigorous civic participation that emerged during the apartheid era—and still seems present—is based on the premise of social change, with the research agenda often considered secondary to this premise. In South Africa, there is the recognition that behavioural research designs *must* include community participation, even if such research designs would not necessarily meet the definition of PHR. Furthermore, there is the understanding that broad sector input is critical and that the community—alongside other key stakeholders, such as frontline healthcare provider staff—must be an integral part of the participatory health approach.

It is also important to consider the dual roles that are often required in PHR: that of participant and researcher. Unlike traditional mainstream research, the fluidity of the participant-researcher boundary provides both opportunities and challenges for research. "Participants" can take on various roles from providing data to informing research questions and instruments, collecting data and even contributing to data interpretation and the implementation of interventions. A similar tension emerges for the primary researcher, in that different roles may be required for collecting data and dissemination of research findings, compared to the tasks and roles required for facilitating interventions that emerge from these findings. This multiplicity of roles also raises ethical challenges for issues like confidentiality, anonymity and informed consent (Williamson and Prosser 2002).

While community member-as-researcher can enrich data by establishing legitimacy within a community and offering an insider perspective of the findings, there are also challenges that must be considered. One such challenge we encountered while training and working with community researchers from a resource-poor and socially fragmented community in South Africa was the mental burden and stress taken on by the community researchers as they managed their own personal struggles "coupled with the emotional stressors induced by their increased exposure to the conditions in their community" (Mosavel et al. 2011, p. 150).

PHR in the Context of Formative Research

PHR is particularly important in the context of formative research in South Africa. Two types of formative research are commonly conducted. First, the more typical formative research which is driven by the local academic-community partnership or agenda where the primary goals are community entrée, needs assessment and facilitating participation. The second type of formative research includes intervention or programme development which seems to be driven by the many different international research collaborations, in particular the implementation and testing of interventions from Northern countries.

Community Entrée

Entrée into the community is an important foundational goal of PHR. During the formative stage, research teams use various participatory strategies to foster trust-building and to mobilize participants. Strategies that have been used in South Africa include information sessions, key informant interviews, focus groups and surveys (Lazarus et al. 2014; Mosavel et al. 2005; Ramjee et al. 2010; Simwinga et al. 2016; Tucker et al. 2013).

In this stage, it is important that "community" be defined broadly to include all stakeholders directly and indirectly affected by any proposed research. Interested stakeholders include, although are not limited to, government officials, civic leaders, community residents, traditional leaders, healthcare providers, etc. Particularly relevant in South Africa is obtaining permission from the community's traditional leaders which is often seen as a critical first step for building a trusting relationship and gaining acceptance for the project (Simwinga et al. 2016; Treves-Kagan et al. 2017). For example, Ramjee et al. (2010) consulted with political and traditional leaders in the community who, in turn, consulted with community members to gain support for their HIV prevention research. Several research projects have also engaged laypersons as ambassadors who can assist in navigating and bridge-building between academic researchers and communities where there may be varying levels of mistrust, scepticism and misalignment of needs. To access an especially difficult-to-reach community, men who have sex with men, Tucker et al. (2013) spent 3 months networking with leaders of the community to gain trust and buy-in and ultimately was able to utilize these leaders as ambassadors to identify and engage other community members. Formative research provides the opportunity to build credibility and research integrity specifically by seeking and incorporating community feedback and identifying or modifying the research focus to address community priorities or anxiety (Mosavel et al. 2005).

Intervention/Programme Design

The other type of formative research in the South African context is that of programme or intervention development. For example, Remien et al. (2013) relied on a local team of researchers, clinicians and patients to address language and cultural differences (such as concepts of illness and treatment) when adapting an HIV intervention from the USA for use in South Africa. Similarly, Wechsberg et al. (2015) used community focus groups to understand the local context which resulted in modifications to the core elements, delivery style and structure of the

HIV prevention intervention they were adapting. While inclusion of youth in the research process has been limited, there are examples where youth have been engaged to help inform intervention design. In one such example, researchers sought to develop tobacco, drug and alcohol prevention materials for adolescents. They utilized a photo-voice methodology in which adolescents representing differing races were provided cameras and were asked to document the people and things they considered important in their lives. Through group discussion of the photos, the researchers were able to gain a better contextual understanding of adolescent lives which was used in the development of educational materials (Strecher et al. 2004).

Formative research that involves the community from the outset of the project as well as addresses issues such as trust, scepticism and the misalignment of agendas increases the likelihood of sustainable research agendas, with mutual benefits for both researchers and community members. For example, when we initiated our participatory health research project in Cape Town, we were narrowly focused on cervical cancer, and it was only due to the many meetings we conducted with varied stakeholders that we learned the importance of expanding our conceptual framework to encompass cervical *health (women's health more broadly)* rather than only *cancer* thus acknowledging that poor women face health challenges beyond just cancer (Mosavel et al. 2005). Unfortunately, it is not uncommon for imported programmes, interventions and research—primarily driven by the need to generalize findings and interventions—to entrench Northern agendas and Western concepts, in spite of the intentions of those conducting the projects (Daniels 2011; Lau and Seedat 2015; Tomlinson et al. 2006).

Partnerships in PHR

Partnerships are essential to facilitate engagement in the translation and dissemination of research outcomes and to ensure sustainability beyond the scope of the research funding. There are many well-documented challenges associated with community-researcher partnerships, not least of which are the power dynamics, differing values and constituents and conflicting perspectives.

Academic Partnerships

Academic institutions in South Africa, not unlike universities elsewhere, are being called to collaborate with government, private sector and communities to address the various health manifestations of social, political and economic inequities (Brown-Luthango 2012). While many academic institutions explicitly specify community engagement as part of their role, it is unclear to what extent equal partnerships are established, and many of the difficulties present in other contexts also seem to be present here.

Collaboration and participation are greatly facilitated when there is a recognition of the varying expertise amongst partners, especially the expertise of community stakeholders (Marks et al. 2015). For some academics, it can be challenging to embrace the expertise of community members as it counters the traditional research paradigm and the way researchers are trained in academic institutions. It can be difficult for researchers to accept or value the insider expertise of community members or to understand how the community perspective can lend validity and scientific integrity to the research (El Ansari et al. 2002; Kearney et al. 2013).

International Partnerships

International research partnerships abound in South Africa, many of which are HIV intervention related (Desmond Tutu HIV Foundation 2015). Communities, researchers and the scientific field, more generally, are greatly benefiting from cross-sector and international collaborations. Partnerships in general, and with international researchers in particular, are invaluable to stakeholders (inside and outside South Africa) and have significant potential to positively impact practice and health outcomes.

However, with international NGOs there is more of a need for researchers to understand the local culture, politics and dynamics amongst the stakeholders (Costella and Zumla 2000; Tomlinson et al. 2006). International researchers often enter the collaboration with a limited understanding of the interplay between stakeholders or the implicit values or expectations of the partners (Nama and Swartz 2002). Furthermore, these international partnerships are characterized by unequal and divergent assets. Most importantly, it is likely that international partners will be in a position to provide financial resources to the partnership. The imbalance of financial contributions can often lead to concerns about power and value and invariably determines who sets the research agenda (Edejer 1999; Jentsch and Pilley 2003). With funding often being generated from Northern international partners, this inequality means that for both the researchers and communities from the South, power is structurally located with the Northern partner and thus can significantly impact on all aspects of the research. In all partnerships, and in particular in international partnerships, it is imperative that roles and responsibilities as well as power dynamics, benefits and burdens of implementation are recognized, deliberated and addressed (Costello and Zumla 2000; Jentsch and Pilley 2003).

Community Advisory Boards (CABs)

The engagement of an advisory group is usually seen as a foundational element for most participatory research (Newman et al. 2011). In general, CABs are established at the discretion of researchers or the funder's requirements. CABs are used in various projects, many of which are HIV/AIDS related (Ramjee et al. 2010; Reddy et al. 2010). CABs usually have diverse roles in participatory research, with the major task being the provision of input to researchers. Within HIV/AIDS research, CABs appear to have an important monitoring role. Reddy and colleagues did a study of CABs in HIV vaccine trials in South Africa. Their findings suggest that the use of CABs in South Africa is primarily researcher-initiated and research-driven, with the overall goal to provide community input and scientific oversight (Reddy et al. 2010). However, there are several questions about the effectiveness and participatory nature of CABs, specifically questions about the selection of CAB members, to what extent they represent community voice, and whether CABs are independent or merely serve as a gatekeeper. Some of these unanswered questions have resulted in a preference for the terminology *community advisory groups* instead of boards (Reddy et al. 2010).

Building Capacity for PHR

Using an asset-based approach which builds on the existing strengths in a community—whether those strengths are people, organizations or social structures—is considered to be an important principle in PHR. Given the focus on social transformation, it is not surprising that capacity building is so prominent in some South African research. In fact, in the South African context, capacity building may be considered as important an outcome as the research itself. Building the research capacity of the community providers can be considered one form of levelling of power and provides a means for local participants to set their research agenda and address issues they see as important (Tomlinson et al. 2006). The engagement of laypersons in participatory health research in South Africa, both in the role of community/peer researcher and as a community health worker (CHW), is ostensibly used as a capacity-building strategy capitalizing on existing community strengths. These strategies also have the effect of addressing the important community need of building research capacity (El Ansari 2005; Mitchell et al. 2005; Mosavel et al. 2005).

The evolution of the CHW is a part of South Africa's economic, political and healthcare response to the HIV/AIDS crisis (Clarke et al. 2008). CHW are usually hired by NGOs and provide outreach to improve access to care and act as the middle person between the healthcare system and the community (Nxumalo et al. 2013; Schneider et al. 2008; Suri et al. 2007). While there is debate about the appropriate training, role and support for CHW, there is consensus that they are an integral interface between the community and the healthcare system (Friedman 2005). CHW are primarily utilized for health promotion purposes (Friedman 2005), and while there is mention of the potential benefit utilizing CHW to collect health data (Suri et al. 2007), their research role is less well-defined. Bradley and Puoane, for example, discuss the important role of CHW in identifying their community's concerns and the benefits of involvement in all aspects of the research process, from collecting data to developing training programmes, and directing the interventions (Bradley and Puoane 2007). While there are arguably various ways to build capacity and utilize the strengths of the community in South Africa, the CHW movement as an engagement strategy has resulted in tangible improvements to health outcomes and health policy (Clarke et al. 2008; Schneider et al. 2008).

Community researchers or laypersons in the role of peer researcher engaging with the community are another key capacity-building and asset-based strategy used in social and behavioural research. There is, however, a distinction between the role of CHW and that of community researcher. Community researchers, or peer researchers, have less of a health promotion role, their tasks being more specifically centred on research. For example, Batist et al. (2013) trained five community members to conduct an HIV prevention intervention for a community of men who have sex with men. In this capacity, the community researchers participated in the planning and facilitation of the research and intervention activities, including recruitment of participants, dissemination of information and healthcare referrals (Batist et al. 2013). Photo-voice projects are another participatory technique for engaging community researchers. In utilizing the photo-voice methodology to improve collaboration between CHW and teachers in preventing HIV in young people, Mitchell et al. (2005, p. 268) have suggested that by engaging in the research, "it has opened up an important space for groups to take action themselves. They are not waiting for the research team to come back to give them answers."

However, the use of community members in participatory research also raises a number of challenges. Mosavel and colleagues, in a cancer prevention community-based needs assessment, trained laypersons as community researchers to recruit and conduct interviews with fellow residents. The authors described various ethical considerations as well as benefits and challenges associated with the role of community researcher (Mosavel et al. 2011). Not often discussed are the tensions and difficulties the community researchers might be experiencing in their role, especially given that they are the "frontline workers" who witness up-close the harrowing and challenging conditions that they might be asked to "research" (Kingori 2013; Nama and Swartz 2002). The emotional support of community researchers is an area that has not received the investigation it warrants. Being the intermediary between the researchers/health professionals and the community is a role that can be difficult, as it underlines unanswered questions about researcher burden, credibility, conflicts and commitments.

Conclusion

The context of huge inequities and a history of citizen participation form the backdrop of participatory research in South Africa. Following the marginalization and virtual exclusion of People of Colour, there has been a far greater attempt in the post-apartheid era to involve these communities. In addition to conducting more community-based research, it would not be inaccurate to conclude that most of the research can be characterized as *research in communities*, rather than the gold standard of *research with communities*. The challenges evident in participatory research globally emerge in South Africa; there are, as well, challenges that may be specific to the local context.

There is some consensus that research is shaped by a global neo-liberal agenda (Bayliss et al. 2011; Roberts and Peters 2008), which creates particular challenges for PHR in developing contexts such as South Africa. South Africa, like other developing countries, has a long history of "parachute" research, whereby researchers from "wealthy" or "Western" countries travel to developing countries to collect data before returning home to analyse and publish their results (Costello and Zumla 2000; Tomlinson et al. 2006). Even in cases where international researchers "embed" in the country of interest, the research agenda is often still controlled by outsiders, and research findings may not be translated into programmes for local benefit (Costello and Zumla 2000; Tomlinson et al. 2006).

At the research partnership level, a particular set of challenges emerge. The inequity and power differentials in North-South partnerships may serve to preserve the notion that developing countries must depend on the wealthier western nations to advance and progress. In the South African context, there are also the racial inequalities between Black and White researchers, as well as between historically White, well-resourced institutions and historically Black under-resourced institutions; North-South collaborations may further serve to maintain these existing inequities. In other words, there is not only a Northern-led agenda but an agenda driven by historically advantaged institutions inside South Africa which are also historically isolated from communities in need.

The potential dominance and reproduction of a Northern agenda have a huge impact on the local community agenda. Attempts to involve the community from the outset, the emphasis on capacity building and the popularity of photo-voice methodologies can all be understood as attempts to engage with power dynamics and social inequities. It serves to give voice to communities under conditions which these voices run the risk of being muted.

A focus on social transformation from the apartheid era reinforces the research vs. service delivery tension. Given the urgent and pressing needs in many communities, research is often seen as a luxury. The emergence of "relevant research" (Long 2013) can be understood as an attempt to manage this tension. The prominence of this debate (Long 2013) highlights the fact that research cannot be decoupled from some kind of action. Current manifestations include asset mapping, engaging with policy and the undertaking that data will eventually be used to improve the living conditions of members of that community. While these are important, the marked tension between social action informed by research and the large-scale civic participation reflected in service delivery protests, characterized as a rebellion of the poor (Alexander 2010), is a distinct feature of South African participatory research. South Africa's history of civic participation precedes attempts at community-engaged research and is helpful perhaps in foregrounding the social action component of PHR.

Entrée into communities remains complex and shaped by colour, class and culture as well as the daily challenges these communities face. While there is certainly greater representation in terms of class, colour and culture, like all other areas of South African society, research profiles and resources remain concentrated largely in the hands of the White minority. Furthermore, Black researchers who may have come from the communities they now serve may by virtue of their class position be quite removed from these communities.

The power-sharing philosophy of PHR resonates well and is particularly helpful for contexts like South Africa. However, the social conditions create both unique opportunities and challenges for this type of research. Perhaps the most important lesson from the South African context is the extent to which it foregrounds the need for research to be informed by a social justice agenda. Indubitably, health research is inextricably linked to social inequities and the transformation of social conditions.

References

Alexander, P. (2010). Rebellion of the poor: South Africa's service delivery protests – a preliminary analysis. *Review of African Political Economy, 37*, 25–40.

Batist, E., Brown, B., Scheibe, A., Baral, S. D., & Bekker, L. G. (2013). Outcomes of a community-based HIV-prevention pilot programme for township men who have sex with men in Cape Town, South Africa. *Journal of the International AIDS Society, 16*(Suppl 3), 18754. https://doi.org/10.7448/IAS.16.4.18754.

Bayliss, K., Fine, B., & Van Waeyenberge, E. (2011). *The political economy of development: The World Bank, neoliberalism and development research*. Chicago: University of Chicago Press.

Bradley, H. A., & Puoane, T. (2007). Prevention of hypertension and diabetes in an urban setting in South Africa: Participatory action research with community health workers. *Ethnicity & Disease, 17*, 49–54.

Brown-Luthango, M. (2012). Community-university engagement: The Philippi CityLab in Cape Town and the challenge of collaboration across boundaries. *Higher Education, 65*, 309–324. https://doi.org/10.1007/s10734-012-9546-z.

Chitiga M., Sekyere E., & Tsonamatsie N. (2015) Income inequality and limitations of the gini index: The case of South Africa. http://www.hsrc.ac.za/en/review/hsrc-review-november-2014/limitations-of-gini-index. Accessed 18 Dec 2017.

Clarke, M., Dick, J., & Lewin, S. (2008). Community health workers in South Africa: Where in this maze do we find ourselves? *South African Medical Journal, 98*, 680–681.

Coovadia, H., Jewkes, R., Barron, P., Sanders, D., & McIntyre, D. (2009). The health and health system of South Africa: Historical roots of current public health challenges. *Lancet, 374*, 817–834. https://doi.org/10.1016/S0140-6736(09)60951-X.

Cornwall, A., & Jewkes, R. (1995). What is participatory research? *Social Science & Medicine, 41*, 1667–1676.

Costella, A., & Zumla, A. (2000). Moving to research partnerships in developing countries. *Bristish Medical Journal, 321*, 827–829.

Costello, A., & Zumla, A. (2000). Moving to research partnerships in developing countries. *BMJ, 321*, 827–829.

Daniels, D. (2011). *Decolonising the researcher's mind about southern research: Reflections from the field*. Stellenbosch: Stellenbosch University.

Deacon, H. (2000). Racism and medical science in South Africa's Cape Colony in the mid- to late nineteenth century. *Osiris, 15*, 190–206.

Desmond Tutu HIV Foundation. (2015) Academic collaboration with national and international institutions. http://desmondtutuhivfoundation.org.za/our-partners/. Accessed 27 Jan 2016.

Edejer, T. T. (1999). North-South research partnerships: The ethics of carrying out research in developing countries. *BMJ, 319*, 438–441. https://doi.org/10.1136/bmj.319.7207.438.

El Ansari, W. (2005). Collaborative research partnerships with disadvantaged communities: Challenges and potential solutions. *Public Health, 119*, 758–770. https://doi.org/10.1016/j.puhe.2005.01.014.

El Ansari, W., Phillips, C. J., & Zwi, A. B. (2002). Narrowing the gap between academic professional wisdom and community lay knowledge: Perceptions from partnerships. *Public Health, 116*, 151–159. https://doi.org/10.1038/sj.ph.1900839.

Friedman, I. (2005). CHWs and community caregivers: Towards a unified model of practice. In P. Ijumba & P. Barron (Eds.), *South African health review*. Durban: Health Systems Trust.

Gouws, E., & Karim, Q. A. (2010). HIV infection in South Africa: The evolving epidemic. In S. S. A. Karim & Q. A. Karim (Eds.), *HIV/AIDS in South Africa* (2nd ed.). Cape Town: Cambridge University Press.

Habib, A., & Taylor, R. (1999). South Africa: Anti-apartheid NGOs in transition. *Voluntas: International Journal of Voluntary and Nonprofit Organizations, 10*, 73–82. https://doi.org/10.1023/a:1021495821397.

International Collaboration for Participatory Health Research. (2013). *Position paper 1: What is participatory health research? Version May 2013*. Berlin: International Collaboration for Participatory Health Research.

Jentsch, B., & Pilley, C. (2003). Research relationships between the South and the North: Cinderella and the ugly sisters? *Social Science & Medicine, 57*, 1957–1967. https://doi.org/10.1016/s0277-9536(03)00060-1.

Kearney, J., Wood, L., & Zuber-Skerritt, O. (2013). Community–university partnerships: Using participatory action learning and action research (PALAR). *Gateways: International Journal of Community Research and Engagement, 6*, 113. https://doi.org/10.5130/ijcre.v6i1.3105.

Kingori, P. (2013). Experiencing everyday ethics in context: Frontline data collectors perspectives and practices of bioethics. *Social Science & Medicine, 98*, 361–370. https://doi.org/10.1016/j.socscimed.2013.10.013.

Lau, U., & Seedat, M. (2015). The community story, relationality and process: Bridging tools for researching local knowledge in a peri-urban township. *Journal of Community and Applied Social Psychology, 25*, 369–383. https://doi.org/10.1002/casp.2219.

Lazarus, S., Naidoo, A. V., May, B., Williams, L., Demas, G., & Filander, F. J. (2014). Lessons learnt from a community-based participatory research project in a South African rural context. *South Africa Journal of Psychology, 44*, 149–161. https://doi.org/10.1177/0081246314528156.

Long, W. (2013). Rethinking "relevance": South African psychology in context. *History of Psychology, 16*, 19–35. https://doi.org/10.1037/a0029675.

Mabunda, J. T., Khoza, L. B., Van den Borne, H. B., & Lebese, R. T. (2016). Needs assessment for adapting TB directly observed treatment intervention programme in Limpopo Province, South Africa: A community-based participatory research approach. *Afr J Prim Health Care Fam Med, 8*, e1–e7. https://doi.org/10.4102/phcfm.v8i2.981.

Marks, M., Erwin, K., & Mosavel, M. (2015). The inextricable link between community engagement, community-based research and service learning: The case of an international collaboration. *South African Journal of Higher Education, 29*, 214–231.

Maxwell, M. L., Abrams, J., Zungu, T., & Mosavel, M. (2016). Conducting community-engaged qualitative research in South Africa: Memoirs of intersectional identities abroad. *Qualitative Research, 16*, 95–110. https://doi.org/10.1177/1468794114567495.

Mitchell, C., DeLange, N., Moletsane, R., Stuart, J., & Buthelezi, T. (2005). Giving a face to HIV and AIDS: On the uses of photo-voice by teachers and community health care workers working with youth in rural South Africa. *Qualitative Research in Psychology, 2*, 257–270. https://doi.org/10.1191/1478088705qp042oa.

Mosavel, M., Simon, C., van Stade, D., & Buchbinder, M. (2005). Community-based participatory research (CBPR) in South Africa: Engaging multiple constituents to shape the research question. *Social Science & Medicine, 61*, 2577–2587. https://doi.org/10.1016/j.socscimed.2005.04.041.

Mosavel, M., Ahmed, R., Daniels, D., & Simon, C. (2011). Community researchers conducting health disparities research: Ethical and other insights from fieldwork journaling. *Social Science & Medicine, 73*, 145–152. https://doi.org/10.1016/j.socscimed.2011.04.029.

Musesengwa, R., & Chimbari, M. (2017). Community engagement practices in Southern Africa: Review and thematic synthesis of studies done in Botswana, Zimbabwe and South Africa. Acta Trop, 175(Nov), 20-30. https://doi.org/10.1016/j.actatropica.2016.03.021

Nama, N., & Swartz, L. (2002). Ethical and social dilemmas in community-based controlled trials in situations of poverty: A view from a South African project. *Journal of Community and Applied Social Psychology, 12*, 286–297. https://doi.org/10.1002/casp.682.

Newman, S. D., Andrews, J. O., Magwood, G. S., Jenkins, C., Cox, M. J., & Williamson, D. C. (2011). Community advisory boards in community-based participatory research: A synthesis of best processes. *Preventing Chronic Disease, 8*, A70.

Nxumalo, N., Goudge, J., & Thomas, L. (2013). Outreach services to improve access to health care in South Africa: Lessons from three community health worker programmes. *Global Health Action, 6*, 19283. https://doi.org/10.3402/gha.v6i0.19283.

Ramjee, G., et al. (2010). Experiences in conducting multiple community-based HIV prevention trials among women in KwaZulu-Natal, South Africa. *AIDS Research and Therapy, 7*, 10. https://doi.org/10.1186/1742-6405-7-10.

Reddy, P., Buchanan, D., Sifunda, S., James, S., & Naidoo, N. (2010). The role of community advisory boards in health research: Divergent views in the South African experience. *SAHARA Journal, 7*, 2–8. https://doi.org/10.1080/17290376.2010.9724963.

Remien, R. H., et al. (2013). Masivukeni: Development of a multimedia based antiretroviral therapy adherence intervention for counselors and patients in South Africa. *AIDS and Behavior, 17*, 1979–1991. https://doi.org/10.1007/s10461-013-0438-8.

Richman, K. A., Alexander, L. B., & True, G. (2012). Proximity, ethical dilemmas, and community research workers. *AJOB Primary Research, 3*, 19–29. https://doi.org/10.1080/21507716.2012.714837.

Roberts, P., & Peters, M. A. (2008). *Neoliberalistm, higher education, and research*. Rotterdam: Sense Publishers.

Rohrer, K., & Rajan, D. (2016). Population consultation on needs and expectations. In G. Schmets, D. Rajan, & S. Kadandale (Eds.), *Strategizing national health in the 21st century: A handbook*. Geneva: World Health Organization.

Schneider, H., Hlophe, H., & van Rensburg, D. (2008). Community health workers and the response to HIV/AIDS in South Africa: Tensions and prospects. *Health Policy and Planning, 23*, 179–187. https://doi.org/10.1093/heapol/czn006.

Simon, C., & Mosavel, M. (2011). Getting personal: Ethics and identity in global health research. *Developing World Bioethics, 11*, 82–92.

Simon, C., Mosavel, M., & van Stade, D. (2007). Ethical challenges in the design and conduct of locally relevant international health research. *Social Science & Medicine, 64*, 1960–1969. https://doi.org/10.1016/j.socscimed.2007.01.009.

Simwinga, M., et al. (2016). Implementing community engagement for combination prevention: Lessons learnt from the first year of the HPTN 071 (PopART) community-randomized study. *Current HIV/AIDS Reports, 13*, 194–201. https://doi.org/10.1007/s11904-016-0322-z.

South Africa Department of Higher Education and Training. (2014). Table 2.13: Number of students who fulfilled the requirements for a degree (African).

Steyn, K., Fourie, J., & Temple, N. (eds) (2006). Chronic diseases of lifestyle in South Africa: 1995–2005. Technical Report. South African Medical Research Council, Cape Town.

Strecher, V. J., Strecher, R. H., Swart, D., Resnicow, K., & Reddy, P. (2004). Photovoice for tobacco, drug, and alcohol prevention among adolescents in South Africa. Paper presented at the Annual Meeting of the American Public Health Association, Washington, DC.

Suri, A., Gan, K., & Carpenter, S. (2007). Voices from the field: Perspectives from community health workers on health care delivery in rural KwaZulu-Natal. *Southern African Journal of Infectious Diseases, 196*(Suppl 3), S505–S511. https://doi.org/10.1086/521122.

Tomlinson, M., Swartz, L., & Landman, M. (2006). Insiders and outsiders: Levels of collaboration in research partnerships across resource divides. *Infant Mental Health Journal, 27*, 532–543. https://doi.org/10.1002/imhj.20105.

Treves-Kagan, S., Naidoo, E., Gilvydis, J. M., Raphela, E., Barnhart, S., & Lippman, S. A. (2017). A situational analysis methodology to inform comprehensive HIV prevention and treatment programming, applied in rural South Africa. *Global Public Health, 9*, 1–19. https://doi.org/10.1080/17441692.2015.1080590.

Tucker, A., de Swardt, G., Struthers, H., & McIntyre, J. (2013). Understanding the needs of township men who have sex with men (MSM) health outreach workers: Exploring the interplay between volunteer training, social capital and critical consciousness. *AIDS and Behavior, 17*(Suppl 1), S33–S42. https://doi.org/10.1007/s10461-012-0287-x.

Wechsberg, W. M., El-Bassel, N., Carney, T., Browne, F. A., Myers, B., & Zule, W. A. (2015). Adapting an evidence-based HIV behavioral intervention for South African couples. *Substance Abuse Treatment, Prevention, and Policy, 10*, 6. https://doi.org/10.1186/s13011-015-0005-6.

Williamson, G., & Prosser, S. (2002). Action research: Politics, ethics and participation. *Journal of Advanced Nursing, 40*, 587–593.

Woodsong, C., Mutsambi, J. M., Ntshele, S., & Modikoe, P. (2014). Community and research staff collaboration for development of materials to inform microbicide study participants in Africa. *Journal of the International AIDS Society, 17*, 19156. https://doi.org/10.7448/IAS.17.3.19156.

Worden, N. (2011). *The making of modern South Africa: Conquest, apartheid, democracy* (5th ed.). Hoboken: Wiley-Blackwell.

Chapter 16
"Home Thoughts from Abroad": Reflections on the History of Participatory Health Research in the UK

Jane Springett

Introduction

Participatory health research (PHR) as understood and practised in the UK is a product of its unique history and culture, building on a rich tradition of participatory action research (PAR) across the four nations that make up the UK. As a former colonial power with connections to many parts of the world, the UK has also attracted migrants from a wide assortment of ethnic groups. Historically, however, there is a deeply entrenched class system which is reinforced by privilege, inherited wealth and contacts resulting in what has been described as an ongoing class struggle manifesting in poor industrial relations as well as social inequalities (McGuiness 2016). The resulting health inequalities became a focus of UK academic interest in the 1970s continuing to the present day (Marmot 2010). Those inequalities have been accentuated more recently by the relentless pursuit of neoliberal economic policies (Craig 2016). Nonetheless, due to the introduction of a welfare state after the Second World War, each of the four countries of the UK has a publicly funded health-care system, the National Health Service (NHS), founded in 1948. Responsibility for health and social care—as well as other functions, including education—was devolved to Scotland, Wales and Northern Ireland in 1998. However, taxation, overall welfare policy and the allocation of funding remain firmly centralised with the UK Government which also exercises strong controls over local government spending in England. Highly centralised tax and spend powers, the uneasy relationship between the local and the central government and the only recent devolution of limited powers to the Welsh Assembly, Scottish Parliament and the Northern Ireland Assembly need to be seen as a backdrop to any understanding of public health and health care and the development of PHR (Callaghan and Wistow 2006).

J. Springett (✉)
School of Public Health, University of Alberta, Edmonton, Canada
e-mail: jane.springett@ualberta.ca

© Springer International Publishing AG, part of Springer Nature 2018
M. T. Wright, K. Kongats (eds.), *Participatory Health Research*,
https://doi.org/10.1007/978-3-319-92177-8_16

This chapter traces the recent history of the development of the approach within the UK exploring some of the main influences on the tradition. In particular, it examines the different factors in public sector funding and the academic environment that over time have impacted on the use and development of this type of research in a health context and the key challenges this has created. It will conclude with a reflection on future prospects in a period of austerity and uncertainty. The positionality of the author lends a certain perspective to this story. As a contributor to the development of PHR within health promotion and public health, she is now living in a different academic and political-economic environment with its own inherited challenges. This has coloured the lens through which developments in the UK are viewed.

Origins of Participatory Action Research in the UK

In the UK the common terminology for this type of research is participatory action research (PAR) reflecting the philosophical roots and origins. There have been three main strands that together contributed to the way PAR has developed in the UK as a whole. Firstly, as a former colonial power, there has been a strong tradition of involvement in development in other parts of the world, both through government funding and also charities and NGOs. It is from these contexts that development workers brought back to the UK experience of working in a participatory way largely outside established institutions. Indeed the first edited volume on participatory research in health was co-authored by two researchers with such a background, while its content reflected that international experience (de Koning and Martin 1996). The driver of this type of participatory research was the need to engage the voices of local populations in development initiatives and their evaluation alongside a deep sense of social justice. A key player was the Institute for Development Studies (IDS) founded in 1966 at the University of Sussex, particularly the work of Robert Chambers who during the 1970s spearheaded participatory approaches to development (Chambers 1997). The methods he and his colleagues pioneered, like participatory rapid appraisal, started being used in the UK context particularly in community health needs assessments (Chambers 2015). For example, it was used in Northern Ireland where unlike elsewhere in the UK, health and social care are under one jurisdiction (Lazenbatt et al. 2001). By the 1990s participatory methods had spread widely to over 60 countries and in the operations of several UN funds and agencies, notably in the World Bank and amongst a number of donors influenced by IDS. The importance of participation as a cornerstone of social change became a key component of the Institute's work, and a Master's programme was started in 2004. The library at IDS remains a rich source of case studies from development contexts (Jolly 2008). It is this development strand that is also reflected in the landmark paper on participatory health research published in *Social Science and Medicine* in 1995 by two UK authors (Cornwall and Jewkes 1995).

Secondly, there was the development of participatory research in the context of management science spearheaded by the work of Peter Reason, a professor of management studies and Director of the Centre for Action Research in Professional Practice at the University of Bath until 2009. Here the focus was not on the poor per se but on a different epistemology strongly connected to ecological thinking (Reason 1998), outlined in detail in the both the first and second editions of the Sage Handbook on Action Research published in 2001 (Reason and Bradbury 2001) and 2008 (Bradbury and Reason 2008) and also in the journal *Action Research* which was founded in 2003. Reason himself was strongly influenced by humanist psychology and incorporated that thinking in his interpretation of PAR. He distinguished between first person, second person and third person action research and promoted collaborative inquiry (Reason and Heron 1994). An early study involved general practitioners of medicine exploring the use of complementary therapies in their practice. Along with John Rowan, he also discussed different forms of knowledge: propositional, practical, experiential and presentational knowing and coined the term "new paradigm research" (Reason 1998; Reason and Rowan 1981).

The third strand comes from community development, itself a product of adult education, which rose to particular prominence in the 1960s when the government funded a number of community development workers in specific inner-city areas across the country. The radical perspective embodied by community development was a product of the community workers' experience of the impact of government policy. This proved to be too challenging politically, leading to the disbandment of community development projects in England (Craig et al. 2011). In Scotland, however, community development and PAR continued to be supported, resulting in a strong investment in terms of education and training which has continued following devolution (Abdulkadir et al. 2016). Indeed the right to participate was part of the Community Empowerment (Scotland) Act 2015. Elsewhere, community development workers continued to operate below the radar within the public sector or in civil society throughout the 1970s and 1980s, resurfacing in strength when the Labour Government took power in 1997 and various area-based policy initiatives were implemented in England and Wales. After civil strife in Northern Ireland culminated in the Northern Ireland Agreement, community development workers played a strong role in the peace process, trying to heal the wounds created by deep divisions and violence which were the result of a long colonial history originating in the seventeenth century (Lundy and McGovern 2006; McIntyre 2003).

During the 1990s and beyond, training in community development was greatly enhanced and a core set of values became the hallmark of community development work: social justice and equality, respect and democratic control, with Freirean notions of empowerment and conscientisation as key components (Ledwith 2015; Ledwith and Springett 2010).

The Halcyon Days of Health Promotion

Developments in PAR impinged on the health sector in the UK from the late 1980s, in part through the rise of health promotion and the "new public health" (Green and Tones 1999). The main driver was the Healthy Cities project led by the European Office of WHO and the Health for All movement fuelled in the UK by local government officers concerned about health inequalities (Berkeley and Springett 2006; Davies and Kelly 2014). Both led to the establishment of the UK Health for All Network, now replaced by the UK Healthy Cities Network. The first Healthy Cities conference was held in Liverpool in 1987. In that city many of those involved with the WHO Healthy City project were advocates of participation and participatory action research and other health promotion principles as laid down in the Ottawa Charter (Dooris and Heritage 2013). Capacity building in relation to participatory approaches flourished in community-focused universities and former polytechnics, particularly in interdisciplinary or social science orientated faculties. Master's courses in health promotion were established across the country (Wills et al. 2008). By the early 1990s, participatory approaches to research were beginning to emerge as key to the type of social change for health required to address inequality (Chiu 2007). At the same time, action research approaches to health-care system change were being more widely used as the result of trends in organisational development as well as in nursing. A Health Technology Assessment Report provides an overview of health-related action research in the UK by 2001. Most projects were conducted between 1988 and 1996 and lasted from 1 to 48 months, mostly involving nurses. There were 21 funded studies (Waterman et al. 2001).

Riding on the tide of enthusiasm for a social approach to health, Health Action Zones were designated by a new Labour Government in 1999 (Judge et al. 1999). Indeed many of the health promotion experiences provided case studies for government policy documents (Department of Health 1999). It is therefore somewhat ironic that during this time, the words *health promotion* disappeared from the policy discourse, replaced by *health improvement* and then *health development*. Within a few years, medical hegemony regained its ground as the Faculty of Public Health Medicine took control of public health training, forcing the many health promotion postgraduate courses to rebrand themselves as Master's in Public Health (Scott-Samuel and Springett 2007; Wills et al. 2008). Nonetheless, participatory approaches to research and evaluation started to become more commonplace and were referenced more often in government documents as well as being subject to evaluation scrutiny. Through the Health Action Zones, many of which built on previous Healthy City projects, an increasing number of public sector decision-makers were exposed to partnership working and PAR, whether in the context of evaluation or other forms of research (Cole 2003; Springett and Young 2002). For example, the Merseyside Health Action Zone invested resources in participatory evaluation training for all participants of its 253 funded projects (Springett 2005; Crawshaw et al. 2004).

Participatory health research, if not mainstreamed, was beginning to be established as an approach to research. Capacity was being built in the academic sector and more was being published, with publications reaching a new peak in 2006

(Boote et al. 2015). However, there were few participatory health research courses in degree programmes, and actual research following this paradigm remained on the margins, receiving funding from largely ad hoc sources. Most projects were still mainly taking place outside the academic sector in many NGOs and charities working to reduce poverty and increase social justice both in the UK and beyond.

The Influence of Teacher Education on Participatory Health Research

At the same time, as PAR was gaining ascendency in development management studies and adult education, it was being advocated for in the area of teacher education as a vehicle for self-inquiry and improvement in classroom teaching. The Classroom Action Research Network (CARN) was founded by John Elliott in 1976 at the University of East Anglia with a small-scale grant from the Ford Foundation to support the activities of teacher-researchers who had engaged in the Ford Teaching Project's action research into "discovery learning". By the 1980s, CARN provided a meeting point and a national and international support network for all those developing action research work in schools, communities and universities. As the network enlarged, not only teachers and teacher educators but also other professionals increasingly became involved, including health-care educators as well as those concerned with inclusive research and education for those with learning difficulties. The name changed to the Collaborative Action Research Network (Somekh 2010). Today CARN, which is coordinated from North West England, is well-established as an international network that supports action researchers in local contexts from a wide variety of backgrounds and strengthens the collaborative relations of the global action research community. Through its annual conferences and study days, CARN provides a forum for all action researchers to present their work and engage in critical discussion of ideas in a safe environment. The journal of CARN, *Educational Action Research*, was founded in 1993 and publishes many papers on PAR and PHR. For many years this network became the main outlet for those working in the health sector doing PAR to share their interest in PAR/PHR. CARN is linked to the recently formed UK Participatory Research Network (Balogh et al. 2017). The latter is affiliated with the International Collaboration for Participatory Health Research (ICPHR).

Buffeted by the Winds of Change in the NHS: PHR in the Twenty-First Century

Government direct funding of health care through the NHS, rather than indirectly through social insurance, has meant that health care as well as public health remains a political football and subject to the whims of politicians. With each new government has come a raft of new organisational changes aimed at reducing health-care costs and increasing efficiency. Until 2012, when it was transferred to local authorities, public health remained a NHS-led function. Historical underlying structures of power permeate the NHS and its decision-making processes as well as how health research is funded. Every attempt to reduce bureaucracy during the twentieth century led to new bureaucratic structures to compensate for the consequences of each reorganisation, with a return to the "old wine being put in new bottles" in terms of those power relations, including a re-emergence of scientific bureaucratism (Harrison 2002). Such relations of power are in turn linked to the relative influences of medical or social models of health. Although the social model was championed strongly and was to some extent reflected in legislation (Crawshaw et al. 2004), its influence as a strong force in public health practice was comparatively short-lived. Historically, scientific rationalism has provided the dominant value structure in an NHS in which medical and associated clinical professions have prevailed even in the face of an emergent consumerism (Harrison 2002; Harrison et al. 2002).

For participatory health research, two elements of reform provided both an opportunity and a threat. Firstly, there was to be an emphasis placed on evidence-based practice; and secondly, there was to be consumer involvement in health-care decision-making. Advocacy for evidence-based practice came from an increasing concern that clinicians often based their clinical decision-making on out-of-date or under-researched interventions and from a concern regarding the failure of research generally to have an impact on practice. A strong influence was the Cochrane Collaboration which had been established in 1993. A central plank of Cochrane has been a hierarchical approach to evidence with the "gold standard" of experimental designs (randomised controlled trials or RCTs) being at the top. Although originating in medical science, those in favour of a positivist paradigm actively promoted this hierarchy for all health research funding and as the basis for discussions on the merits of different types of research including health promotion and other non-medical areas. This view did not go uncontested, for example, by disability groups, but it re-established the dominance of the medical model, and the mantra of evidence-based practice began to pervade the health service lexicon (Hammersley 2005; Devisch and Murray 2009).

However, although a threat to PHR in terms of funding, the focus on evidence could be seen as an opportunity. The need for evidence-based decision-making generated a number of openings for evaluation, including participatory evaluation, providing spaces for health professionals and decision-makers to have experience of the approach (e.g. Springett 2001; Springett et al. 2007).

Patient and public involvement was also central to the British government's modernisation of the National Health Service. A "patient-centred service" it was argued is necessary to improve health outcomes, provide a better experience of care for patients and reconnect the health service with the communities it serves. New structures were put in place to enable and promote these changes. Public involvement within the hierarchical structure of the NHS had historically consisted of limited agendas and formal advisory roles aimed at securing consumer feedback and advice (Wistow and Barnes 1993). Although the public involvement policy embodied in earlier policy documents advocated the importance of listening to local communities, in practice the focus initially was primarily on developing methods of consultation about satisfaction with existing services (NIHR 2015). The new arrangements introduced in 2001 were an attempt to change this, being a response to a whole series of social movements in health care—from breast cancer to mental health and disability—by patients seeking greater control over the type and nature of health services. Significantly, the new policy directive extended this involvement into health research, developing a training infrastructure called INVOLVE. Opening the door to citizen engagement in research also held potential dangers, as the notion of consumer as a passive recipient in a market economy could prevail, rather than an empowered citizen who takes active control, the central plank of PAR/PHR (Beresford 2002). Citizen engagement in research also challenges the dominant epistemology that research should be done at arm's length from the patient (Beresford 2003; Gillard et al. 2010).

Nevertheless, when the main health service research funding body, the National Institute of Health Research (NIHR), was established in 2006, it announced its commitment to "involving patients, carers and the public at all stages of the research process". This has meant requiring researchers to demonstrate how members of the public have been involved in the design and development of their grant applications and how the public will be actively involved in managing the research undertaking, the analysis and disseminating the findings (NIHR 2006). INVOLVE defined the public as "patients and potential patients; people who use health and social services; informal carers; parents/guardians; disabled people; members of the public who are potential recipients of health promotion programmes, public health programmes and social service interventions; and organisations that represent people who use services". Moreover, public involvement in research is conceptualised as "doing research 'with' or 'by' the public rather than 'to' 'about' or 'for' the public" (Evans et al. 2014).

Suddenly the door into the mainstream had been opened for participatory researchers. Increasingly, research papers exploring the whole issue of patient and public involvement (PPI) started to reference action and participatory research in the search for ways to implement PPI, while participatory researchers were increasingly present at conferences and meetings debating and reporting their experiences. But PPI is not the same as participatory health research. A number of writers recognise PAR as an approach that was true to the INVOLVE definition of PPI, unlike the most common types of research that were practised under the PPI umbrella (Boote et al. 2002, 2010, 2011; Marston and Renedo 2013; Mockford et al. 2012; Brett et al. 2014; Staniszewska et al. 2011). In common with policy directives in general, the reality can obfuscate the intention (Blencowe et al. 2015; Staley et al. 2014). Institutional practices and structures still act as barriers to change, for example, through the blocking of PAR research in NHS ethics committees which are largely populated by positivists (Goodyear-Smith et al. 2015). A number of challenges remain before it can be said that marginalised groups, such as people with learning difficulties, are commonly included in an empowering way in the mainstream of research affecting their lives (Aldridge 2015; Baxter et al. 2001; Okereke et al. 2007; Bennett and Roberts 2004; Cawston et al. 2007). These challenges include the attitudes of some professionals, the diversity and complexity of lay groups' knowledge, power relationships, resources (both personal and financial) and values. Moreover, while many UK participatory researchers have aspirations at the emancipatory end of the spectrum of PAR which emphasises social justice and transformation, the reality related to funders' requirements firmly places the practice at the pragmatic end. Thus the emphasis is more often on improving research outcomes through engagement (Cook 2013; Holland et al. 2010; (Gilbert 2004; Hynes et al. 2012; Wimpenny 2013).

Public Engagement, Universities and Research Impact

While public engagement was being encouraged in NHS research in universities, the need for accountability has also been driving research funding, again presenting both a challenge and an opportunity for PHR. Apart from various research councils, British universities currently receive block funding for research. The level of funding is determined by a process of peer review every 6 years; whereby, each subject is ranked across universities, the criteria changing every ranking period. In the 2014 cycle, research impact was a new criterion, and, following the rejection of a purely bibliometric approach, a whole industry has developed on measuring research impact as universities scramble for resources and prestige. Since impact on the wider society was one of the dimensions, public engagement has been placed further up the agenda (Brett et al. 2014; Oliver et al. 2015; Pain et al. 2016). The UK Research Councils, Higher Education Funding Councils and the Welcome Trust had funded the establishment of the National Co-ordinating Centre for Public Engagement (NCCPE) as part of a £9.2 m project to inspire a culture change in how UK universities engaged with the public alongside six "Beacons for Public Engagement". These were partnerships between higher education institutions (HEIs) and civil society organisations (NCCPE 2009). At the heart of the initiative was an active commitment to learning and reflection. The NCCPE invested in a national action research process which drew on action research methodology to develop a systemic inquiry process (Burns 2007). Six parallel learning streams were established, and participants with different organisational relationships to public engagement (PE) were drawn into small inquiry groups. The findings identified a number of barriers to change as well as ways these barriers might be overcome (Burns and Squires 2011). This with experience distilled from the Beacons projects informed the creation of a new PE Concordat (RCUK 2011) signed by all the major research funders. It articulated their expectations of institutions they funded: (1) UK research organisations should have a strategic commitment to PE; (2) researchers should be recognised and valued for their involvement with PE activities; (3) researchers should be enabled to participate in PE activities through appropriate training support and opportunities; and (4) the signatories and supporters of this Concordat will undertake regular reviews of their and the wider research sector's progress in fostering PE across the UK. A recent report indicates there is much more to be done and significant barriers remain. Certainly, with a few exceptions, the notion of engaged scholarship or of community-university partnerships like those which exist in North America, is rare in the UK. Nonetheless, the NCCPE has provided a further communicative space for PHR and PAR within the academic sector and is contributing to the building of intellectual and social capital around the issues[1]. It now has its own peer review journal *Research for All*.

This concern for impact mirrors the knowledge translation trend in Canada (Bowen and Graham 2013). There, despite the "discovery" of integrated knowledge translation with its similarity to an older tradition of participatory action research (Kothari and Wathen 2013; Kothari and Armstrong 2011), the pipeline model of impact as something that happens in a linear fashion after research still dominates. In the UK recent work on impact in PAR in general (Pain et al. 2016; Greenhalgh et al. 2016) and in PHR in particular (Cook et al. 2017) potentially will mean the criteria for measuring impact are widened.

Types of PHR Projects in the UK

The complex and disparate history of PAR and PHR in the UK has meant that those wishing to develop this type of approach have found themselves ducking and diving as well as riding some waves of change. This has resulted in a wide variety of types of projects, so it is difficult to highlight specific projects as representative.

PHR has remained largely the remit of a raft of committed individuals with a concern for social justice and democratic knowledge production, supporting learning through research undertaking largely small-scale projects whose numbers have ebbed and flowed over the years. Occasionally some have coalesced in specific institutions, but there is no centre dedicated to this methodology within health faculties, although a number of interdisciplinary centres in social science and interdisciplinary networks within universities explicitly value this type of research (Kindon et al. 2007). The diverse and scattered nature of this type of research, embedded as it is in the local, is reflected in the published papers as well as unpublished reports and theses from the UK. The written record almost certainly hides a wealth of projects that go unreported or are found scattered across the websites of independent researchers working outside academia. The majority of publications focus on more marginalised populations. With no recent history of indigenous oppression, these marginalised groups include mainly black and ethnic minority groups, mental health service users, people with learning difficulties, gypsy/travellers as well as groups with a specific health need and children. Projects that take place in community settings, including primary care, tend to be more participatory in terms of the level of involvement of people than those in a hospital setting where participatory research amongst health professionals (often called practitioner research) is more common, if present at all. INVOLVE hold a database of projects on which people from

[1]www.nccpe.org

England can register their projects as well as a bibliography from their own library (INVOLVE 2014). Participatory research projects where involvement is on the higher levels of participation represent about 15% of all the projects registered.

One initiative in Wales deserves mention. This was the highly innovative Sustainable Health Action Research Project (SHARP) which was funded by the Welsh Assembly. It remains the only example of an attempt to go to scale in an action research type of project which was geared towards the social determinants of health. It was unusual in that it was funded for 5 years (2001–2006) and it had an in-built evaluation component with an emphasis on reflection and learning. While all the seven project clusters were subject to financial control governance by the Assembly, this was facilitative rather than controlling, enabling local people to drive the co-inquiry process through the cycles of research and action. This one-off experiment has unfortunately never been repeated, but its experience is explored in depth in a book (Cropper et al. 2007).

The much richer community development and health experience in Scotland is reflected in the Community Health Exchange (CHEX) part of the Scottish Community Development Centre (SCDC) which brings together various community development initiatives across sectors in Scotland. However, there is no reference to research on the entire CHEX website despite acting as resource for community-led health across the nation. What the SCDC website does house are the 130 community-led action research projects supported between 2002 and 2009 by the Scottish Community Development Action Research Fund (SCARF). Many of the projects could be classified under the banner of the social determinants of health, and nine are explicitly labelled as health. More recently, *What Works Scotland*, a collaborative initiative to improve the way local areas in Scotland use evidence to make decisions about public service development and reform, has been using collaborative and participatory research methods in keeping with Scotland's commitment to co-production of research and services (Bennett 2017).

Looking Back and Looking Forward

A repeated experience with (participatory research) has been the tension and contradiction between top down bureaucratic cultures and requirements tending as they do to standardise simplify and control and demands generated at the local level tending as they do to be diverse and complex and to require local-level discretion. (Chambers 1998)

The above quote illustrates a constant tension in PR which is also reflected in the history of PHR in the UK. With each government there have been new NHS reforms and each has had an influence beyond the term of that government. The reforms on PPI in England, for example, instituted in 2001 have continued to have influence beyond 2010. The rich community development tradition and its funding history in Scotland have influenced developments today in public service reform and community participation. However, the politically driven forms of involvement which have resulted in research institutions apparently sympathetic to public involvement are different from the longer-standing emancipatory movements where people who are directly affected by the issues seek to bring about change (Beresford 2002). With institutionalisation comes dangers. A number of critiques of the "top-down" drive for involvement argue that they encourage tokenistic approaches where involvement is perceived as an "add on" rather than being embedded from the outset (Beresford 2005). This is certainly the case in Northern Ireland where self-rule through unstable power-sharing, following on from very centralised control through direct rule and a history of violence and division, has inhibited any community-led initiatives (Lundy and McGovern 2006).

Quality of involvement remains a key issue (Van Bekkum and Hilton 2015) throughout the UK. If you look at health research funding decisions and the membership of panels in the four nations of the UK, the medical model continues to dominate. Outside the health sector, PAR continues to flourish in the arts, humanities, design, natural resource management, agriculture and overseas development. This is reflected in the membership of the UK Participatory Research Network as well as a study group on participatory research in the Institute for British Geographers. The Scottish Development Centre supports a Scottish Co-production Network[2]. Beyond the academic sector, charities and small NGOs and consultancies still extend this type of work. Thus while the landscape has many flowers, much fewer seeds have flourished in the bed of health. Moreover, while opportunities for learning and exposure to new ways of doing research are more frequent, the prospects for a more explicit emancipatory approach remains rare (Jordan and Kapoor 2016).

More fundamentally, although participation experiments such as participatory budgeting are written into Scottish legislation on empowerment, the lack of institutionalised participatory democratic structures remain an ongoing issue, particularly in the other three nations of the UK. Political events after 2015, cuts to public funding and welfare particularly at the local level including public health and a disdain for evidence and democracy suggest that the continued advance of this type of approach could slow or even retrench, as it has in the past. On the other hand, with health inequalities and poverty ever increasing, calls for a renewed democracy may reinvigorate those who practise PHR to become more explicit about the values of social justice and emancipation which underpin PHR as a vehicle for change (Jordan and Kapoor 2016). Moreover, social movements such as Momentum, which at the time of writing is using many participatory democratic methods to try and reform the Labour Party, are likely to create further support for this type of approach amongst a younger generation. Time will only tell. As ever, the diverse and contradictory forces at play within the PHR movement in the UK will play out sometimes fettered by institutional practices and sometimes empowered to challenge the status quo. It is up to the pioneers of the last 30 years to pass the baton to a new generation of participatory researcher, whether marginalised in society or in academia, so they too can experience the process such that they can never go back to doing research in the same way again. In doing so, they can further progress the democratisation of knowledge and society through deliberation and reflection.

---

[2] http://www.coproductionscotland.org.uk/

References

Abdulkadir, A., et al. (2016). *What do you mean I have a right to health ? Participatory action research on health and human rights*. Glasgow: University of Strathclyde.

Aldridge, J. (2015). *Participatory research: Working with vulnerable groups in research and practice*. Bristol: Policy Press.

Balogh, R., McAteer, M., & Hanley, U. (2017). Maintaining a network of critical connections over time and space: The case of CARN the collaborative action research network. In: Rowell, L., Bruce, C., Shosh J M, Riel M (eds) The Palgrave international handbook of action research 403–418 Springer, New York.

Baxter, L., Thorne, L., & Mitchell, A. (2001). *Small voices big noises. Lay involvement in health research: Lessons from other fields*. Exeter: Washinton Singer Press.

Bennett, F., & Roberts, M. (2004). *From input to influence: Participatory approaches to research and inquiry into poverty*. York: Joseph Rowntree Foundation.

Bennett, H. (2017). Fife collaborative action research programme: An overview of the process. What works Scotland research report. Edinburgh.

Beresford, P. (2002). User involvement in research and evaluation: Liberation or regulation? *Social Policy and Society, 1*(2), 95–106.

Beresford, P. (2003). *It's our lives: A short theory of knowledge distance and experience*. London: OSP for Citizen Press.

Beresford, P. (2005). Developing the theoretical basis for service user/survivor-led research and equal involvement in research. *Epidemiologia e Psichiatria Sociale, 14*(1), 4–9.

Berkeley, D., & Springett, J. (2006). From rhetoric to reality: Barriers faced by health for all initiatives. *Social Science and Medicine, 63*(1), 179–188.

Blencowe, C., Brigstocke, J., & Noorani, T. (2015). Theorising participatory practice and alienation in health research: A materialist approach. *Social Theory and Health, 13*(3–4), 397–417.

Boote, J., Baird, W., & Beecroft, C. (2010). Public involvement at the design stage of primary health research: A narrative review of case examples. *Health Policy, 95*(1), 10–23.

Boote, J., Baird, W., & Sutton, A. (2011). Public involvement in the systematic review process in health and social care: A narrative review of case examples. *Health Policy, 102*(2), 105–116.

Boote, J., Telford, R., & Cooper, C. (2002). Consumer involvement in health research: A review and research agenda. *Health Policy, 61*(2), 213–236.

Boote, J., Wong, R., & Booth, A. (2015). Talking the talk or walking the walk? a bibliometric review of the literature on public involvement in health research published between 1995 and 2009. *Health Expectations, 18*(1), 44–57.

Bowen, S., & Graham, I. (2013). Integrated knowledge translation. In S. Straus, J. Tetroe, & I. Graham (Eds.), *Knowledge translation in health care: Moving from evidence to practice* (2nd ed., pp. 14–23). London: BMJ Books.

Bradbury, H., & Reason, P. (2008). *The Sage handbook of action research: Participative inquiry and practice*. London: Sage Publications.

Brett, J., Staniszewska, S., Mockford, C., Herron-Marx, S., Hughes, J., Tysall, C., & Suleman, R. (2014). Mapping the impact of patient and public involvement on health and social care research: A systematic review. *Health Expectations, 17*(5), 637–650.

Burns, D. (2007). Systemic action research: A strategy for whole system change. Bristol: Policy Press.

Burns, D., & Squires, H. (2011). Embedding public engagement in higher education: Final report of the national action research programme, NCCPE (https://www.publicengagement.ac.uk/sites/default/files/publication/action_research_report_0.pdf)

Callaghan, G., & Wistow, G. (2006). Governance and public involvement in the British national health service: Understanding difficulties and developments. *Social Science and Medicine, 63*(9), 2289–2300.

Cawston, P. G., Mercer, S. W., & Barbour, R. S. (2007). Involving deprived communities in improving the quality of primary care services: Does participatory action research work? *BMC Health Services Research, 7*, 88.

Chambers, R. (1997). *Whose reality counts? : Putting the first last.* London: Intermediate Technology.

Chambers, R. (1998). Beyond "whose reality counts?" new methods we now need? *Studies in Cultures Organizations and Societies, 4*(2), 279–301.

Chambers, R. (2015). PRAPLA and pluralisms: Practice and theory. In H. Bradbury (Ed.), *The SAGE handbook of action research* (3rd ed., pp. 31–46). London: Sage.

Chiu, L. (2007). Health promotion and participatory action research: The significance of participatory praxis in developing participatory health intervention. In H. Bradbury & P. Reason (Eds.), *Handbook of action research: Participative inquiry and practice* (pp. 534–549). London: Sage.

Cole, M. (2003). The health action zone initiative: Lessons from Plymouth. *Local Government Studies, 29*(3), 99–117.

Cook, T. (2013). Where participatory approaches meet pragmatism in funded (health) research: The challenge of finding meaningful spaces. Forum Qualitative Sozialforschung/Forum: Qualitative Social Research 13.

Cook, T., Boote, J., Buckley, N., Vougioukalou, S., & Wright, M. (2017). Accessing participatory research impact and legacy: Developing the evidence base for participatory approaches in health research. *Educational Action Research, 25*(4), 473–488.

Cornwall, A., & Jewkes, R. (1995). What is participatory research? *Social Science and Medicine, 41*(12), 1667–1676.

Craig, G. (2016). Community development in the UK: Whatever happened to class? A historical analysis class inequality and community development. In M. Shaw & M. Mayo (Eds.), *Class, inequality and commuity development* (pp. 39–51). Bristol: Policy Press.

Craig, G., Mayo, M., Popple, K., Shaw, M., & Taylor, M. (2011). *The community development reader: History themes and issues.* Bristol: Policy Press.

Crawshaw, P., Bunton, R., & Conway, S. (2004). Governing the unhealthy community: Some reflections on UK health action zones. *Social Theory and Health, 2*(4), 341–360.

Cropper, S., Porter, A., Williams, G., Carlisle, S., Moore, R., O'Neill, M., Roberts, C., Snooks H. (eds). (2007). *Community health and wellbeing: Action research on health inequalities.* Bristol: Policy Press

Davies, J. K., & Kelly, M. (2014). *Healthy cities: Research and practice.* London: Routledge.

De Koning, K., & Martin, M. (1996). *Participatory research in health.* London: Zed Books.

Devisch, I., & Murray, S. J. (2009). 'We hold these truths to be self-evident': Deconstructing 'evidence-based' medical practice. *Journal of Evaluation in Clinical Practice, 15*(6), 950–954.

Dooris, M., & Heritage, Z. (2013). Healthy cities: Facilitating the active participation and empowerment of local people. *Journal of Urban Health, 90*(1), 74–91.

Evans, D., Coad, J., Cottrell, K., Dalrymple, J., Davies, R., &Donald, C., ... Sayers R. (2014). *Public involvement in research: Assessing impact through a realist evaluation.* Health Services and Delivery Research NIHR Library 236.

Gilbert, T. (2004). Involving people with learningdisabilities in research: Issues and possibilities. *Health and Social Care in the Community, 12*(4), 298–308.

Gillard, S., Turner, K., Lovell, K., Norton, K., Clarke, T., Addicott, R., & Ferlie, E. (2010). "Staying native": Coproduction in mental health services research. *International Journal of Public Sector Management, 23*(6), 567–577.

Goodyear-Smith, F., Jackson, C., & Greenhalgh, T. (2015). Co-design and implementation research: Challenges and solutions for ethics committees. *BMC Medical Ethics, 16*, 78.

Green, J., & Tones, K. (1999). For debate towards a secure evidence base for health promotion. *Journal of Public Health, 21*(2), 133–139.

Greenhalgh, T., Jackson, C., Shaw, S., & Janamian, T. (2016). Achieving research impact through co-creation in community-based health services: Literature review and case study. *The Milbank Quarterly, 94*(2), 392–429.

Hammersley, M. (2005). Is the evidence-based practice movement doing more good than harm? Reflections on Iain Chalmers'case for research-based policy making and practice. *Evidence and Policy, 1*(1), 85–100.

Harrison, S. (2002). New labour modernisation and the medical labour process. *Journal of Social Policy, 31*(03), 465–485.

Harrison, S., Moran, M., & Wood, B. (2002). Policy emergence and policy convergence: The case of 'scientific-bureaucratic medicine'in the United States and United Kingdom. *The British Journal of Politics and International Relations, 4*(1), 1–24.

Department of Health. (1999). *Reducing health inequalities: An action report*. London: DH.

Holland, S., Renold, E., Ross, N. J., & Hillman, A. (2010). Power agency and participatory agendas: A critical exploration of young people's engagement in participative qualitative research. *Childhood, 17*(3), 360–375.

Hynes, G., Coghlan, D., & McCarron, M. (2012). Participation as a multi-voiced process: Action research in the acute hospital environment. *Action Research, 10*(3), 293–312.

INVOLVE (2014). Evidence Bibliography 5. http://www.invo.org.uk/wp-content/uploads/2014/11/Bibliography5FinalComplete.pdf. Accessed 4 Jan 2018.

Jolly, R. (2008). *A short history of IDS: A personal reflection*. Brighton: Institute of Development Studies at the University of Sussex.

Jordan, S., & Kapoor, D. (2016). Re-politicizing participatory action research: Unmasking neoliberalism and the illusions of participation. *Educational Action Research, 24*(1), 134–149.

Judge, K., Barnes, M., Bauld, L., Benzeval, M., Killoran, A., Robinson, R., & Zeilig, H. (1999). *Health action zones: Learning to make a difference*. Essex: PSSRU.

Kindon, S., Pain, R., & Kesby, M. (2007). *Participatory action research approaches and methods: Connecting people participation and place*. London: Routledge.

Kothari, A., & Armstrong, R. (2011). Community-based knowledge translation: Unexplored opportunities. *Implementation Science, 6*(1), 59.

Kothari, A., & Wathen, C. N. (2013). A critical second look at integrated knowledge translation. *Health Policy, 109*(2), 187–191.

Lazenbatt, A., Lynch, U., & O'Neill, E. (2001). Revealing the hidden 'troubles' in Northern Ireland: The role of participatory rapid appraisal. *Health Education Research, 16*(5), 567–578.

Ledwith, M. (2015). *Community development in action: Putting Freire into practice*. Bristol: Policy Press.

Ledwith, M., & Springett, J. (2010). *Participatory practice participatory practice*. Bristol: The Policy Press.

Lundy, P., & McGovern, M. (2006). Participation truth and partiality: Participatory action research community-based truth-telling and post-conflict transition in Northern Ireland. *Sociology, 40*(1), 71–88.

Marmot, M. (2010). Fair society health lives: The marmot review. http://www.instituteofhealthequity.org/resources-reports/fair-society-healthy-lives-the-marmot-review. Accessed 4 Jan 2018.

Marston, C., & Renedo, A. (2013). Understanding and measuring the effects of patient and public involvement: An ethnographic study. *The Lancet, 382*, S69. https://doi.org/10.1016/s0140-6736(13)62494-0.

McIntyre, A. (2003). Through the eyes of women: Photovoice and participatory research as tools for reimagining place. *Gender Place and Culture: A Journal of Feminist Geography, 10*(1), 47–66.

McGuiness, F. (2016). Income inequality in the UK. http://www.instituteofhealthequity.org/projects/fair-society-healthy-lives-the-marmot-review. Accesed 4 Jan 2018.

Mockford, C., Staniszewska, S., Griffiths, F., & Herron-Marx, S. (2012). The impact of patient and public involvement on UK NHS health care: A systematic review. *International Journal for Quality in Health Care: Journal of the International Society for Quality in Health Care/ISQua, 24*(1), 28–38.

NCCPE. (2009). The beacons project. http://www.publicengagement.ac.uk/beacons. Accessed 4 Jan 2018.

NIHR. (2006). Best research for best health: a new national health research strategy How the NHS in England will contribute to health research and development over the next 5 years. London: DH

NIHR. (2015). Going the extra mile: Improving the nation's health and wellbeing through public involvement in research. https://www.nihr.ac.uk/patients-and-public/documents/Going-the-Extra-Mile.pdf. Acessed 4 Jan 2018.

Okereke, E., Archibong, U., Chiemeka, M., Baxter, C. E., & Davis, S. (2007). Participatory approaches to assessing the health needs of African and African-Caribbean communities. *Diversity in Health and Social Care, 4*(4), 287–301.

Oliver, S., Liabo, K., Stewart, R., & Rees, R. (2015). Public involvement in research: Making sense of the diversity. *Journal of Health Services Research and Policy, 20*(1), 45–51.

Pain, R., Askins, K., Banks, S., Cook, T., Crawford, G., Crookes, L., & Houston, M. (2016). *Mapping alternative impact: Alternative approaches to impact from co-produced research.* Durham: Centre for Social Justice, Universty of Durham.

Reason, P., & Heron, J. (1994). Three approaches to participatory inquiry. In N. K. Denzin & Y. S. Lincoln (Eds.), *Handbook of qualitative research.* London: Sage.

Reason, P. (1998). Political epistemological ecological and spiritual dimensions of participation. *Studies in Cultures Organizations and Societies, 4*(2), 147–167.

Reason, P., & Bradbury, H. (2001). *Handbook of action research: Participative inquiry and practice.* London: Sage.

Reason, P., & Rowan, J. (1981). *Human inquiry: A sourcebook of new paradigm research.* Chichester: Wiley.

Scott-Samuel, A., & Springett, J. (2007). Hegemony or health promotion? Prospects for reviving England's lost discipline. *The Journal of the Royal Society for the Promotion of Health, 127*(5), 211–214.

Somekh, B. (2010). The collaborative action research network: 30 years of agency in developing educational action research. *Educational Action Research, 18*(1), 103–121.

Springett, J. (2001). Appropriate approaches to the evaluation of health promotion. *Critical Public Health, 11*(2), 139–151.

Springett, J. (2005). Geographically-based approaches to the integration of health promotion into health systems: A comparative study of two health action zones in the UK. *Promotion and Education, 12*(3_suppl), 39–44.

Springett, J., Owens, C., & Callaghan, J. (2007). The challenge of combining 'lay'knowledge with 'evidence-based'practice in health promotion: Fag ends smoking cessation service. *Critical Public Health, 17*(3), 243–256.

Springett, J., & Young, A. (2002). Comparing theories of change and participatory approaches to the evaluation of projects within health action zones: Two views from the north west on engaging community level projects in evaluation. In L. Bauld & K. Judge (Eds.), *Learning from health action zones.* Chichester: AeneasPress.

Staley, K., Buckland, S. A., Hayes, H., & Tarpey, M. (2014). 'The missing links': Understanding how context and mechanism influence the impact of public involvement in research. *Health Expectations, 17*(6), 755–764.

Staniszewska, S., Brett, J., Mockford, C., & Barber, R. (2011). The GRIPP checklist: Strengthening the quality of patient and public involvement reporting in research. *International Journal of Technology Assessment in Health Care, 27*(4), 391–399.

RCUK. (2011). Concordat for engaging the public with research. http://www.rcuk.ac.uk/pe/Concordat/. Accessed 4 Jan 2018.

Van Bekkum, J. E., & Hilton, S. (2015). UK research funding bodies'views towards public particpation in health related research decisions: An exploratory study. *BMC Health Services Research, 14*(1), 318.

Waterman, H., Tillen, D., Dickson, R., & de Koning, K. (2001). Action research: A systematic review and guidance for assessment. *Health Technology Assessment (Winchester England), 5*(23), iii–157.

Wills, J., Evans, D., & Samuel, A. S. (2008). Politics and prospects for health promotion in England: Mainstreamed or marginalised? *Critical Public Health, 18*(4), 521–531.

Wimpenny, K. (2013). Using participatory action research to support knowledge translation in practice settings. *International Journal of Practice-based Learning in Health and Social Care, 1*(1), 3–14.

Wistow, G., & Barnes, M. (1993). User involvement in community care: Origins purposes and applications. *Public Administration, 71*(3), 279–299.

Index

Printed in the United States
By Bookmasters